A WOMAN'S GUIDE TO MENOPAUSE AND PERIMENOPAUSE

Yale University Press Health & Wellness

A Yale University Press Health & Wellness book is an authoritative, accessible source of information on a health-related topic. It may provide guidance to help you lead a healthy life, examine your treatment options for a specific condition or disease, situate a healthcare issue in the context of your life as a whole, or address questions or concerns that linger after visits to your healthcare provider.

Ruth Grobstein, M.D., Ph.D., *The Breast Cancer Book: What You Need to Know to Make Informed Decisions*

James Hicks, M.D., *Fifty Signs of Mental Illness: A Guide to Understanding Mental Health*

Mary Jane Minkin, M.D., and Carol V. Wright, Ph.D., *A Woman's Guide to Menopause and Perimenopause*

Mary Jane Minkin, M.D., and Carol V. Wright, Ph.D., *A Woman's Guide to Sexual Health*

Catherine M. Poole, with DuPont Guerry IV, M.D., *Melanoma: Prevention, Detection, and Treatment*, 2nd ed.

A Woman's Guide to

Menopause & Perimenopause

Mary Jane Minkin, M.D.

Carol V. Wright, Ph.D.

YALE UNIVERSITY PRESS   NEW HAVEN & LONDON

Designed by Rebecca Gibb.
Set in Minion type by The Composing Room of Michigan, Inc.
Printed in the United States of America by R. R. Donnelley & Sons.

Library of Congress Cataloging-in-Publication Data

Minkin, Mary Jane.
   A woman's guide to menopause and perimenopause / Mary Jane Minkin, Carol V. Wright.
      p.   cm.
   Includes bibliographical references and index.
   ISBN 0-300-10435-9 (paperbound : alk. paper)
      1. Menopause—Popular works.   2. Perimenopause—Popular works.   3. Middle-aged women—Health and hygiene.   I. Wright, Carol V.   II. Title.
   RG186.M573   2004
   618.1′75—dc22

                                                                        2004014636

A catalogue record for this book is available from the British Library.

The paper in this book meets the guidelines for permanence and durability of the Committee on Production Guidelines for Book Longevity of the Council on Library Resources.

10 9 8 7 6 5 4 3 2 1

The information and suggestions contained in this book are not intended to replace the services of your physician or caregiver. Because each person and each medical situation is unique, you should consult your own physician to get answers to your personal questions, to evaluate any symptoms you may have, or to receive suggestions on appropriate medications.

The authors have attempted to make this book as accurate and current as possible, but it may nevertheless contain errors, omissions, or material that is out of date at the time you read it. Neither the authors nor the publisher have any legal responsibility or liability for errors, omissions, outdated material, or the reader's application of the medical information or advice contained in this book.

Although the case histories have been drawn from Dr. Minkin's medical experience, the names of the patients have been altered to protect their privacy.

▶ CONTENTS

▶ **ILLUSTRATIONS**

FIGURES

TABLES

BOXES

I AM a man, and therefore will not experience menopause; based on my wife's up-close-and-personal experience with the topic, I will be forever grateful for this accident of fertilization. Through my wife, however, I have managed to experience firsthand the joys of hot flushes, night sweats, and sleep disruption. I learned that each woman responds to hormone replacement therapy (HRT) in unique physiological and psychological ways. I observed her logically integrate reams of conflicting scientific reports on the risks and benefits of such therapy, peppering me with insightful questions along the way and ultimately opting to forego hormone therapy. She has since moved comfortably through this milestone along a woman's life journey.

Fortunately, or unfortunately, for daily consults my wife had the benefit of a husband who is a Yale professor of obstetrics, gynecology, and reproductive sciences. For the vast majority of women who do not have such ready and immediate access to "expert" advice, I am happy to offer up the next best thing: *A Woman's Guide to Menopause and Peri-*

menopause. This outstanding book gives a woman all the information she needs to know when facing both perimenopause and menopause.

Chapter 1 fittingly addresses the history of HRT, culminating in the release of the results of the Women's Health Initiative (WHI) hormone replacement trial study. This landmark clinical trial was designed to evaluate the risks and benefits of hormone replacement therapy with Prempro (a combination of the estrogen Premarin and a progestational drug, Provera) versus placebo. The National Institutes of Health halted the study when it was concluded that after an average of five years of combined estrogen-progestin therapy there was a statistically significant, but incredibly small, increase in the occurrence of breast cancer, heart disease, and stroke. Conversely, the study showed a significant reduction in osteoporotic fractures and colon cancer among HRT users.

But the authors first tell the story of hormone therapy, which for practical purposes began in 1965 with the publication and publicity surrounding Dr. Robert A. Wilson's book *Feminine Forever,* which viewed estrogen replacement therapy as a veritable fountain of youth. A decade later the Food and Drug Administration warned that giving women estrogen therapy alone was associated with an increased risk of endometrial cancer. This first crisis was overcome with the introduction of combined estrogen-progestin therapy. The pendulum then swung back in favor of widespread HRT use when studies abounded suggesting that such therapy not only relieved the signs and symptoms of menopause but prevented osteoporosis and coronary heart disease, and perhaps colon cancer and Alzheimer's disease.

By 1990, the accumulated data was sufficient for Premarin's manufacturer, Wyeth Ayerst, to petition the FDA for labeling indicating that HRT was protective against heart disease. The FDA requested clearer evidence derived from randomized clinical trials. The results of these studies have appeared in the past three years, starting with the Heart and Estrogen/Progestin Replacement Study, which found no protective effect of hormone therapy on the occurrence of heart disease, and ending with the Women's Health Initiative finding of a slight increase in the risk of heart disease among HRT users. But more concerning was the WHI's finding that HRT increased the risk of breast cancer.

What is missing from these studies, however, is why most women take HRT in the first place—the signs and symptoms of menopause. Those readers who have experienced these effects firsthand will understand instantly how complex the issues are. The insomnia, flashes and sweats, irritability, and physical changes associated with menopause can be absolutely intolerable to many women.

What, then, should women do? Well, I would suggest they start by reading this book.

The chapters that follow tell you how menopause comes about and what to expect in terms of physical changes and symptoms. Mary Jane Minkin, M.D., and Carol V. Wright, Ph.D., describe the changes menopause makes on your body and brain and offer a range of options to minimize these symptoms and potential adverse health effects. The chapters cover a vast array of women's health topics—from bone loss to hysterectomy to cancers of the reproductive organs—and honestly and clearly address the complex issues surrounding HRT, giving each woman enough information to make up her own mind.

I have known Mary Jane Minkin since I came to Yale as a young trainee in 1985. In the ensuing two decades I can affirm that she has lost none of her humor, energy, and enthusiasm for learning or dedication to her patients. She is a doctor's doctor who is both respected by her colleagues and loved by her patients. She regularly lectures the Yale medical students and obstetrics and gynecology residents about menopause and presents both formal and informal talks to various medical and community groups. Her great skill as a teacher shines across the pages of this book and will illuminate your own journey through menopause.

Charles J. Lockwood, M.D.
Anita O'Keefe Young Professor and
Chair, Department of Obstetrics, Gynecology, and Reproductive Sciences
Yale University School of Medicine

ABOUT ten years ago, we wrote an earlier version of this book from which portions of the present text have been adapted. Since that time, menopause has come out of the closet. A generation ago women did not talk about the "change of life," as it was euphemistically called; menopause was concealed as if it were shameful. Women were comfortable talking about childbirth, surgery, or even cancer, but many were unwilling to discuss menopause with friends or family, or even to articulate their feelings about it to themselves.

Because of this wall of silence and the influence of a culture that has often valued women primarily for their sexuality and fertility, myths have long surrounded menopause. Menopause is said to signal the end of youth and sexuality, and to lay waste to women's minds, memories, and emotional stability. Menopause is thought to bring instant wrinkles, extra weight, and overall dowdiness, consigning anyone over fifty to the scrap heap—or at least to the sidelines.

In the past few years, however, the barrier of silence has crumbled, and the topic of menopause has leapt onto the front pages. A woman approaching menopause today may not even have known when her mother was going through "the change," but she can open the newspaper and see the latest scientific results about hormone replacement and read conflicting editorials about its risks and benefits. Whereas once there may have been too little information, now there may be too much conflicting research. We have scientific studies suggesting that estrogen replacement is good for our bones and heart. We also have studies stating that estrogen replacement therapy has risks that outweigh its benefits.

Amid this controversy, women still need to know about this stage of life in order to pass through menopause as comfortably as possible and to protect their health for the years that lie beyond. In 1900, the average woman died only a few years after the end of her childbearing years (at age forty-eight). Today the same average American woman—the beneficiary of antibiotics, better nutrition, better public health measures, and better medical care—can look ahead to thirty or even forty postmenopausal years. Despite the cultural bias against older women, these years may be among the most productive and enjoyable of her life. It is crucial, however, that every woman know how to maintain her health if she is to optimize this time of life.

Our increasing body of scientific knowledge about menopause and the maintenance of health throughout life tells us, incontrovertibly, that exercise basically is good for everyone. Stopping smoking and limiting drinking are good for everyone. Some calcium intake is good for almost everyone. In other areas, the choices have become increasingly complex and difficult. Since the results of the Women's Health Initiative hit the headlines in 2002, estrogen replacement therapy has become an even more controversial topic than it was formerly. It may benefit many women, but it is not necessarily right for all. For many women, the risks or the psychological consequences will outweigh the benefits. For others the discomforts of menopause or the long-term effects of losing estrogen's protective action may tip the scales in the other direction.

If hormone replacement is not a reasonable option for a particular woman, what other choices does she have? Will other approaches help with hot flashes? Are herbal medicines safe? Are the heavy periods she is experiencing dangerous or merely a sign of approaching menopause? Will exercise protect her bones from osteoporosis? Is heart disease a risk she should consider?

And although many women have pressing questions about menopause, the traditional annual office visit of fifteen minutes hardly allows time for answering them. In the past decade, changes in the health care system pressuring doctors to see more and more patients in less and less time have made the situation worse.

If you are approaching midlife and menopause, or perhaps are already there, the chapters that follow have been written for you. One of us (MJM) has been a practicing gynecologist for about twenty-five years, talking with and listening to thousands of women as they go through menopause. This book is based on what these women have wanted to know—on their concerns, questions, and experiences at midlife. We have written this book in a question-and-answer format, trying to anticipate what you might ask your own physician, given the luxury of time. (Although there are two authors, the "I" who answers and discusses the questions is MJM, the physician.)

We hope that this volume will help you understand the physical and emotional changes that you are probably feeling as you approach menopause. It will tell you why you feel as you do, if medical science has the answer. It will inform you about what we know scientifically, and it will tell you what we do not know. It will try to sort out the controversy surrounding the newest studies on estrogen replacement therapy. Obviously there are important questions you will have to answer for yourself, but we hope that this book will give you the information you need to make wisely the decisions that will ultimately affect the rest of your life.

Because research into women's health care is ongoing, new studies will be published that offer new insights into our understanding of menopause. In fact, not long after the manuscript for this book went to our editors, the results of new studies on hormone replacement therapy began appearing in the media. Although we have made this book as up-to-date as possible at the time of writing, we can't guarantee that it will remain so, but we hope that it will give you a framework for evaluating new studies as they emerge.

Think about the design of the new research. Were many women involved in the study or just a few? Were these women typical of menopausal women in the United States? Did the study go on for many years or was it short-term? If hormones were being evaluated, were they identical to the ones used in the United States or were they different? What is the reputation of the institution that published the study? Is it respected? Well known?

Even though you may not be a trained statistician, you can use common sense in evaluating results. Try to put the numerical data in a form you can readily understand. What does it mean if a study shows that taking some medication increases (or decreases) your risk by a certain percentage? For example, a Harvard study published in 1995 showed that women aged fifty-five to fifty-nine who had been taking hormone replacement therapy for five or more years had a 40 percent higher risk of breast cancer than women who had never used hormone replacement. Forty percent sounds frightening, but if you look at the figures another way, the increased risk seems less alarming. Statisticians expect about thirty-five cases of breast cancer per thousand women in this age group who don't use hormone replacement. If the women used hormone replacement for at least five years, then statistically there would be fifty cases of breast cancer instead of thirty-five, an increase of fifteen cases.

Another perhaps misleading statistic is the well-known one-in-eight breast cancer figure: during the 1980s an American woman's risk of getting breast cancer rose from one in nine to one in eight. Does this mean that of every eight women in the United States, one will get breast cancer? No, it means that at birth each woman has a one-in-eight lifetime risk of getting breast cancer if she lives to be 110. The jump from one in nine to one in eight during the 1980s happened in part because the National Cancer Institute decided to broaden its statistical pool to include women over eighty-five, a very high risk group.

If the results of a study do concern you, it is a good idea to discuss your feelings with your doctor.

Many people assisted us in preparing this book. We thank Dr. Kristen Zarfos for helping with the section on breast cancer. Doctors Donna Criscenzo and Mary Scheimann suggested the guidelines on general medical care. Doctor Fred Naftolin, who read the manuscript of the earlier version, pencil in hand, made thoughtful suggestions on the sections devoted to the physiology of menopause. Without our agent and friend, Mildred Marmur, this project would never have gotten off the ground. Jean Thomson Black of Yale University Press has provided continuing enthusiasm and encouragement as well as judicious editorial advice over the years.

Closer to home, we would like to acknowledge the important, sometimes extrascientific contributions of our families, Allie, Max, and Steve Pincus, and Fred and Catherine Wright.

1 The Women's Health Initiative and What It Means to You

WHEN I arrived at work on July 10, 2002, the phone was ringing. It rang constantly all that day and all day for the next several weeks. Hundreds of our patients were calling the office, deeply worried because they had been taking hormone replacement therapy and feared that they were at increased risk for breast cancer. The same thing was happening all over the country. Some doctors, overwhelmed by the volume of calls, took their phones off the hook.

The day before, July 9, the National Institutes of Health (NIH) had abruptly halted the part of the Women's Health Initiative (WHI) that assessed the risks and benefits of

Note: In this chapter as elsewhere in the book, "hormone therapy" refers to estrogen combined with a progestin (synthetic progesterone). "Estrogen therapy" refers to estrogen alone; it is usually given to women who have had hysterectomies and don't need the protection of progestin against endometrial cancer.

Although the North American Menopause Society now endorses the term "hormone therapy" instead of "hormone replacement therapy," the abbreviation "HT" does not seem to have replaced "HRT" in the common parlance. Since my patients still refer to "HRT" instead of "HT," we've decided to retain the older abbreviations "HRT" and "ERT."

hormone replacement therapy for women who were taking combined estrogen and progesterone. The designers of the study, supported by the NIH, the governmental department for medical research and one of the foremost such centers in the world, had concluded that the risks of estrogen-plus-progestin hormone replacement therapy outweighed the benefits. Specifically, the researchers found that the use of hormone therapy caused small increases in rates of breast cancer, heart attack, stroke, and blood clots, which outweighed small decreases in the rates of hip fracture and colorectal cancer. Letters were mailed to women in the study who were taking the hormones, telling them to stop doing so. Unfortunately for both women and their doctors, the NIH did not alert physicians and other health care providers, who were unprepared for the deluge of phone calls and did not know immediately how to respond.

Even more information about the negative effects of hormone replacement has appeared since then, and many of the previously believed benefits of hormone therapy are now in doubt. Its positive effects on women's quality of life were questioned after analysis of data from the WHI suggested that hormonal therapy did not improve women's energy level, sexual pleasure, restful sleep, emotional functioning, mood swings, cognitive functioning, or memory. Another substudy of the WHI, called WHIMS (Women's Health Initiative Memory Study), reported in May 2003 that women older than sixty-five who took HRT had a higher rate of dementia, much of it possible Alzheimer's disease, than women who did not take hormones.

To understand why the WHI results were such a bombshell and, more important, to understand what those results mean for you, let's look at the background leading up to the release of the WHI data.

A SHORT HISTORY OF ESTROGEN REPLACEMENT THERAPY

Hormone therapy of one kind or another has been with us for generations. In the 1920s, laboratory researchers isolated estrogen and progesterone, the two most important female hormones. Estrogen became commercially available in the 1930s, and in 1942 the federal Food and Drug Administration (FDA) approved Premarin, a form of estrogen developed from the urine of pregnant mares, to relieve hot flashes. Its introduction radically altered the choices available to women going through menopause.

During the 1950s and 1960s, hormones continued to get good press. In 1960, birth control pills, which made use of synthetic hormones to block ovulation and prevent pregnancy, became available. Oral contraceptives found wide acceptance in the 1960s. For the first time in history, women had an effective and convenient means of contraception, something they did not need to think about each and every time they had intercourse.

In 1966, a book entitled *Feminine Forever* claimed that by taking estrogen postmenopausal women could remain young, healthy, and vibrant all their lives. Written by a physician named Robert Wilson, who was born in 1895, this book reflected the cultural attitudes of a seventy-one-year-old male doctor. Wilson pointed out that there was nothing "unnatural" about taking hormones, that doing so merely "restores a natural harmony between the rate of aging and life expectancy." Women who chose not to take estrogen after menopause were "prematurely aging castrates." In addition, Wilson stated that there was no causative link between cancer and hormones and, in fact, that taking estrogen might prevent cancer. Wilson's book was received with great enthusiasm, and the postmenopausal use of estrogen increased considerably.

In the 1970s, however, studies began to show a link between estrogen use (or ERT, estrogen replacement therapy, which then was given without the balancing action of progesterone) and cancer of the uterus (endometrial or uterine cancer). To balance the estrogen, doctors began adding progestins (synthetic forms of progesterone), mimicking the action of these two hormones during women's reproductive years.

Unfortunately, progestins caused several problems. When used intermittently with estrogen to imitate the menstrual cycle, they cause bleeding that resembles menstrual periods—and menopausal women, who are generally thrilled not to have periods, begin to have them again. To counteract this side-effect, researchers proposed giving the progestins daily instead of cyclically. This approach, too, was not entirely successful, since it turned out that many women bled or at least spotted on this regimen. Nevertheless, by 1996, when the estrogen-plus-progestin pill Prempro came on the market, combination hormone replacement therapy (HRT) was becoming increasingly popular.

No one questioned the effectiveness of combination hormone therapy for relieving menopausal symptoms—hot flashes, night sweats, vaginal dryness, and so on—and even today, no one questions their effectiveness for these purposes. Other benefits of HRT began to be noted in the 1980s, when studies appeared suggesting that women who took HRT significantly reduced their risk of developing coronary artery disease and heart attacks. This made intuitive sense, because coronary artery disease is rare in women before menopause but becomes much more common later. Women whose ovaries were removed at a young age are also at increased risk for heart disease.

At about this time, it was becoming clear that HRT was good for bones, helpful in preventing osteoporosis, a condition in which bones lose their strength and density. As women lived longer, osteoporosis emerged as a health risk, and statistics showed that the aftereffects of bone fractures were a major cause of death among older women.

Did scientific data support the good news? It seemed so. Observational studies had compared women who took estrogen with those who did not. The problem with these studies, however, is that women who chose to take estrogen tended to be healthier than those who chose not to—better educated, less likely to be overweight or to smoke, more attentive to their general health. Did estrogen make these women healthy? Or were they healthy to begin with?

In addition to the observational studies, laboratory studies showed positive effects on animals and on body cells, suggesting that estrogen prevents the deposits of plaque in the arteries that cause them to harden and that it improves blood circulation to the brain. The evidence that estrogen replacement therapy might prevent heart disease seemed convincing, though it was indirect.

But even as these encouraging data about cardiac and bone health were emerging, a few studies began to suggest that women who took estrogen long-term increased their risk for breast cancer, a disease American women dread above all others. In 1994, when a team of Gallup pollsters asked a group of women aged forty-five to sixty-five to estimate the mortality rate of various diseases, the participants indicated that 40 percent of American women died of breast cancer and 4 percent of cardiac disease. The truth is just about the opposite: 36 percent die of heart disease and 4 percent of breast cancer. The poll results suggest how frightening breast cancer is to most women.

All these developments led in the early 1990s to the Women's Health Initiative (WHI). Because the data on estrogen replacement and heart disease looked promising, Wyeth Ayerst, the pharmaceutical company that manufactures Premarin (and Prempro) asked the FDA to approve Premarin as a preventive for coronary artery disease. The FDA turned down the request, asking for randomized placebo-controlled double-blinded studies showing that Premarin really did help prevent coronary artery disease.

Randomized, placebo-controlled, double-blinded studies are the gold standard of clinical investigation, far more scientifically reliable than observational studies. The people in the study (or trial, as it is sometimes called) are divided into two random groups. One group takes the medication being tested; the other takes placebos (inactive pills). Neither doctors nor patients know who is getting the medication and who is getting the placebo.

Confident of the outcome, Wyeth Ayerst agreed to randomized studies. In 1993, with Wyeth Ayerst providing the medications, the National Institutes of Health began the

Women's Health Initiative, a long-term, massive undertaking of more than twenty-six thousand women, aged fifty to seventy-nine. The study had two separate "arms," or sections. In one, sixteen thousand postmenopausal women who had never had a hysterectomy were randomized to get either Prempro (a combination of estrogen and medroxy-progesterone, a commonly used synthetic progesterone) or a placebo. In the other arm, ten thousand women who had undergone hysterectomy received either Premarin or a placebo. (These women did not need the protection of a progestin against uterine cancer.) The investigators set out to study not only coronary artery disease but also the rates of breast cancer, strokes, blood clots in the veins, fractures caused by osteoporosis, and colon cancer.

Wyeth Ayerst also sponsored a trial of HRT for what is known as "secondary prevention." In this study, women who had already had a heart attack and/or severe angina—chest pain caused by insufficient blood flow to the heart muscle—were given Prempro in hopes of preventing future heart attacks. This study was called the HERS trial (the Heart and Estrogen/Progestin Replacement Study). The results published in 1998 stunned most health care providers. Not only did the Prempro fail to lower the rate of repeat heart attacks, it actually increased the rate of heart attacks in the first year of taking the medication, though over a three-to five-year period the rate of heart attack decreased slightly.

The American Heart Association (AHA) responded quickly, pronouncing HRT an inappropriate medication for preventing a second heart attack or death among women who already had heart disease. If a woman was already taking HRT and doing well with it (whether she had heart disease or not), then the AHA found it medically acceptable for her to continue.

All these events set the stage for July 9, 2002. The *Journal of the American Medical Association,* where the crucial research results were to appear on July 17, established an embargo to keep the news secret until the official publication date. Somehow the results were leaked to the press and the story hit the front pages of newspapers all across the country. When the study was designed, it included an automatic stop if the researchers perceived any increased risk in breast cancer, and on May 31, when women on the study drug had been taking Prempro for an average of 5.2 years, the safety monitoring board of the study recommended stopping the study, three years before its planned conclusion in 2005.

The arm of the study that involved estrogen only (Premarin) was allowed to continue until 2004, when it, too, was halted, because data showed a slight increase in the number of strokes but no decrease in risk for heart disease. Data did not show the increase in breast cancer for women who were not taking progestin as well as estrogen. This seemed to implicate progestin (synthetic estrogen) as a culprit, but no studies since the WHI have announced results that either confirm or deny this hypothesis.

Deluged by calls from anxious patients, doctors and other health care providers tried to reach a consensus in interpreting the study. Some doctors simply told all their patients to stop taking HRT immediately. Many others, however, including the group of medical professionals who wrote up the WHI study, agreed that hormone replacement therapy is the most effective treatment for the symptoms of menopause and agreed to the use of HRT for at least several years. The American College of Obstetricians and Gynecologists (ACOG), the professional group for physicians in these specialties, recommended that HRT be used only to relieve the symptoms of menopause and that it be used for as short a time as possible. The North American Menopause Society reached a similar conclusion.

Many gynecologists, however, believe that the results of the WHI study were not as stunning as the press reports suggested. These doctors found that the initial WHI results showed nothing that was not known previously, and they plan on continuing to prescribe HRT, though they will certainly talk over the risk-benefit equation with their patients. And while the official stance of North American Menopause Society is that HRT use should be limited to relief of postmenopausal symptoms, papers presented at recent meetings of the society have stressed the importance of estrogen in maintaining sexual function and for women who have had their ovaries surgically removed.

While recognizing the importance of the WHI results, many gynecologists commented on design flaws in the studies. First, the average age of women selected for the study was well past menopause. Thus, they had been postmenopausal for about fifteen years, during which time their arteries could be accumulating plaque and their bones could be deteriorating without the benefits of estrogen. Half of the study subjects were current or former smokers. The average weight of the women was high: they had an average body mass index of 28+ (which translates into a weight of 170 pounds for a woman five feet, five inches tall). A third of the women had high blood pressure and were taking medications for it. In many ways the study subjects were not typical women going through menopause.

Even so, on January 8, 2003, just six months after the announcement that the WHI would be abruptly ended, the FDA pronounced that all estrogen medications in the United States—whether or not they included progestins—had to be labeled with a boxed warning (the highest level of warning information in labeling) showing the WHI results. Since then, all labels describe the increased risks of breast cancer, stroke, and heart disease; the labels recommend the use of the lowest possible dose of estrogen for the shortest time; and they warn against the use of estrogen for protecting against heart disease.

The sections of the WHI on the risks and benefits of hormone therapy are only part of this vast study. In its entirety, the WHI is a multimillion dollar, fifteen-year project that involves more than 161,000 women between the ages of fifty and seventy-nine. The WHI has both clinical trials (in which women are randomly selected to receive either HRT or a placebo) and observational studies (in which the medical history and health habits of more than 100,000 women are tracked for eight to twelve years). The goal of the WHI is to provide practical information not only on hormone replacement but also on such matters as dietary patterns and calcium and vitamin D supplements on the prevention of heart disease, cancer, and osteoporosis.

So far the WHI has published results only on hormone therapy, in particular on HRT (estrogen-plus-progestin therapy) as it relates to risk for breast cancer, cardiovascular disease, osteoporosis, mental functioning, and quality of life. The studies on the effects of diet and calcium supplements and other factors are yet to come.

Many health care professionals have been reevaluating the data, realizing that the WHI did not study women actually going through menopause. Statistical reevaluation of the same WHI data has shown that the cardiovascular risks were overrated. Researchers looking at the WHIMS trial have begun to emphasize that starting HRT in women over sixty-five may not be beneficial, although there is still a considerable possibility that early intervention (that is, giving HRT right at the time of menopause) may still be helpful for Alzheimer's and is unlikely to cause any harm.

▶ *What do the results of the WHI mean to you?*

In the face of all the recent negative evidence on HRT, some of it in direct contradiction to studies that had been previously published, you may well wonder what you should do to protect your well-being as you approach menopause and for the rest of your life thereafter. Is it safe to take HRT for a short time to minimize the hot flashes and other discomforts that plague many women in the years around menopause? How can you protect your bones throughout your lifetime? How can you remain sexually active through your postmenopausal years? What strategies can you use to maximize your cardiovascular health? Can you ward off dementia or Alzheimer's disease?

The purpose of this book is to guide you toward making sensible and informed decisions—not just on the subject of hormone replacement therapy but on a wide range of health issues that surround midlife and beyond. We hope that the book will give you a thorough understanding of what happens during and after menopause, so that when you make choices about your health, you can make decisions that enhance both your well-being and your peace of mind.

2 The Physiology of Menopause

HOW IT HAPPENS

MENOPAUSE is not something that happens but something that stops happening, not an event but a nonevent. By definition, menopause is the cessation of menses caused by the cessation of ovarian function—in other words, the end of your menstrual cycles caused by the shutdown of your ovaries. It represents the end of about forty years of monthly menstrual cycles. After producing, nurturing, and sending out an egg cell every month—except during pregnancies—your ovaries finally wear out and cease functioning. Unlike labor, a process that has three well-defined stages, menopause has only one well-defined endpoint, your final menstrual period. The changes leading up to this event, however, may make themselves evident to you for as long as ten years.

"Perimenopause," which means "around menopause," describes these years, the time when you may start to notice menopausal symptoms: hot flashes, sleep disruptions, mood swings, and other signs, many of them annoying.

In order to understand the changes that lead up to menopause, you need to understand something about the years that preceded it. Understanding basic female physiology

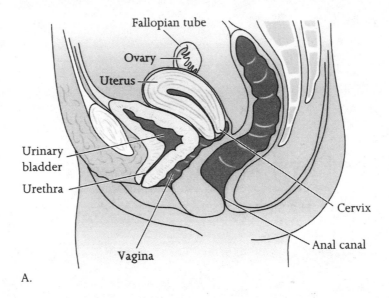

A.

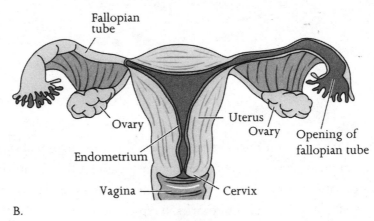

B.

FIGURE 1. The internal female reproductive organs. A, lateral view; B, frontal view.

will also help you appreciate why certain symptoms occur and how various treatments work. This brief refresher should get you up to speed, if you've forgotten what you learned many years ago.

THE OVARIES AND THEIR FUNCTIONS

The main players in the process of menopause are your ovaries. The ovaries have two functions: to make eggs and to make sex hormones—mainly estrogen and progesterone, but also a few others.

The ovaries make estrogen in several forms, of which the most important is estradiol. Other forms are estriol and estrone, but all three are usually grouped under the single name "estrogen." This hormone is important in changing a girl into a woman, in contributing to the growth spurt of adolescence, in the maturation of the uterus and other reproductive organs, and in the development of female sex characteristics. Estrogen also plays a major part in regulating the menstrual cycle, and it influences other organs that are seemingly unrelated to reproduction. The second important ovarian hormone is progesterone, which along with estrogen regulates the menstrual cycle.

In addition to estrogen and progesterone, generally known as the female sex hormones, the ovaries produce small amounts of male sex hormones called androgens, including testosterone. In women, testosterone seems to have a role in the female sex drive and in assertiveness, and it may account for certain "masculine" traits (such as facial hair) in postmenopausal women.

The other important function of the ovaries is to produce eggs. The ovaries are formed during fetal life, as are the egg cells within them. Early in fetal life, the future baby girl carries within her immature ovaries about a million eggs, her full complement for a lifetime; at birth, this number has dwindled to perhaps four hundred thousand. Only a small fraction of these, perhaps four hundred, are destined to reach maturity; the others degenerate at some point in their development, and at menopause only a few remain.

This state of events means that a woman's egg cells are the same age she is, a fact that is important to older women who are seeking to bear children. Consequently, the eggs that are available to be fertilized when a woman is forty-five are twenty-five years older than the eggs that were available for fertilization when she was twenty. Statistics have confirmed that certain birth defects, in particular Down syndrome, result from chromosomal changes that take place in the eggs as they age.

THE PHYSIOLOGY OF THE MENSTRUAL CYCLE

By the time a girl reaches puberty, more than half of the million eggs that were formed prenatally have been lost. The others are at rest, encapsulated in structures that will form the ovarian follicles. In their simplest or primordial state, the follicles consist of the egg cell surrounded by a single layer of cells called granulosa cells. When the ovaries become more active at puberty, the eggs begin to develop. Every month some of the follicles start growing. In each growing follicle the granulosa cells divide and reproduce many times so that soon, instead of a single layer, layers and layers of them surround the egg cell; these granulosa cells make most of the estrogen in the body.

The cells in the ovary around the outside of the follicle contribute to the process, too, causing the outer layer of the follicle to grow and its cells, in turn, to differentiate. Then when the follicle reaches a certain size, it develops a fluid-filled pocket, which gets bigger and bigger as the cycle continues.

About a week into the menstrual cycle, a selection process takes place. The biggest follicle of the group that is growing and differentiating is chosen to be "follicle of the month"—in scientific terminology, the dominant follicle. It continues to increase in size while the other follicles degenerate and die off. (Once in a while the signals get crossed and more than one follicle continues to develop, creating the possibility of fraternal twins.)

When the dominant follicle reaches a certain size, it ruptures. The egg cell and some of the surrounding granulosa cells burst through the wall of the ovary, an event that is known as ovulation. This happens on about day fourteen of the twenty-eight-day menstrual cycle. If all goes well, the egg cell is swept into the fallopian tube. The ends of the tube have specialized cells whose hairlike projections sweep back and forth, beating in waves and propelling the egg cell toward the interior of the tube. Once in the tube, the egg

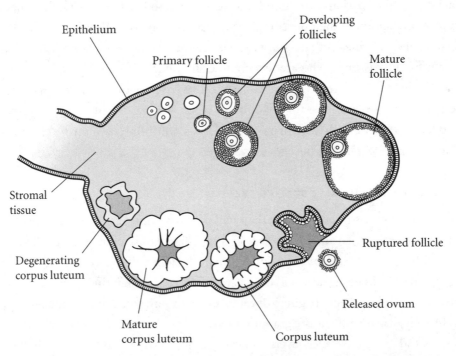

FIGURE 2. The ovary, with follicles developing and degenerating during the menstrual cycle.

may or may not be fertilized. This part of the cycle, which deals with the development of the follicles, is called the follicular phase.

Meanwhile, back in the ovary, what is left of the follicle starts to become active again. It changes into a glandlike structure called the corpus luteum, Latin for "yellow body," which indeed is the color of the follicle remnant. If the egg cell in the fallopian tube does not meet any sperm and get fertilized, the corpus luteum reaches its maximum growth in about ten days (day twenty-four of the cycle) and in its turn begins to degenerate. But during its short life span (in a nonpregnant woman), the corpus luteum is very active and secretes large amounts of both progesterone and estrogen.

All of this action in the ovaries brings about changes in the uterine lining, or endometrium. As the follicles within the ovaries enlarge and develop, the lining of the uterus begins to thicken and proliferate in response to the estrogen produced in the ovaries. After ovulation takes place, roughly on day fourteen, the estrogen level again rises. The additional progesterone produced by the corpus luteum acts on the endometrial tissue to stabilize it and turn it into a hospitable environment, ready to receive an egg should fertilization occur.

If fertilization does not occur and the once-active corpus luteum degenerates (on about day twenty-eight of the cycle), there is a sudden shutdown in the production of both progesterone and estrogen and the endometrium is deprived of its support system. The uterine blood vessels constrict, so that the lining has a diminished supply of oxygen and of nutrients. The muscular tissue of the uterus begins to contract rhythmically. Soon the uterine lining disintegrates and is sloughed off as menstrual blood, except for a thin deep layer that will start regenerating the endometrium for the next cycle. This part of the menstrual cycle, from ovulation on day fourteen to the onset of menstruation on day twenty-eight, is called the luteal phase.

This routine is complex, at least as carefully organized as an intricately plotted murder mystery. The organizers or controllers—the agents that start and stop the different actions of the cycle—are hormones, and in fact the very name "hormone" comes from a Greek verb meaning "to urge on" or "rouse." Although the ovaries are the chief producers of the female sex hormones estrogen and progesterone, they do not do their job in isolation but are part of a chain of command that begins (to the best of our knowledge) in the brain.

The remotest roots of the sequence seem to be in the cerebral cortex, the mass of gray matter that is known to play a role in memory, language acquisition, and motor control. The exact action of the cerebral cortex in the hormonal regulation of the menstrual cycle is not yet known, but the cortex seems to influence such changes as the loss of periods during times of stress.

The next player in the sequence is the hypothalamus, a small region of the brain that lies above the pituitary gland (and below an area called the thalamus, as the name suggests). Though tiny, the hypothalamus has a role in regulating the internal environment of the body, for example influencing the water balance within the cells and tissues, eating behavior, and the daily sleep and waking cycle. The hypothalamus also releases the hormones that will trigger menstruation.

Starting around the time of puberty, the hypothalamus initiates the ovarian cycle every month by secreting a hormone called GnRH, gonadotropin-releasing hormone. The gonadotropins, which are luteinizing hormone (LH) and follicle-stimulating hormone (FSH), control the ovaries, the female gonads. (The word "gonad" simply means an organ that produces reproductive cells—eggs or sperm.)

The chemical messenger GnRH alerts the appropriate region of the pituitary gland, geographically a close neighbor of the hypothalamus, to secrete its hormones, LH and FSH. The hormones from the pituitary will in turn stimulate the ovaries. The FSH does just what its name suggests: it stimulates the follicles to develop. The LH, whose presence in the blood surges at midcycle, causes the dominant follicle to release the egg cell, culminating in ovulation.

All of this regulation is governed by a control system called negative or reciprocal feedback, which works more or less like a thermostat. After you set the thermostat in a room at the desired level, the device senses the temperature and turns the furnace off or on to keep the level where you want it. Within your body the regulating factors are chemical, rather than thermal, but the principle is the same. There is a constant reciprocal feedback loop between the brain and the ovaries, and the brain continuously responds to the levels of estrogen that it senses. For example, a lack of estrogen in the blood causes the LH and FSH to rise, during the menstrual cycle and also after the menopause.

WHAT HAPPENS AT MENOPAUSE

Your ovaries, like many of your other organs, peak at some time in your late twenties or early thirties. Thereafter their production of estrogen and progesterone begins to decline gradually and finally stops altogether. Researchers surmise that this has to do with the depletion and finally the absence of follicles. It is estimated that you have five thousand to ten thousand follicles left when you are forty; the number declines precipitously after that. Researchers also know that with aging either the follicles become less responsive to

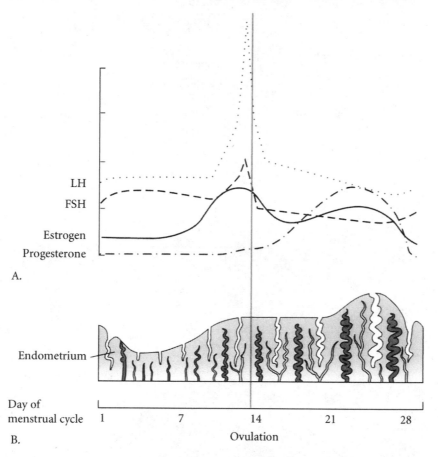

LH
FSH
Estrogen
Progesterone

A.

Endometrium

Day of
menstrual cycle   1   7   14   21   28

B.   Ovulation

FIGURE 3. Hormone levels and changes in the uterine lining during the normal menstrual cycle. A, levels of pituitary and ovarian hormones in the bloodstream; B, maturation and thickening of the lining of the uterus and its blood supply.

the gonadotropins that formerly urged them to action or the smaller number of follicles started at each cycle results in lower estrogen and increased LH and FSH.

At some point, most likely when you are in your early forties, your menstrual periods will probably become irregular in response to these declining estrogen and progesterone levels. You will begin having occasional anovulatory periods, that is, periods in which no egg is released from a follicle. (Your ovaries are producing enough estrogen to build up the endometrium, but not enough to fully mature a follicle.) Because ovulation does not occur, there is no corpus luteum to make progesterone. And because there is no proges-terone, there is no way to stabilize the uterine lining; nor is there a signal (the withdrawal

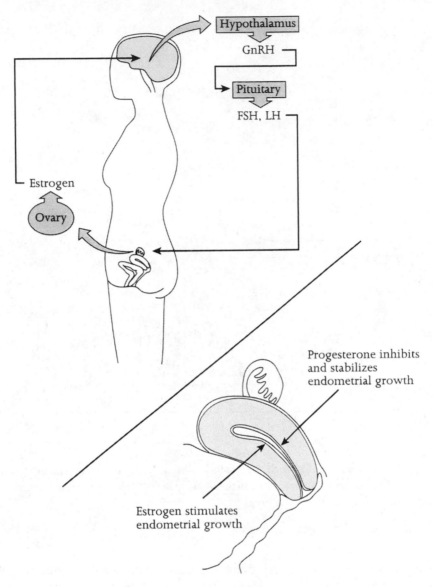

FIGURE 4. Hypothalamic-pituitary-ovarian feedback loop. The hypothalamus manufactures GnRH, which stimulates the pituitary to make FSH and LH. These in turn stimulate the ovaries to make estrogen. The presence of estrogen inhibits further production of GnRH. When estrogen levels fall, the hypothalamus makes more GnRH.

of progesterone) for the shedding to take place in an orderly, controlled manner. Instead, the uterine lining keeps on building and building, eventually breaking down only because it outgrows its blood supply.

Another scenario for the menopause is that your ovaries may be producing some estrogen and progesterone, but not enough to keep the cycle going at its usual rate; the process may take longer than usual, and while you may still have ovulatory cycles, your periods may be more widely spaced. Sooner or later you will have your last menstrual period. A year afterward, you can safely say that you are menopausal.

3 Signs and Symptoms

A decade ago, menopause was a mysterious and somewhat taboo subject. Women who came into my office knew what menopause was, but they wondered what it was like. They knew that menopause, the conclusion of menstruation, was a milestone that marks the end of a woman's reproductive life, just as menarche, the onset of menstruation, marks the beginning of a woman's childbearing years. Most knew about hot flashes, but few women connected sleeplessness, mood swings, fatigue, crawly skin, or increased menstrual flow with the beginning of menopause.

This chapter will help you identify the signs of approaching menopause and suggest ways for dealing with the changes that come about during the five to ten years before and after menopause.

In the medical literature, as we saw in Chapter 2, menopause has a clear definition: the cessation of ovarian function, which results in the permanent cessation of menstrual periods. In life things are seldom as straightforward as they are in literature, and so this definition is not entirely helpful. In the first place, it is useful only after the fact. Because most women skip a few menstrual periods before they cease altogether, you can't be sure that you are truly menopausal, that your periods have stopped and will never return, until you have gone for a year without one. In other words, you don't even know that you are menopausal until a year after the "event" has happened.

In the second place, the medical definition suggests (as do some of the afternoon television talk shows) that menopause is a single event, something that happens once and is over. Actually, the process that ends in menopause, the decrease of ovarian function to the point that menstruation ceases, happens over a period of years beginning in your midthirties and continuing for many years.

What concerns most women is not that final menstrual period or the time thereafter but the changes in long-established physical and psychological patterns that come about in the five to ten years on either side of menopause—the period known medically as the perimenopause. Also important to women and to their medical caregivers are the long-term issues, after the acute menopausal symptoms have passed.

▶ *At what age can I expect to go through menopause?*

The average age of natural menopause in this country is about fifty-one, a statistic that has remained remarkably constant over the years. The normal range of age at menopause is about forty-five to fifty-five, but among my patients I see a range from about age thirty-five to fifty-nine. Any individual woman can begin experiencing the symptoms of perimenopause as early as her midthirties or as late as her early fifties.

The relative stability of the average age of menopause has a couple of interesting implications. First, it stands in contrast to the average age of menarche, which decreased slightly between the turn of the twentieth century and the 1950s, probably because of improved nutrition; for girls in Western industrialized countries a plateau seems to have been reached in the age of menarche, which has remained stable for the past five decades or so. Menstruation doesn't usually begin until a girl weighs somewhere between ninety-five and one hundred pounds. Since children in financially comfortable families nowadays are likely to be optimally nourished, girls probably reach their adult weight sooner than their mothers did. Body-fat percentage also plays a role in triggering the onset of menstruation, so lean, athletic girls may begin menstruating later than rounder, plumper girls.

Second, while the age of menopause has remained the same, the life expectancy of

American women has gone up to about age eighty for white women and to about age seventy-five for women of color. Thus the average American woman, who begins menstruating at age twelve and goes through menopause at fifty-one, spends more than a third of her life as a postmenopausal woman. The significance of this fact to her health is tremendous and will reflect the care she takes of herself during the perimenopausal years. Doctor Fred Naftolin, former chair of the department of obstetrics and gynecology at the Yale University School of Medicine, has correctly pointed out that "the perimenopause casts a long shadow."

Each year hundreds of thousands of American women, many of them not near the age of natural menopause, experience surgical menopause—that is, removal of the ovaries—at the time of hysterectomy. Surgical menopause, if not followed by estrogen replacement, often leads to more profound menopausal symptoms than does natural menopause.

▶ *How can I predict when I might experience menopause?*

The best way to predict the age of your own menopause is to check your family history. If your mother was menopausal at age forty-two, then it is likely that you will have a relatively early menopause (though not necessarily at forty-two). If she had a late menopause, you can probably count on having yours later than the average.

The onset of perimenopausal symptoms, hot flashes for example, does not necessarily predict the actual coming of menopause. If you begin noticing perimenopausal symptoms at forty-two, there is a chance that you might not be fully menopausal until you are fifty, especially if your mother and older sister did not experience menopause until that age.

The classic dogma used to be that if you began menstruating late, say between the ages of fourteen and sixteen, you would reach menopause early. Conversely, if you began your periods early, before twelve, you would reach menopause relatively late. The notion behind this theory, presumably, was that if your ovaries weren't robust to begin with (accounting for late onset of menstruation), they would give up and stop functioning early. Although some gynecologists still find some relevance in this theory, my own clinical practice does not support it.

Studies have shown that smokers have an earlier menopause than nonsmokers. To put it bluntly, smoking destroys your ovaries. That is the bad news; the good news is that if you stop smoking, you may buy yourself a few extra years of ovarian function. So if you are concerned about preserving your fertility, perhaps wanting to delay childbearing until you get your career on track, you should quit smoking immediately.

▶ *Can a sudden, stressful event bring on menopause all at once?*

I have talked to many women who said that menopause came on them suddenly without any warning symptoms.

> Natalie F. started menstruating when she was ten. Unlike most girls, she began with the pattern she would follow for her entire reproductive life, her periods coming like clockwork every twenty-eight days. She never missed a period (except when she was pregnant or nursing) and never was either late or early. When she was fifty, her mother died. Natalie never had another period.

Often the traumatic event is not of such magnitude as the death of a parent. I have had women call me to say that they stopped menstruating after their dog died.

▶ *What are the reasons for early menopause?*

Early menopause, also called premature menopause or premature ovarian failure, is menopause that occurs for any reason before age forty; it happens to about 1 percent of American women. About 30 percent of these women have a female relative who is also affected, suggesting that in many cases they have inherited a genetic predisposition for it. The exact reasons are unknown. Researchers have hypothesized that women with premature ovarian failure were born with fewer egg follicles, or perhaps their follicles simply had a shorter life span. New research, however, has revealed that a genetic mutation may be involved. The mutated gene seems to cause women to produce fewer eggs, either because it halts normal egg follicle development or brings about some action that destroys the eggs.

Factors other than inheritance can also play a role. In some autoimmune diseases, a woman's immune system makes antibodies against her own ovaries. The situation is analogous to diabetes, where the immune system attacks the pancreas. Early menopause can, of course, be caused by surgical removal of the ovaries. The ovarian function of women who have had chemotherapy and/or radiation as treatment for cancer often is either temporarily or permanently altered or destroyed. In some women ovarian function comes back fully after the therapy is completed; in some women it comes back partially;

and in some women it never comes back. Although younger women, in their thirties for example, have a better chance of ovarian recovery than do older women, it is not easy to ascertain the outcome ahead of time. Smoking, as we have seen, shortens the number of years the ovaries continue to function.

Although there is no ironclad evidence, some data suggest that women who have had hysterectomies many years before menopause (but have retained their ovaries) may also have a somewhat earlier onset of menopausal signs. It has been suggested that surgery alters the blood supply to the ovaries, causing them to age more quickly.

Other reasons for early menopause include several rare conditions. One is Turner's syndrome, a genetic disease that involves chromosomal abnormalities.

▶ What problems are associated with early menopause?

Whatever its cause, premature ovarian failure, especially if abrupt, is associated with more symptoms and more serious medical consequences than menopause at the usual age. Early menopause leads to immediate inability to conceive children. It is also associated with increased rates of osteoporosis and coronary artery disease, and with incontinence. Of course, these problems respond favorably to ERT. It is just possible that there is a correlation between early menopause and other concerns of aging, such as Alzheimer's disease.

▶ Can anything be done about premature menopause?

You can certainly avoid compromising your ovaries by not smoking. With some diseases that require radiation therapy, such as Hodgkin's lymphoma, the surgeon can take protective measures, moving the ovaries out of the field of radiation, which makes damage and subsequent ovarian failure less likely.

If genetic inheritance is at the root of the problem, all the critical events have occurred in fetal development, and although this kind of premature menopause currently can't be prevented, its symptoms can be managed and many of its long-term consequences can be avoided, especially if treatment begins early.

In this area, I believe, the Women's Health Initiative studies are way off base. Women who have premature ovarian failure should talk to their doctors about the importance of hormone therapy in maintaining bone strength, vaginal lubrication, and other benefits. At the September 2003 meeting of the North American Menopause Society (a professional organization of physicians specializing in this field), the WHI review panel encouraged women with premature ovarian failure not to pay attention to the WHI findings, since the study specifically excluded women under age fifty. Women who undergo menopause early are now strongly encouraged to consider HRT.

▶ *Can women who have had premature menopause ever have children?*

The advances in assisted reproductive techniques may help women who have had premature menopause to bear children. These are the very women for whom technologies involving donor eggs were developed.

▶ *What signs or symptoms suggest the approach of menopause?*

A classic group of physical signs suggest menopause is approaching. These signs (they are not really symptoms in the pathological sense of the word, because menopause is not a disease but a normal condition of life) include hot flashes, night sweats, and changes in the frequency, length, and amount of flow of your periods. Many women experience sleeplessness or broken sleep, even if they do not have night sweats and hot flashes. Some women report psychological symptoms that include depression, mood swings, and irritability. Others comment on their poor memory or inability to focus mentally. Headaches, sometimes migraines, can be associated with menopause.

You may notice some of these changes, all of them, or none of them. You may have some of them occasionally but not all the time. Or, if you are lucky, you may be among the 15 to 20 percent of American women who simply stop menstruating one day without any noticeable evidence to suggest that they have just had their last period. If you are among the majority of American women, some 65 to 70 percent, you will find these perimenopausal changes troublesome in degrees that vary from mildly annoying to seriously disruptive. If you are very unlucky, you might be among the 10 percent who find the changes surrounding menopause overwhelmingly difficult to cope with. Fortunately, even if you are in the group with more severe menopausal signs, modern medicine should be able to help you.

There are also physical and psychological changes that simply go along with getting older. They come at about the same time as menopause and may (or may not) be associated with it. In fact, one of the problems associated with menopause is that it is sometimes hard to separate changes that are caused by growing older from changes that are caused by decreased hormone production. As we age, our hair (including pubic hair, eyebrows, and leg and arm hair as well as the hair on our head) gets sparser and may change in texture. In contrast, hair on the lower face increases. Skin becomes thinner and less elastic; we tend to accumulate fat around our middle and to gain weight on the upper arms, back, abdomen, and breasts. Studies show that a significant proportion of perimenopausal and postmenopausal women experience a decline in sexual interest, although it is not clear whether these changes in attitude come from menopause itself or simply from growing older.

▶ *Are the signs of early menopause different from those of regular menopause?*

The signs are the same, except of course that they occur earlier: hot flashes, night sweats, irritability, and mood swings. Menstrual periods may become lighter, less frequent, or stop altogether. You might consider the possibility of premature menopause also if you or someone in your family has an autoimmune disease (hypothyroidism, Addison's disease, Graves' disease, diabetes, lupus, rheumatoid arthritis, inflammatory bowel syndrome).

▶ *If I think I am having premature menopause, what should I do?*

You should see your doctor sooner rather than later. If your premature menopause is being caused by some other disorder, the underlying condition can be dealt with.

▶ *Is there any way to predict whether menopause will be easy or difficult?*

Unquestionably, some women pass through menopause with fewer symptoms and less discomfort than others. In the bad old days, it was generally believed that women brought discomfort on themselves by their neurotic responses to the physiological changes that were occurring.

Some older studies showed that married women were more distressed than single women and that mothers were more distressed than women who had not had children, perhaps because married women and mothers were more likely to feel the pangs of loneliness and the so-called empty nest syndrome when their children left home. But modern research has not targeted any group of women as likely to experience extreme distress and any other group as likely to sail through menopause without any symptoms whatsoever.

Today most physicians are willing to acknowledge that the discomforts of menopause are caused physiologically rather than psychologically. It is true, however, that the mind shapes and refines our responses to the physiological changes that underlie

TABLE 1. Could It Be Menopause?

SYMPTOM	NEVER	SOMETIMES	FREQUENTLY
Irregular menstrual periods			
Hot flashes			
Night sweats			
Vaginal dryness			
Vaginal itching or burning			
Depression			
Memory lapses			
Fatigue			
Painful intercourse			
Insomnia			
Heart palpitations			
Joint aches or pains			
Mood swings			
Tingling skin			
Headaches			
Decreased sexual desire			
Anxiety			
Irritability			
Crying spells			
Frequent urination			
Leaking of urine			
Weight gain			

Note: All these symptoms can have causes other than menopause, but all of them can also be associated with the approach of menopause.

menopausal discomforts. My experience as a physician is that there does seem to be a familial predictor, but one that results from conditioning rather than from inherited genetic traits or physiological problems. Women whose mothers described their own menopause as "terrible" and "really almost unbearable" are likely to experience more discomfort than women whose mothers did not complain of such severe symptoms. I find an analogue in menstrual discomfort: mothers who say they "nearly died" during their periods are likely to condition their daughters to have uncomfortable periods.

I do tell menopausal women who are concerned because their mothers had such an unfortunate menopausal experience that in today's world we have therapies that can probably relieve discomfort completely. A woman who is fifty-one years old in the twenty-first century need not be overwhelmed with symptoms, as her mother was before her.

▶ Are there laboratory tests for diagnosing menopause?

The answer to this question is a rousing yes and no. Yes, there are tests; no, they won't tell you absolutely whether you are menopausal or how far along in the process you are.

▶ What are these tests?

Physicians usually rely on one of two tests: the first measures estrogen in the bloodstream, the second measures blood levels of follicle-stimulating hormone. In general, the tests look for low estrogen levels in the bloodstream and high levels of FSH.

Of the several kinds of estrogen normally circulating in the bloodstream, estradiol tends to be the easiest to measure. The test for menopause looks for an estradiol level lower than 50 pg/ml (picograms per milliliter). During the normal premenopausal menstrual cycle, estradiol varies widely, ranging between 50 and 400 pg/ml. (A picogram is one one-trillionth of a gram; a milliliter is one one-thousandth of a liter.) Physicians generally agree that an estradiol of 20 or 30 confirms menopause. Menopause happens because the ovaries no longer produce estrogen, so it is reasonable and indeed correct to assume that a menopausal woman will have lower blood estrogen levels than someone who is menstruating regularly.

The other lab test for menopause is a blood test for follicle-stimulating hormone, which in a premenopausal woman is sent by the pituitary to stimulate the ovary to cause follicles to develop. The postmenopausal ovary cannot make estrogen in response to the FSH, so more and more FSH is produced by the pituitary in hopes of stimulating the ovary to its former function. Thus what physicians are looking for as confirmation of menopause is a high level of FSH. During the menstrual cycle of a premenopausal woman blood levels of FSH vary but generally remain below 30 (that is, 30 milli-international units per milliliter of blood). Menopausal women have FSH levels higher than 30, sometimes even in the 100s. So if your FSH level turns out to be 67 and you have other signs and symptoms, by laboratory indicators you are menopausal.

▶ *Why don't these lab tests always accurately diagnose menopause?*

Women generally want to have blood estradiol levels and FSH levels taken for one of two reasons: they are partway through the menopausal process and want to know how far along they are, or they think they are menopausal and want to be sure. Unfortunately lab tests won't give a definitive answer to either question 100 percent of the time.

The problem with taking a blood estradiol level, and one reason why the utility of this test is controversial, is that during the menstrual cycle the normal estradiol level fluctuates anywhere between 50 and 400. Without knowing where a woman is in her cycle, the level alone does not mean much. Since a perimenopausal woman frequently has irregular ovulatory cycles and irregular periods, it is often difficult to decide where she is in her cycle. Is she just about to ovulate? Or did she ovulate several weeks ago? Her low estradiol level may simply indicate that she is very early or very late in her cycle.

> Louisa W., in her late forties, comes in to me experiencing occasional hot
> flashes, irregular periods, and some episodes of insomnia. A blood test shows
> that her estradiol level is 40 and her FSH is 67. Based on these tests, it looks as
> though Louisa is menopausal. I tell her and she feels relieved. Two months later
> she has a period. So she is not menopausal yet.

In fact, the tests didn't tell more than the history and the physical exam did. What did the numbers mean? Did that 40 represent a peak of estrogen for this cycle, or was it measured at a low point in the cycle? If she were ten years younger, would that 40 have been a 400? Was Louisa in the late part of her ovulatory cycle when the blood was drawn, in which case we would expect low estradiol levels, or was she just about to ovulate, in which case we would expect that 40 to be much higher? Since perimenopausal women have highly irregular cycles, it is difficult from any one assessment to know just where Louisa is in her cycle.

If her estradiol level had come back at something like 20, we could have said yes, certainly this is low; premenopausal women do not normally have estradiol levels that low at any time during their cycles.

The same kinds of problems interfere with the accuracy of the FSH test. Like estradiol levels, FSH levels fluctuate both in premenopausal and in perimenopausal women, so the test is not necessarily conclusive. Louisa's FSH level is higher than we would expect in a premenopausal woman, whose normal FSH maximum is no more than 30.

> Marian A. is fifty-three. She has gone almost a year without a period. She has hot flashes at regular intervals and wants to know whether she is fully menopausal. To my way of thinking, there doesn't seem much reason to do an estradiol or an FSH level to confirm that yes, Marian is menopausal. Her age, the length of time she has been without a period, and the presence of hot flashes all suggest that she is very nearly menopausal. These signs do not mean, however, that she will never have another menstrual period. Many women do have one or two after a significant time without one.

In most cases, then, estradiol and FSH levels aren't really worth checking, because they will not tell you what you want to know any better than can be determined without the tests. Even if you do have an FSH level that is substantially elevated and an estradiol level that is very low, there is no guarantee that you are forever finished with your periods.

Many physicians will biopsy women like Marian if they go about a year without a period and then suddenly have one, because of concern about the possibility of cancer. What most biopsies show is normal, proliferative endometrial tissue, the type one sees in regularly menstruating women. A biopsy showed with certainty that what was happening to Marian was normal ovarian activity, not some pathological condition.

▶ How much do FSH and estradiol tests cost?

These are expensive tests. In the area where I work they cost about one hundred dollars apiece and are not always covered by insurance. Given the direction in which health care seems to be moving, they are unlikely to be covered in the future. So if your test is inconclusive and your doctor wants it repeated in six months, you could be faced with a bill for about two hundred dollars, a substantial amount. Some women feel that it is definitely worth two hundred dollars to learn whether their estradiol and FSH levels are high or low. But at a time in history when many people are trying to keep down medical costs, it is worth thinking twice about drawing estradiols and FSHs.

▶ *What is the physiological explanation for these hormone levels?*

We know that as a woman ages, her ovaries produce less and less estrogen, until at menopause they produce virtually none. This decline causes the lower estradiol levels in the blood. Although levels fluctuate during a perimenopausal woman's cycle, rebounding upward now and again, the trend is definitely downward. Perimenopausal women produce less estrogen than women who have not begun the menopausal process.

The mechanism that accounts for the high levels of FSH in menopausal women is more complex. The ovaries do not independently decide how much FSH or estrogen to produce, or when, as we have seen; instead, they are driven and regulated by the pituitary gland through a process of feedback. When the pituitary senses low blood estrogen, it sends a message to the ovaries, in the form of a burst of follicle-stimulating hormone, to increase estrogen production. If the ovaries cannot make much estrogen because of their planned obsolescence, the pituitary continues to secrete more and more FSH, signaling the ovaries to step up their estrogen production. Blood levels of FSH rise and rise, sometimes quite high. A newly discovered hormone called inhibin, which is secreted by follicles, has been shown to control FSH. So not having normal amounts of estrogen or inhibin in the blood is a kind of double whammy, giving a disproportionate increase in FSH in comparison to LH.

▶ *When do these perimenopausal changes appear?*

Although ovarian function begins to decline when women are in their midthirties, signs of menopause usually become evident in the early to middle forties. But they can start as soon as the early thirties or appear as late as the midfifties. The age at which these changes begin does not necessarily indicate when menopause will actually take place, for the perimenopausal period in general lasts somewhere between five and eight years. Occasional women get their first hot flash at age forty-two and are not fully menopausal until they are fifty-five.

▶ *What variations in the menstrual cycle occur during the perimenopausal years?*

One of the first things that many women notice as they approach menopause is a variation in the pattern of their periods, a pattern established perhaps thirty years before in early adulthood. Periods may change in length, frequency, or amount of flow. The key word here is "change," because individuals vary widely. Menstrual periods can become heavier or lighter; they can be longer or shorter. Some women find themselves bleeding two or three weeks out of every month, while others notice that their periods are spaced further and further apart. Some women have light periods every couple of months; others have very heavy periods every couple of weeks. Some women skip periods for several months and then have very heavy flows. In short, there are many patterns of change, and no one pattern seems to predominate.

Patterns may also change for a single individual. For a while, a woman may have very heavy periods that may then taper off and become more widely spaced. Conversely, after a period of light and infrequent periods, she may experience heavy, frequent bleeding. All these changes are normal. However, heavy and frequent bleeding, especially after intercourse, can raise the possibility of cancer and should trigger a visit to the doctor.

▶ *Are heavy periods a sign of approaching menopause?*

Many women experience heavy bleeding, medically known as menorrhagia, during the perimenopausal period. For some women menorrhagia is merely an inconvenience, but others find that it can disrupt their everyday lives, interfere with their work schedules, or at the very least ruin their vacations. For some women, loss of blood is itself worrisome.

▶ *How heavy is so-called heavy bleeding?*

In general, women tend to overestimate the amount of blood they lose during a normal period. Doctor Ian Fraser, a researcher at the University of Sydney in Australia, weighed tampons and pads to determine blood loss during periods. He divided the test group into heavy and light bleeders and found that the women in the heavy group lost between 70 and 130 ml of blood each month. Thirty ml is one fluid ounce, so the average blood loss for the "heavy" group was about four and a half ounces of blood per cycle. In common household terms, the heavy bleeders in the study lost about half a cup, or a fourth of the pint usually given at a blood-donation center.

You are unlikely to measure your blood loss this way, so doctors offer various ways to gauge how heavily you are bleeding. Some suggest that you can consider yourself to be bleeding heavily if you have to change a super tampon every hour for twenty-four hours; other physicians suggest a standard of every half-hour for six hours. While this rate of loss could be considered "heavy," it is not life threatening.

A relatively small proportion of perimenopausal women really do experience worrisome blood loss. On rare occasions women have come into my office with a towel between their legs because they were hemorrhaging so badly.

Cathy H., forty-eight years old, called me from the grocery store in a nearby town one Saturday morning. She was having a heavy period and had gone to buy tampons; while she was standing in the feminine products aisle, she suddenly started to hemorrhage, quickly soaking through her clothes. I told her to get to the emergency room immediately. We performed an emergency D&C (dilatation and curettage), the only measure that would control her flow. This kind of bleeding, however, is uncommon.

▶ *Is heavy bleeding dangerous?*

Heavy bleeding is apt to be more of a nuisance and a concern to the women who experience it than it is a serious threat. On rare occasions, however, heavy periodic bleeding can be dangerous because it leads to significant anemia, in which the red-blood-cell count falls drastically. And strangely enough, women who become anemic tend to bleed more heavily with their periods, which creates a vicious cycle. Most of the time we think of the body as being "smart," that is, responsive to its own needs; but in this case, for reasons that are not understood, the body is "dumb."

For women the normal hematocrit (a measure of the percentage of red blood cells in the blood) is about 40; for men it is in the mid- to high 40s. A small percentage of women bleed so heavily that their hematocrit drops two or three points every time they have a period, but if the hematocrit remains somewhere in the range of 35 or 36, that level does not interfere with their health or curtail their activities.

A significant degree of anemia does occur in the woman whose hematocrit drops to the high 20s or low 30s. Her symptoms might include fatigue, light-headedness, and even shortness of breath with exercise. One of my patients, a woman in her midforties, bled so much that she lowered her hematocrit to 16, which means that she has only a little more than one-third of her normal measure of red blood cells. She obviously needs treatment—first, because she will feel better, and second, because if she has a sudden, very heavy bleed, she is not well supplied with hemoglobin. If someone who has plenty of hemoglobin loses a pint or two of blood, the situation is not life threatening. But if she starts with a borderline hematocrit, she has a serious problem. So women who have very heavy periods should have their hematocrits checked periodically.

▶ *Does heavy bleeding have any pathological or dangerous causes?*

Although much of the heavy bleeding women experience at midlife has hormonal causes, other factors, both anatomical and psychological, can be involved. Psychological stress, which can interfere with regular ovulation, may cause heavier bleeding. If the cause of stress is temporary or transient, then it stands to reason that the heavier bleeding should disappear along with the stress. But since this time of life is stressful for many women who are caught between aging parents and young adult children, or who are experiencing all kinds of changes personally and professionally, the stressful situations may be a long time resolving themselves.

Fibroids, which are fairly common, and endometriosis, which is less common, can also cause heavy bleeding and clotting even in women who are nowhere near menopause. Other causes are polyps and uterine cancer.

▶ *How can I distinguish between hormonally caused heavy bleeding and heavy flow caused by some pathological condition?*

Unfortunately there is no simple answer; symptoms alone are not enough to tell you whether heavy bleeding is caused by changes in hormone levels or by something else. Women who are developing anatomical problems (for example, fibroids) that can cause heavy bleeding are likely to be in the same age group as women approaching menopause. Indeed, both fibroids and endometriosis, which are uncomfortable but not life threatening, often become symptomatic in women in their midforties, while uterine cancer seems to peak at about age fifty. If you are concerned about heavy flow, you should talk to your gynecologist so that together you can determine if anything pathological or dangerous is involved.

▶ *Is any danger or risk associated with lighter periods as menopause approaches?*

Many women experience lighter periods as they approach menopause, and most of them are pretty happy with this arrangement; but occasionally a patient comes in, worried about diminished flow. I assure her that if she wants heavy periods, medical science can give them to her. Most of the time, once a woman knows that lighter periods are simply a sign of approaching menopause, she is content with the situation. Certainly there is no medical reason to have periods identical to those she had earlier in life.

▶ *Are there problems associated with either frequent or infrequent menstrual periods?*

While it obviously is inconvenient to be bleeding three weeks out of four, it is not necessarily dangerous—unless the periods are very heavy as well as frequent. In that case the danger, as we have pointed out, is anemia. In rare instances, heavy flow can be associated with cancer, so it does need to be discussed with your caregiver.

The only difficulty associated with less frequent periods is that sometimes a woman's periods may space out for two, three, or four months and then, when a period does occur, she will get very heavy bleeding, what I informally call Niagara Falls flooding. Usually such a woman is not far along in the menopausal process. Her ovaries are still producing estrogen, and in response the lining of her uterus is building up. If she is not ovulating, the lining will continue to build for a month or two; then suddenly, either she will ovulate spontaneously or her uterine lining will have built up so much that it reaches the saturation point and starts pouring out. The problem is that the bleeding is uncontrolled; there is no progesterone to make sure that the period tapers off and ends after an appropriate time. Usually the hematocrit of such women drops several points and they may lose as much as a pint or two of blood with a period.

▶ *Is bleeding between periods dangerous?*

We have seen that many women experience erratic menstrual periods as they approach menopause, and most of these irregularities can be considered normal. With perimenopausal women, changing levels of hormones are most often the culprit, but since spotting between periods is one of the indications of uterine cancer, it can be a cause for concern. Spotting can also be a manifestation of cervical cancer, though bleeding from the cervix generally takes place in the context of bleeding after intercourse, whereas bleeding from the uterus is apt to be spontaneous, unassociated with any particular activity.

▶ *How do I differentiate between the harmless spotting that is related to normal changes in my ovaries and the potentially dangerous spotting that might indicate something abnormal or pathological?*

The answer is that in general, you can't. If you spot once and the problem goes away, there is a good chance that nothing pathological is happening. One episode of spotting in a perimenopausal woman is usually nothing to worry about. But if you start spotting repeatedly or routinely, even though the spotting is just a little bit here and there, you should call your gynecologist and keep track of what is going on.

Many women are ovulatory spotters and bleed a few drops every time they ovulate. In most cases nothing is wrong. This bleeding will recur regularly, around day fourteen in a woman who has a normal twenty-eight-day cycle and less predictably in a woman whose cycles are less regular.

But perimenopausal women who have irregular cycles cannot count on day fourteen as being the time of ovulation. Thus, it is important to pay attention if you do spot. When in your cycle does the bleeding occur? How much bleeding is there? Does it happen after intercourse or is it spontaneous?

Spotting in postmenopausal women may well be a different matter. If you have gone for longer than a year without a period and suddenly begin to spot, you should inform your physician right away. I tell my patients that if something is wrong, if they have a polyp or uterine cancer, it will probably bleed more than once—so that, again, a single episode of postmenopausal bleeding usually does not indicate something terribly wrong. Nevertheless, many (but not all) gynecologists will perform a biopsy on the basis of just one episode of spotting in a postmenopausal woman in order to make sure that it doesn't represent something dangerous.

Gynecologists who choose to biopsy the lining of the uterus make that decision because a routine pelvic exam is not particularly helpful in revealing what is happening inside the uterus. Even a Pap smear, which gives information about the condition of the cervix, does not tell enough about the lining of the uterus itself to rule out cancerous changes. New techniques used to assess the uterine lining are relatively noninvasive and can give helpful information.

▶ *Are blood clots in the menstrual flow a sign of trouble?*

Another thing that concerns many women is clotting. It is generally more troubling to the perimenopausal woman than to her doctor, for clotting is just a manifestation of heaviness of flow. Clots may be startling if you have never had them before; they may be unpleasant and messy, but they are a medical concern only because clots signal a greater blood loss and because they sometimes can cause pain. If a clot forms in the uterus, the uterus may try to expel it by contracting as if the clot were a fetus; these contractions can cause strong cramps.

► *Do perimenopausal women suffer from menstrual cramps?*

Cramping is not a classic menopausal phenomenon. The kind of cramping that women sometimes experience with their periods, the ordinary garden-variety primary dysmenorrhea (menstrual pain that begins early in life), is actually caused by the manufacture of prostaglandins by the lining of the uterus.

Prostaglandins are chemical substances that serve as messengers and, like the hormones to which they are related, act in a number of ways. They cause the uterus to contract; this action restricts blood flow to the uterine muscle, causing pain. Prostaglandin production is highest in those cycles in which ovulation occurs, so if a woman is not ovulating, she doesn't usually make much prostaglandin and tends not to feel much or any discomfort.

This process explains why at the beginning of the menstrual spectrum young girls just getting their periods seldom have cramps. Perhaps after they have been menstruating for a year or so they will begin to have cramps, because they are then beginning to ovulate regularly. The dysmenorrhea is a result of the ovulatory cycles. Just the opposite is happening in a woman at the other end of the menstrual spectrum. As she approaches menopause, some of her cycles are ovulatory, but many of her periods occur without ovulation.

I get a phone call on this subject about once a day. A perimenopausal patient will tell me that she had her regular period two weeks ago, a normal period with her customary cramps. Two weeks later she finds herself again bleeding heavily but with no cramps. She wants to know what's going on. Because she is not ovulating, she is not making prostaglandins. The lining of her uterus has built up in response to the estrogen she is producing, but what she is experiencing in the second, cramp-free period is a kind of breakthrough bleeding uncontrolled by progesterone, which would have been produced in larger amounts after ovulation. Loss of cramping is more characteristic of menopause than cramping.

Still, if you find yourself having cramps, especially when you have not had them regularly before, you should pay attention and alert your gynecologist. Cramps are not necessarily worrisome, but they may be an indication of some other condition such as fibroids or endometriosis.

► *What causes all these irregularities in the menstrual cycle?*

The menstrual changes that women notice at midlife are basically related to changes in ovulatory patterns, which vary as ovarian function decreases. A woman in her late thirties or in her forties does not ovulate as well, and often not as frequently, as she did ten years earlier. Although her ovaries are still making a significant amount of estrogen, her production of progesterone after ovulation is not as copious as it was when she was, say, twenty-five.

Progesterone, a vital hormone in preparing the lining of the uterus to receive a fertilized egg, functions in three ways. It limits the buildup of the lining of the uterus, it stabilizes the lining until fertilization can take place, and if fertilization does not occur, its level drops rapidly, triggering the shedding of the lining. When a woman in her twenties has a normal cycle, she produces an adequate amount of estrogen followed by an adequate amount of progesterone. The progesterone stabilizes the lining of the uterus; but if the egg that leaves the ovary that month is not fertilized, then the part of the ovary that makes progesterone (the corpus luteum) dies. When progesterone levels fall, the lining of the uterus (the endometrium) is shed in a nice, controlled way.

If your ovaries are not making progesterone, there is no hormone to trigger the shedding of the uterine lining, so you don't have a period. If you are making small amounts of progesterone, you may have an early period because your hormone level is too low to keep the endometrium intact. If you are making some progesterone but not enough to limit the growth of the endometrium or prevent excessive buildup, then you may bleed heavily.

▶ What are hot flashes?

Hot flashes, which in Great Britain are called hot flushes, are one of the most common features of menopause. About 70 to 75 percent of women get them to some degree. The classic hot flash is a feeling of heat over the face, shoulders, head, and upper torso; it is usually accompanied by sweating. Often hot flashes are preceded by a premonition that a flash is on the way. Women describe this feeling as one of anxiety or illness, or a tingling sensation or pressure in the head.

What happens in a hot flash is much like what happens whenever the body feels overheated, whether from strenuous exercise on a hot day or from fever. Overheating triggers the body to respond with vasomotor changes, changes in blood vessels that in turn cause changes in blood flow. This process is intended to cool the body to its normal resting state. The blood vessels near the surface of the skin dilate and blood flow to the skin increases, which makes the skin feel hotter and look flushed. Then the skin begins to perspire, and the evaporation from sweating cools the body. This is exactly what happens in a hot flash, although the trigger is not heavy exercise or elevated body temperature.

The usual hot flash is restricted to the face, neck, and upper torso, yet the feelings of flushing and heat can occur in any part of the body. One of my patients says that hot flashes affect only her ears, which turn bright red and feel as if they are on fire. Other women feel hot all over.

Often hot flashes are accompanied by profuse sweating, classically from the neck up, though some people sweat all over and some do not sweat at all. Some women have "cold sweats" instead of hot flashes. They feel chilled or clammy but sweat profusely and often shake and shiver. Many women alternate between hot and cold. The pattern of feeling hot, sweating, and then feeling cold is so predictable for many women that their husbands have been known to ask them, a few minutes after they have thrown back the blankets at the beginning of a flash, whether they are ready yet to have the blankets back.

Hot flashes are not figments of the menopausal imagination. Scientific studies using sensors have shown that skin temperature actually rises one to four degrees, although internal body temperature does not. In a series of experiments published as early as 1975, researchers monitored physiological changes during hot flashes and discovered that they included increased heart rate and profuse sweating.

In addition to the flushing, sweating, and sense of heat, some women notice prickly skin sensations, a feeling that ants are crawling on their skin. The scientific name for this phenomenon is formication, from the Latin word for "ant." Some women experience other odd vasomotor symptoms including palpitations, fluttering or racing sensations of the heart. Others feel tingling sensations like "pins and needles" in their hands or fingers.

Still other women have hypotensive sensations, as if their blood pressure had suddenly plummeted; they feel dizzy and light-headed and fear that they will faint. An occasional woman has showed up in the emergency room feeling that she is about to pass out, because her hot flashes have made her weak and giddy; these women get so vasodilated from the flushing that their blood pressure actually falls. Some, especially small, slim women with low blood pressure, may pass out from hot flashes if they get overheated or dehydrated.

Hot flashes will not kill you; they will not even harm you seriously, but they can be extremely uncomfortable. They are also one of the most dreaded indications of approaching menopause, perhaps because they are so visible. No one knows, unless you tell them, that your period is heavy to the point of flooding or that your skin feels as if it is crawling with ants; but everyone, at least so it seems, can notice your dripping red face. The professional women I see in my practice, especially those in situations where dress and grooming are very important, are particularly embarrassed by this feature of menopause.

In some ways the stigma attached to hot flashes is like the shame a generation or two ago of being visibly pregnant. If you were pregnant, obviously you had engaged in sex. If you have hot flashes, obviously you are menopausal and are getting to be an old woman—not an admirable status in a society that idealizes and cultivates youth. Although modern medicine cannot reverse the clock or change societal outlooks, it can at least make women more comfortable when they are experiencing hot flashes. In most cases the hot flashes can be banished altogether, so that no one will know you are menopausal.

▶ *What factors trigger hot flashes?*

The most obvious culprit is external heat, which can range from torrid weather (especially with high humidity) to a warm room, heavy clothing, a hot shower, or a scorching hair dryer. Women notice that they get hot flashes more frequently in the summer than in the winter; they also notice that the insomnia that often accompanies hot flashes is worse in the summer.

Drinking hot beverages, especially tea and coffee, which contain caffeine, can bring on hot flashes. And alcohol is a well-known inducer of hot flashes.

Patty L. is director of nursing at a major hospital and as a medically educated person is very aware of changes in her body. She is fifty-two and takes estrogen replacement therapy, 0.625 mg of Premarin daily, to control her hot flashes. The other day she came to me and said that she knew she had her estrogen dosage right, because if she had one glass of wine she was fine. If she had two or three, she would turn bright red unless she took an extra Premarin the night before the occasion when alcohol was to be served.

Karen G., a nurse, activist in women's causes, and local officeholder, came home from the hospital after a total hysterectomy. Because her ovaries had been removed, she was surgically menopausal. She was taking ERT to control menopausal symptoms and generally getting along very well. Karen's housekeeper regularly cooked foods from her native country, a rich spicy cuisine that was heavy on black pepper and tomato sauce. Although Karen had enjoyed this food before her operation without any consequences, she discovered that the highly seasoned food now gave her hot flashes; lobster fra diablo in fact made her resemble a well-boiled lobster. To cope with the problem, Karen had to adopt a blander diet and increase the level of her ERT.

The relation between hot flashes and eating is problematic. Often when you have a really large meal, the kind you indulge in at Thanksgiving, you may be in a stressful situation—for example, cooking dinner for twenty relatives. Or you may have wine with dinner and coffee or tea with dessert.

Certain medications are known to bring on hot flashes—for example, Sudafed and other over-the-counter sinus remedies that contain the chemical cousins of adrenaline. If you are taking sinus medications, you should not be alarmed if you start flashing.

Another cause is stress or nervousness. You may be in a situation where you have to get up and give a speech, and suddenly you find yourself red in the face and sweating, doubling your anxiety. Or you start to worry about having a hot flash while you are giving the speech, and lo and behold, there you are with a red face, sweat dripping from the end of your nose, and anxiety beyond your wildest nightmares. Fatigue, too, can bring on hot flashes, just as fatigue heightens stress.

▶ *Do other conditions cause hot flashes?*

Certain diseases, like hyperthyroidism, can look like menopause. Women with this condition have irregular periods, they get hot, their hair does strange things; in many ways they resemble perimenopausal women. Some other rare ailments can give you hot flashes; for example, a tumor of the adrenal glands called pheochromocytoma, or carcinoids, a tumor of the appendix.

Occasionally women experience hot flashes after childbirth. These women also have low blood estrogen levels, so it is not surprising that they have symptoms similar to those of menopause.

▶ *How long do individual hot flashes last?*

Classically, hot flashes are said to last a few minutes, maybe as long as five minutes. But sometimes a woman comes into the office and describes what she has been feeling and says that the feelings of heat and flushing have gone on for two hours. Was it a two-hour hot flash? Probably it was. Was she maximally vasodilating for two hours? Probably not.

But certainly it is possible that she was vasodilating enough so that those two hours were uncomfortable.

▶ *How frequently do they occur?*

I have had people tell me that they get one a day. I have had people tell me that they get fifty a day. There is no simple answer, because women have such widely different experiences.

Hot flashes and other menopausal symptoms do seem to follow a bell-shaped curve for most women. As you enter the perimenopausal period, you may notice a few relatively mild hot flashes. They may increase in intensity and frequency, peaking in the year when menstruation ceases. Most women at their peak experience no more than fifteen a day, though that may not be a comforting statistic. Gradually the flashes begin to taper off.

If your menopause is brought on suddenly, say by chemotherapy or by surgery that removes your ovaries, your hot flashes will probably begin immediately and be intense.

▶ *When do hot flashes start during the perimenopausal period, and how long do they last?*

Again, there is no one answer. Some women begin to experience hot flashes and the insomnia that sometimes accompanies them when they haven't even skipped a period. Perhaps they have noticed lighter flow and suspect that they are heading toward menopause; but perhaps they have noticed nothing different about their periods.

Hot flashes may be transient, lasting for perhaps a month and then disappearing, probably coinciding with temporary levels of ovarian function. Or they may continue at a significant level for several years. Classically, most women's hot flashes will subside within a year or two. In my clinical experience, five years is perhaps the outside limit for significant insomnia and hot flashes. But five years is a long time. Whether you are vice president of a bank or have heavy responsibilities taking care of a sick parent or a couple of perfectly healthy but demanding teenagers, five years is a long time to be flashing all day long and sleeping poorly at night.

I have had some women in their eighties report that they still get an occasional hot flash. But they also report that it doesn't really bother or incapacitate them; it simply reminds them of when they were going through menopause. The medical profession does not know exactly why this happens to women in this age group.

► *Do hot flashes cause insomnia?*

While many women are aware of hot flashes as a sign of menopause, they are unaware that insomnia is another classic sign that menopause is on the way. Indeed, these two phenomena are physiologically linked, though the hot flashes do not necessarily cause the insomnia. Hot flashes plus insomnia probably also contribute to the mood swings and emotional instability that have been attributed to menopause.

Many women are awakened by their hot flashes, which often occur more frequently at night than during the day. In a classic example of a nocturnal hot flash, a woman wakes up sweating, often with the feeling that she can't breathe. Sometimes her nightgown feels too hot or else is so drenched with sweat that she has to change into a fresh one. She may sweat on the sheets or the pillowcases and have to change the bedclothes. Her hair may be wet. If she shares the bed, she and her partner may have real temperature wars. Unless they have a dual-control electric blanket, she throws off the covers and opens the windows while he complains that he is freezing.

Some women can toss off their covers, take a deep breath of fresh air at the window, and go right back to sleep. Others wake up but cannot fall back to sleep. A third group goes back to sleep, only to wake again in half an hour and continue that routine for the rest of the night. These women clearly become deficient in REM sleep, the kind that researchers feel is necessary for satisfactory rest.

If you can organize your schedule so that you can nap or rest during the day, perhaps nighttime sleep disruption is not so punishing. But if you must work according to someone else's schedule, you may have real difficulty in coping with the demands of your life.

► *What causes menopausal sleep disruption and hot flashes?*

Unfortunately, we don't really know. Neuroendocrinologists have discovered that the activity of the pituitary gland and the hypothalamus, and almost every endocrinologic hormonal system for that matter, peaks between one o'clock and three o'clock in the morning, which probably has something to do with the fact that many women have their worst or most frequent hot flashes at night. Researchers have not been able to show that high or low levels of particular hormones trigger hot flashes; nor have they been able to demonstrate that fluctuation in hormone level is responsible.

▶ *If I am having hot flashes and other perimenopausal symptoms, can I still get pregnant?*

Although fertility is very much diminished at the age when hot flashes and menstrual irregularities start appearing, someone who is forty-five can still become pregnant. Women who are trying to get pregnant at this time of life may find it difficult, but I have brought a few "cabooses" into this world.

> Martha D. was forty-seven. She had been getting hot flashes and putting on weight, but since she had always been on the chubby side, she thought she was just getting a little thicker. She also attributed the weight gain to approaching menopause. Martha's elder daughter was getting married, and Martha figured that the additional weight came along too because of extra eating caused by the stress of planning a wedding. When she came into my office, she was five months pregnant.

So while fertility is greatly diminished at this time of life, it is not absolutely zero.

▶ *Is emotional instability a characteristic of perimenopause?*

In former times menopausal women were thought to go through a period of extreme instability that in some cases resulted in mental derangement. Even today, women come to me feeling extremely anxious about what will happen to them psychologically when they hit menopause. They are afraid of turning into someone like Great-Aunt Tilly, who, according to family mythology, became a virtual lunatic when she reached the age of fifty-one. Indeed, many people can recall close or distant family members or friends who have had psychological or psychosocial problems when they were perimenopausal, and although there is no way to know retrospectively just what did happen to Tilly, several factors might have contributed to her instability. Her problem may have been sleep deprivation, which by itself can make you pretty irritable. Or she might have been afflicted with depression that was indeed caused by fluctuating hormone levels.

Most women going through menopause do not experience significant and lasting emotional changes. Some do have feelings of depression, anxiety, tearfulness (even when there is no real reason to feel like crying), low energy, and excessive worry. Other women have mood swings, feel irritable, and have trouble concentrating.

▶ *Is loss of short-term memory a menopausal symptom?*

Many women in the perimenopausal period complain of loss of short-term memory. They suddenly start misplacing their eyeglasses, their pocketbooks, their car keys. According to their teenagers, they repeat the same stories or remarks over and over. They can remember their own Social Security number and their husband's, but not their children's, which they memorized at a later time in life.

Others suffer from the "what am I here for?" syndrome. They walk into a room with a specific purpose, then stand there wondering why they have come to the living room or the kitchen or the supply closet at the office. One of my patients ruefully recalls leaping into her car and racing five miles from her home to the center of town on an urgent errand; when she got there, she could not remember why she was there. On returning home, she suddenly recalled that her mission had been to pick up her daughter at the town green.

Other women feel themselves falling victim to a kind of mental vagueness or fuzzy thinking, when in the past they have known themselves to be alert, rational, even witty.

Both men and women can have problems with short-term memory as they age, but there is certainly anecdotal evidence that these problems become more severe during perimenopause.

▶ *Can headaches be a sign of menopause?*

Although headaches certainly can occur at any time of life, they can be a menopausal symptom. Headaches, sometimes migraines, seem to be connected with changing—and especially with low—estrogen levels. Many menstruating women have cyclic headaches, particularly during the part of their cycle when their estrogen is low premenstrually. As they approach menopause and their estrogen levels begin to taper off, they can experience significant headaches. Philip Sarrel, a physician studying menopause at Yale University, treats these women with estrogen pills under their tongue, the method of delivery used with nitroglycerin tablets for heart patients. The advantage is that the estrogen gets into the bloodstream quickly, and some of the women who get these estrogen deprivation headaches have reported relief in as little as twenty minutes.

▶ *Can aching joints be a sign of menopause?*

Many perimenopausal women experience sore, aching joints and muscles. No one knows whether these are caused by approaching menopause (that is, falling estrogen levels) or simply by growing older. I suspect that these aches and pains may be hormonal in origin because over the years many of my patients have volunteered that after estrogen replacement therapy their joint pains have disappeared. These women have noticed in passing that HRT seemed to help with a discomfort they had not even associated with perimenopause.

4 Perimenopause or PMS?

PREMENSTRUAL syndrome (PMS) is a wastebasket diagnosis: probably ten or twelve disorders are grouped under that title. Some of the symptoms categorized as PMS can also be associated with perimenopause, so that if you are in your forties it can be difficult to sort out which symptoms are attributable to PMS (which you may or may not have had before) and which are indicators of approaching menopause. Nowadays, fortunately, PMS is a recognized disease and is no longer considered to be a figment of women's imagination.

The American Psychiatric Association (APA) has developed a list of symptoms for diagnosing and categorizing different kinds of mental illness. One of these is called "premenstrual dysphoric disorder" (PMDD) or "late luteal phase dysphoric disorder," and it seems more or less equivalent to severe PMS, though the APA's diagnostic handbook (understandably) emphasizes psychological symptoms: anger or irritability, mood swings, depression, anxiety or tension, fatigue, difficulty in concentration, loss of sleep, appetite changes; a few are physical: breast tenderness and headaches. To be diagnosed with late luteal phase dysphoric disorder, you must have at least five of the symptoms on the list, and they must recur cyclically.

▶ *What are the symptoms of PMS? How can I differentiate between PMS and perimenopause?*

The two most frequently reported symptoms of PMS are bloating and irritability. A close third is premenstrual sleeplessness. Women approaching menopause typically experience sleeplessness most of the time, not just before their periods, whereas women suffering from PMS report that they have difficulty sleeping a few days or perhaps a week before the onset of menstruation. Some women suffering with PMS have breast discomfort. Others report mental changes, such as lapses in memory and shortened attention span or difficulty in concentrating; others experience depression as well as irritability. These mental changes are also reported by women approaching menopause who do not consider themselves to be suffering from PMS. Some women have cravings for certain

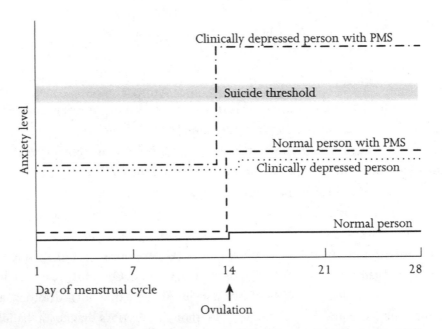

FIGURE 5. Anxiety levels and PMS. Everyone has some baseline anxiety, but the level differs significantly from one individual to another. Premenstrually, most women experience some increase in their baseline level. A few women have a very significant increase.

kinds of food, especially sweets (the chocolate phenomenon is well known), salty items such as potato chips, and caffeine.

The level of anxiety and emotional distress that women feel depends to some extent on what I call their baseline level of agitation. Some individuals are fairly calm most of the time; but if they have mild PMS they feel agitated or anxious premenstrually. Then there are more volatile women who are often agitated; when their baseline level of anxiety gets worse premenstrually, they feel really tense and overwrought. These are the people who are likely to need significant intervention.

The classic PMS pattern, however, describes women who are normally rather serene but spike wildly before their periods. For some of these women the emotional effects of PMS are intolerable.

▶ What causes PMS?

No one knows, unfortunately. There are many theories and no real proof that any of them is correct. For every study showing that one particular chemical imbalance causes PMS, another says no, that's not the cause. Current thinking suggests that changes in the levels of serotonin (a chemical messenger used by nerve cells to communicate with other nerve cells or their targets) are the likely culprit for the most severe mood changes. Formerly leading theories include too much prolactin (a hormone secreted by the pituitary that stimulates milk secretion and is often produced in greater amounts during stress), too little progesterone, or too much estrogen accompanied by too little progesterone.

Since there is no accepted theory about which chemical imbalance causes PMS, there is no laboratory test for PMS. If someone tells you that if you give them four hundred dollars, they will test your blood for PMS, don't do it. Use the money to buy a membership at a gym (or maybe something great to wear).

▶ What can I do to control PMS?

PMS is a complex of symptoms and therefore difficult to treat, so you are probably wise to start at the most basic level: try approaches that may help you and certainly cannot hurt you.

Many women are helped merely by charting their lives and realizing when things happen. If you have the luxury of organizing your own time, you can set up your schedule so that on the days you know you are going to feel irritable or bloated, you will not be performing activities that increase stress. You can say, okay, I know I'm not going to be the most delightful person starting next Tuesday, so I'm just going to stay home. If your life is not within your control to that degree, you can at least not schedule a potentially aggravating meeting with an unsatisfactory employee, or a job interview, or whatever, on those days. In this way charting can be therapeutic.

But charting can also be diagnostic. Suppose that you are keeping track of your symptoms to observe cyclic changes. You notice that in fact you feel awful, depressed, irritable, and anxious every day. Because PMS is a popular ailment, because it's on the airwaves and therefore on everyone's mind, you automatically assume that your bad moods are cyclic. But when you begin charting, you may discover that there's nothing cyclic at all about your mental state. You may have garden-variety depression, which is socially a less acceptable disease than PMS. Furthermore, the usual simple PMS measures are not going to make you feel any better.

We are fortunate in this day and age that a number of effective medications are available for depression; if you have charted your symptoms and find that you are depressed every day of the month, you can take an antidepressant. It will work a lot better than your treating the depression as if it were PMS.

▶ Can diet help my PMS?

One major step to helping yourself get through PMS is controlling your diet. The closer anyone is to her ideal body weight, the better she will feel—whether she is perimenopausal, menopausal, or premenstrual. To achieve ideal body weight, I suggest a relatively low-fat, general weight-loss diet. Keep the calories adequate to maintain health, and lose weight gradually if you need to.

I encourage people to avoid concentrated carbohydrates, forget the chocolate bars, and keep fat intake low. Cut down on salt and caffeine. Reducing salt intake decreases the bloating associated with fluid retention, and limiting caffeine helps both with breast discomfort and with caffeine-induced jitters.

If your body, like Audrey, the carnivorous plant in the *Little Shop of Horrors,* shouts "Feed me! Feed me!" you've got to respond negatively. If you eat the candy bar, you will feel worse with the extra sugar on board. If you eat the salty potato chips, you will increase your tendency to bloat.

▶ *Does exercise have any effect on PMS?*

For any number of reasons, it is a good idea to exercise regularly. Whether or not it helps your PMS, it is good for you. Researchers have discovered substances called endorphins, produced endogenously by the brain, that are natural opiates; they make you feel better, just as drugs do. Endorphins are produced in greater amounts during exercise and account for the phenomenon known as runner's high. Premenstrual depression is an issue for many women who have PMS, and the endorphins generated through exercise will probably help them feel better. The goal is half an hour of aerobic exercise intense enough to get your heart rate up to about 75 percent of its maximum capacity three times a week. This is a goal, not a limit; if you feel like exercising more frequently, so much the better.

> Lucy D. was forty-five when she began feeling out of sorts premenstrually. She decided to start running to see if it would help her control her negative feelings. Lucy found that the more she ran, the better she felt. Eventually she became a marathoner and participated several times in the New York marathon. She then took up karate. Now she is seventy and just finished the Boston Marathon in about seven hours, in the process raising thirty thousand dollars for the Leukemia Foundation.

Lucy is an extreme case. Not every woman who takes up exercise to control PMS will become a marathoner, but her improvement does show clearly what other patients of mine have also demonstrated, that exercise can have a positive effect on PMS.

▶ *Do vitamins help with PMS?*

Beyond the two simple approaches we've discussed, the management of PMS is very controversial. For every scientific paper that tells us something works, others say the same thing doesn't work. The next treatment I suggest is vitamin B6, at a dosage level of 100 to 200 mg daily. This dosage is much higher than the normal daily requirement, which is only about 2 mg; it is higher even than the amount in prenatal vitamins (which contain about 10 mg a day), but it is still safe. Although B6 taken in huge dosages, perhaps 1,500 to 2,000 mg daily, can be associated with neurotoxicity and produce symptoms such as tingling in the fingers, 100 to 200 mg daily is not a harmful amount. As with any kind of vitamin supplement, a lot is not necessarily better than a little. Just because B6 seems to make you feel better, don't take more than 100 to 200 mg daily.

How does vitamin B6 work? For one thing, it is a natural diuretic. For another, it seems to antagonize a couple of brain hormones, particularly one called prolactin, which may be involved in PMS (although researchers are not sure).

In my own practice I see a 60 to 70 percent response rate with vitamin B6, certainly much higher than the placebo effect. But as I have said, PMS treatment is controversial, and in some scientific research, vitamin B6 has no greater effect than a placebo. All the same, because B6 is helpful for breast discomfort, because it is readily available, and because it is not harmful, it is worth trying.

A second substance useful in treating the breast discomfort that often accompanies PMS is vitamin E. I suggest supplementation at about 400 to 600 units a day. Even though vitamin E currently has a reputation as being useful in preventing cancer and promoting cardiac health, it is fat soluble and you have to be careful not to overdose on it. Vitamins that are soluble in fat can be stored easily in the body's fatty tissues and thus can readily accumulate to undesirable levels; water-soluble vitamins are more easily excreted.

Recent research has suggested that calcium can help. Try supplements of calcium (1,000 to 1,200 mg daily) and magnesium (200 mg daily) during the last half of the menstrual cycle. Of course, all women should be getting calcium regularly to keep their bones in shape.

▶ *Do herbal remedies help with PMS?*

Therapies beyond diet, exercise, and vitamins B6 and E get a little esoteric and even more controversial. For many of my patients, evening primrose oil seems to be useful. Evening primrose is a garden plant that happens to be rich in an essential fatty acid called gammalinolenic acid—GLA in the health food business. Some women supposedly develop a deficiency in their fatty acid metabolism, a deficiency involving an enzyme called delta 6 desaturase. According to this theory, the women who develop such a defect cannot metabolize linoleic acid to gammalinolenic acid. By taking the gammalinolenic acid orally, they bypass the "deficient enzyme" and improve their fatty acid metabolism. What this has to do with PMS, no one is quite sure. However, I do get a 50 to 60 percent response with evening primrose oil, which is better than a placebo effect (generally about 30 percent). That is, in any drug trial the placebo helps about 30 percent of the people who try it, so to show that a medication is effective, you have to demonstrate an effect greater than 30 percent.

Evening primrose oil is expensive. You buy it at health food stores, and in my hometown, it costs about twenty-six dollars for a two-month supply. Standard dosage is 500 units per capsule. The dose I recommend to women just starting is two capsules a day, though many of the practitioners who recommend evening primrose oil suggest up to six capsules daily.

One of the advantages of evening primrose oil is that it has no negative side effects. The only way it can hurt you is via your pocketbook, since it's more expensive than vitamins B6 and E or other common therapies.

▶ *Are hormones useful in treating PMS?*

If someone has tried all the simple therapies—diet, exercise, vitamin B6 and vitamin E, evening primrose oil—and still feels awful, it may be time to consider hormonal intervention. The question is, what kind of hormonal intervention will work? Is estrogen a worthwhile consideration?

If sleep disorder is really becoming manifest as a prominent symptom, perhaps estrogen is a viable choice. I sometimes suggest trying it for a month to see whether it is effective.

Another option is progesterone. The initiative for using this drug comes from the work of a woman named Katharina Dalton, an English general practitioner who published her first articles in the 1940s and early 1950s. She was not a gynecologist, nor did she do laboratory research or basic science, yet her work has been influential. Dalton's theory on PMS was that it is a progesterone deficiency disorder, an idea that makes sense intellectually, especially with premenopausal women who also have bleeding disorders. Since, as a woman approaches menopause, progesterone production often falls before estrogen production does, and since progesterone is important in controlling the heaviness of the menstrual flow, Dalton's idea was to prescribe progesterone to replace what a woman was not producing on her own.

In clinical trials Dalton treated thousands of women and got good responses; that is, her patients improved. Her approach was to give women afflicted with PMS supplements of natural progesterone for ten days or two weeks before their periods, to see whether they responded.

To be well absorbed by the digestive system, progesterone must be specially processed, broken down into minute particles. When Dr. Dalton first started using natural progesterone, this process had not yet been invented. She recommended vaginal suppositories, because natural progesterone can be easily absorbed across the mucous membranes.

Although Dalton's published results indicated that her patients got better, researchers have not been able to replicate her work. Most of the studies from the United States show no significant difference in response between placebo and progesterone.

Even though this research does not corroborate Dalton's work, American gynecologists do use progesterone supplements as a therapy for PMS. Progesterone supplementation in appropriate doses is completely safe and seems to help some people. I have patients who have been taking it for years and find it very useful. Other patients have been responsive to synthetic progesterones such as Provera, which are more readily accessible. Some women who have "flunked" synthetic progesterones do well with natural progesterone. There are many variations from one individual to another.

Progesterone as a therapy for PMS is also available in a long-lasting injectable form, something like the contraceptive Depo-Provera. The drawback to injecting progesterone (aside from the inconvenience) is that it is deposited in body fat; once it is on board, it remains there for three months. Because some people do not do well with it, injected progesterone is not a treatment to rush into; nor should it be used without supervision.

Progesterone does have side effects. Although Depo-Provera obliterates most women's periods, many women get breakthrough bleeding, spotting, or staining. Some women who take it get depressed. Some gain weight; women who remain on Depo-Provera for years often put on an unwanted, permanent ten pounds. Other women, however, respond well. They are happy with the loss of periods. Because progesterone can act as a sedative, it calms many women who suffer anxiety premenstrually.

▶ Do birth control pills help?

It stands to reason that birth control pills might help with PMS. If PMS is a disorder of ovulation, then if you wipe out ovulation (as birth control pills do), won't you wipe out PMS?

For some women, birth control pills do suppress PMS. If a woman comes to me with PMS symptoms, and she needs contraception and perhaps gets severe menstrual cramps, I suggest that she try the pill for a month or so and see how she feels. She may find that for her the pill is very effective.

So I do have women in their forties taking birth control pills because the pill solves several problems: it provides contraception, it helps with menstrual cramps, and it lessens bleeding problems caused by irregular or inadequate ovulation. Women who are approaching menopause will also find that the estrogen in birth control pills, though it is a low dose, serves as adequate estrogen replacement therapy. Furthermore, as I have mentioned elsewhere, the low-dose birth control pills used nowadays are considered safe for women in their thirties and forties, as long as they are not smokers.

A recently introduced oral contraceptive called Yasmin has been found to help with PMS symptoms. It contains a new form of synthetic progesterone, drospirenone, which has diuretic properties and decreases bloating.

Yet birth control pills do not work for all women with PMS. For reasons that are not at all understood, they make some women feel much worse. A doctor prescribing birth control pills for PMS should always suggest trying them to see what happens. If you feel worse, stop taking them and try something else.

If none of these therapies relieves the PMS symptoms, it is possible to think in terms of hormone therapy even for women who have not done well on birth control pills. The amount of estrogen used in HRT is considerably smaller, only about one-sixth the amount of the estrogen in birth control pills.

If someone comes to me, menopausally or perimenopausally, and we start talking about estrogen, she may point out that she did poorly on birth control pills many years ago. First of all, if it was many years ago, she was taking high-dose birth control pills. Even if she couldn't tolerate a 30- or 35-mg low-dose pill, the estrogen in ERT is much less. Furthermore, the estrogens we use for HRT are naturally occurring estrogens. All those in birth control pills are synthetic.

To control ovulation, which is what birth control pills do, you need enough estrogen and progesterone to shut down the hypothalamus. But with HRT you need only a small dose, because you are not shutting down ovulation.

If I am treating a woman who is perimenopausal, as opposed to postmenopausal, I still have to give her contraception protection with HRT. A woman aged forty-six or forty-seven may be skipping periods, perhaps having a few hot flashes, perhaps not feeling well in general. But unless she has gone a full year without a period, she should still be thinking of contraception. If she goes on HRT, she must realize that it will not provide contraceptive protection, and she should still be sure she is protected some other way.

▶ *Are there other hormonal ways of controlling PMS?*

If neither birth control pills nor HRT controls your PMS, certain hormonal medications can shut down your ovaries altogether, rendering you chemically menopausal. Lupron, one of the major drugs traditionally used to treat endometriosis, does this. Lupron is a very satisfactory diagnostic tool for PMS, and a number of gynecologists throughout the country use it for this purpose.

Suppose that you are feeling really irritable and depressed. Is your problem PMS, or is it clinical depression caused by something else? In order to distinguish between PMS and "something else," we can shut down your ovaries altogether for a month or two, give you a little estrogen to prevent hot flashes and other discomforts, and see whether your PMS symptoms go away. If they do not, then clearly your problem is not PMS; if the symptoms disappear, at least you know what the problem is. Some physicians use Lupron plus estrogen, long term. The problem with this add-back therapy is that it is extraordinarily expensive, costing more than five hundred dollars a month.

▶ How about treatments to reduce bloating?

Among my patients are women who gain ten pounds during their menstrual cycles. This is certainly not the norm, but it happens to some women and they are quite uncomfortable. I have patients who own one set of clothes for their follicular phase and another set for their luteal phase. Controlling the bloat is really important to them. I think vitamin B6 helps, and I think evening primrose oil helps. When these aids are inadequate, a diuretic, taken premenstrually for a week or two, may provide relief.

The diuretic recommended for PMS is a medication called spironolactone, sold under the trade name Aldactone. It seems to have other effects, too, on the symptoms of PMS, perhaps lessening irritability. Aldactone is a relatively mild diuretic that is potassium sparing—that is, it does not deplete your body of potassium as certain other diuretics do. It is relatively safe both because of its potassium-sparing nature and because, not being superstrong, it will not lower your blood pressure so much that you pass out.

No diuretic is totally safe, however, and there is a danger of becoming addicted. If you have mild bloating and take a diuretic regularly, then suddenly you stop taking it, you may get much more severe bloating. Yet some people, for example those with hypertension, have to take diuretics every day for long periods. If someone comes to my office with mild hypertension and some bloating, a diuretic can take care of everything. But patients should be fully aware that they are going to be on this medication for a long time, that they cannot stop and start whenever they like.

Diuretics are not intended as weight-control pills. Their use must be carefully monitored.

Susanna Y., a very attractive woman in her early forties, was deeply concerned about her appearance and particularly about her weight. Her story is very sad and a dramatic example of how not to approach weight control. She came to me as a patient needing a hysterectomy for fibroids and pain.

One day, years after she had recovered from her hysterectomy, she called me complaining of belly pain. I happened to be at the hospital and saw her in the emergency room. I examined her and found nothing, though her abdomen was clearly sore. Although I might not normally do so under these circumstances, I asked for a round of blood tests.

Blood tests requested routinely from the emergency room often include tests for the amount of sodium and potassium. Her potassium, which normally would be in the 3.5 to 5.5 range, came back at 1.8, which is exceptionally low. Certainly that level could give her plenty of belly pain. It also could give her significant cardiac arrhythmias, which she was also experiencing.

We admitted her immediately into the intensive care unit and put her on a heart monitor. Initially we thought that she had a rare metabolic illness, because a potassium level this low is very unusual. I had never prescribed diuretics for her, so she had no prescription to purchase them. Still, someone on the staff did ask her whether she was taking diuretics and she said no, that she knew it was wrong and could be dangerous. But in fact, she was lying. We ran tests to screen her blood and urine for diuretics, and they turned out positive for Lasix, a diuretic that had been prescribed for her mother, who was taking it for a heart condition.

Susanna had apparently been taking the Lasix for a reasonably long period, though of course we couldn't tell exactly how long. Only a few weeks of it will bring your potassium way down. Susanna was even taking it in the hospital; she had it in her handbag, it turned out. Confronted with the fact, she denied it strenuously and signed out of the hospital against medical advice.

She came back to me several years later, for a routine gynecological checkup. As we were chatting, I asked whom she was seeing as an internist. She mentioned a friend of mine who works in a town nearby. Although gossip about patients is usually unacceptable, I felt that in this case the internist should know that she had done something that could have killed her, so I called and informed him.

When I told him about the episode in the hospital, he replied, "Oh no! She's doing it again."

I said, "What are you talking about?"

"I haven't been able to figure out why she has these very abnormal thyroid function tests." She was overdosing, getting thyroid extract somewhere, and taking it to try to make herself skinny. She even had tremors. Thyroid is available only on prescription, so she couldn't just walk into the drugstore and buy it, but somehow she had found a source. (She believed, incorrectly, that it would slim her down; it has this effect only on people with hypothyroidism.)

I never saw her again. Two or three years after her last visit to my office, however, I read her obituary in one of the local papers. Obviously I don't know what caused her death (the obituary wasn't specific), but she was a woman in her late forties. She had no medical problems that were life threatening. So I assume that she died of some medication that she was surreptitiously taking. Whether she got back on Lasix and managed to kill herself with that, or whether she put herself into a toxic condition by taking extra thyroid medication, I don't know. The sad part is that she wasn't even obese; in fact, she was slender.

So while diuretic therapy may be helpful in controlling bloating and the breast discomfort related to bloating, it must not be regarded lightly. It is not a magic bullet for instant weight loss; diuretic abuse can be life threatening.

▶ Can PMS be treated with antidepressants?

Recent studies have shown the effectiveness of SSRIs (selective serotonin reuptake inhibitors) for PMS. Prozac is an SSRI, as is its relative, Sarafem, which the FDA approved in 2000 for treating PMDD, the severe form of PMS.

These drugs can be taken daily for a week or two before your menstrual period. They don't seem to have serious side effects, and they work quickly in relieving PMS symptoms. SSRIs taken for clinical depression take two to three weeks to have an effect, but for PMDD they work in a day or two.

We know that Prozac, Sarafem, and similar drugs affect brain chemistry, particularly serotonin levels, but we don't know the precise nature of the effects. Nor do we know precisely what changes in brain chemistry cause PMS. Although physicians may be treating such symptoms as depression when they prescribe Prozac or Sarafem, they may also be getting at the root of the problem, the changes in brain chemistry that cause PMS.

In recent years a lot of negative talk about Prozac has suggested that people who take it have an increased likelihood of committing suicide or, less commonly, committing violence against others. Most psychiatrists of my acquaintance believe that Prozac is basically a safe drug, that its bad reputation arises from poorly designed studies and from excessive media attention. People taking Prozac are often depressed or disturbed individuals to start with. So a study that compares suicidal or aggressive behavior in a group of generally depressed and disturbed people who are not treated with a group of depressed and disturbed people who are being treated may find little or no difference. In fact, large-scale studies show that individuals being treated with Prozac commit fewer violent crimes against themselves and against others. Because people being treated with Prozac are already in trouble, it is their baseline illness, not the Prozac therapy, that makes them behave violently. The worst that can be said about Prozac is that does not effectively cure these people of their underlying illness.

As an antidepressant, Prozac is safe when a physician monitors its use. Some of the older antidepressants can have cardiac side effects, but Prozac does not. It is not addictive. It may depress your libido or sexual desire, but only while you take it. When you stop taking Prozac, your libido will return to normal.

5   Menopause and Your Body

THE most obvious effect of menopause on your body is that because your ovaries are no longer producing significant amounts of estrogen, you stop having menstrual periods. Most women are aware of estrogen as a female sex hormone and associate its action with the development of female sex characteristics during adolescence and with the regulation of menstrual periods during their fertile years. But estrogen does more than regulate female sexuality. It is a potent hormone whose effects are far-reaching and whose actions are only partly understood. Its presence affects the heart and cardiovascular system, the bones, the skin, the bladder, the breasts, the uterus, even the brain. Researchers can count hundreds of different actions of this hormone.

Since estrogen is so sweeping in its effects and plays a role in so many body systems and functions, it is not surprising that menopause, whose prime component is the loss of ovarian function, affects your body in lots of ways.

Other physical changes come with aging and are not specifically related to estrogen loss or to menopause. For example, the gradual lowering of basal metabolic rate that can contribute to weight gain as people age occurs in both men and women. It is important to remember that although loss of estrogen causes many changes, it does not cause them all. You cannot blame every negative effect of middle age on menopause.

▶ *What is the effect of menopause on my heart?*

Estrogen, it appears, is good for your heart. It seems obvious from observing our friends and acquaintances that young men are more prone to heart disease than young women. Probably everyone can recall at least one male friend or family member under age fifty who has suffered a heart attack.

Scientific studies bear out this informal observation. According to estimates made by the epidemiologists at the National Heart Lung and Blood Institute, each year in the United States about 34,000 men but only 10,000 women between the ages of twenty-nine and forty-four have heart attacks. During the next twenty years of life, the decades that normally bracket menopause (age forty-five to sixty-four), an estimated 257,000 men have heart attacks, whereas only 86,000 women do. But in the sixty-five-plus age group,

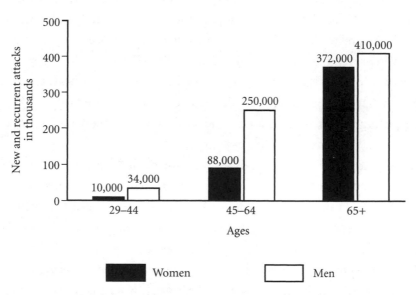

FIGURE 6. Annual number of Americans having heart attack, by age and sex, 1987–2000. Clearly, older women "catch up" with men in terms of vulnerability to heart attack. Source: American Heart Association, *Heart Disease and Stroke Statistics—2004 Update* (Dallas: American Heart Association, 2003).

women begin to catch up to men; 430,000 men and 314,000 women each year suffer heart attacks. These figures do not include "silent" heart attacks (those without symptoms).

▶ *Could blood loss during menstruation have some positive effect on the heart or blood vessels?*

A Finnish study published in the *New England Journal of Medicine* in 1993 suggested that one of the reasons premenopausal women have a lower risk of heart disease is that they have lower hematocrits because of their monthly bleeds. This study did not find complete acceptance in the United States, and supporting studies have not backed it. Since most women lose no more than a couple of ounces of blood during each menstrual cycle, and since during the five or six days following a menstrual period women's bodies replenish the blood loss, it seems unlikely lower hematocrit levels could be the major reason premenopausal women have fewer heart attacks than men.

▶ *Is there a relation between estrogen and cardiovascular disease?*

For many years epidemiological studies and biological experiments suggested that taking hormone replacement therapy after menopause protected women from coronary artery disease. Then the Heart and Estrogen/Progestin Replacement Study (1998) and later the section of the Women's Health Initiative devoted to cardiac issues (2002) questioned the role of HRT in preventing coronary artery disease. The HERS trial showed that HRT did not prevent a second heart attack in women who had already had a heart attack, and the WHI showed that women taking HRT who had not been diagnosed with cardiac disease had a slightly higher risk of heart attack and stroke than women who did not use hormones.

Although the final answers are not yet in, some cardiologists and other physicians believe that estrogen may provide a safeguard for women who do not yet have vascular or cardiac problems, if women receive it immediately after menopause. Estrogen is known to increase the level of HDL (high-density lipoprotein), or good, cholesterol (thereby preventing the formation of plaque) and to relax blood vessels.

For women who have had a heart attack or damage to their blood vessels, however, estrogen may have a negative effect. This may be because when plaque is already present, the estrogen helps dislodge plaque from the blood vessels, creating an inflammatory reaction, which in turn increases the amount of plaque. The women in the WHI study were, by and large, many years past menopause and had been living, in cardiovascular

BOX 1.   Cardiovascular Disease Facts and Figures

Cardiovascular diseases are the number-one killer of women and men.

Cardiovascular diseases kill more than half a million females every year—about a death a minute, which is more lives than the next seven causes of death combined.

About 250,000 people each year die of coronary heart disease without being hospitalized. Most of these are sudden deaths caused by cardiac arrest, usually resulting from ventricular fibrillation.

From 1990 to 2000, the death rate declined 25 percent, but the actual number of deaths declined only 7.6 percent.

The average age of people having a first heart attack is 65.8 for men and 70.4 for women.

Within one year of having a heart attack, 25 percent of men and 38 percent of women will die.

In part because women have heart attacks at older ages than men do, they're more likely to die from them within a few weeks.

About 80 percent of people who die of coronary heart disease are 65 or older.

Within 6 years after a recognized heart attack, 18 percent of men and 35 percent of women will have another heart attack.

Since 1984, more women than men have died of cardiovascular disease. The difference in deaths is now more than 65,000 per year.

In 2000, cardiovascular disease killed 505,661 women; while all forms of cancer together killed 267,009. Of the cancer deaths, 41,872 were caused by breast cancer and 65, 052 by lung cancer.

Each year about 40,000 more women than men have a stroke. This is because the average life expectancy in women is greater than in men and the highest rates for stroke are in the oldest age groups.

Up until age 55, a higher percentage of men than women have high blood pressure. From ages 55 to 74, the percentage of women is slightly higher; thereafter it is much higher. African American women have significantly higher rates of high blood pressure than white women.

Source: Adapted from American Heart Association, *Heart Disease and Stroke Statistics—2003 Update.*

terms, without the benefits of estrogen for years. Many of them had the classic risk factors: they were older (age in itself is a risk); many were overweight or even obese; many were sedentary; many smoked.

▶ What is cholesterol? What effect does estrogen have on it?

Cholesterol is a fatty compound present in meat and dairy products in the diet. The body also manufactures cholesterol. Even though you may be a strict vegetarian and avoid all animal foods, including milk and eggs, you do make your own cholesterol.

Cholesterol has a reputation as a contributing factor to coronary artery disease, but it does a great deal more than that. It plays a significant role in producing certain hormones, it is a building block of cell membranes and other body structures, and it is necessary for the digestion of fats.

Although cholesterol consists of several components, LDL (low-density lipoprotein) and HDL (high-density lipoprotein) are the most important in determining risk of heart disease. LDL is often dubbed "bad" cholesterol because it seems to play a role in forming fatty deposits inside the arteries, whereas HDL is called "good" cholesterol because it appears to help clean out deposits from the artery walls and carry them off to be excreted from the body. Thus high levels of LDL increase the risk of heart disease; high levels of HDL appear to protect against it.

Researchers believe that the presence of estrogen stimulates the liver to produce more HDL. Studies show that women on ERT experience a rise of up to 20 percent of HDL in their blood. Exercise also has a protective action and can increase HDL in the blood up to about 20 percent, so that women on ERT who also exercise can expect a significant boost in their HDL levels. By contrast, progestins such as Provera, which was used in the Women's Health Initiative, lower HDL.

▶ What is homocysteine? What effect does estrogen have on it?

Homocysteine, an amino acid normally present in small amounts in all cells of the body, is beginning to get attention as one of the contributing players in cardiovascular disease. Homocysteine is produced by the metabolism of one of the essential amino acids—the ones you must include in your diet because your body can't produce them on its own. In healthy cells, homocysteine is quickly metabolized into other less harmful substances with the help of a B vitamin known as folate (folic acid) and vitamin B12.

High homocysteine levels in the blood are thought to increase the risk of heart attack

TABLE 2. Effects of Estrogen on Factors Influencing Heart Disease

| | HDL CHOLESTEROL | LDL CHOLESTEROL | TRIGLYCERIDES | HOMOCYSTEINE | C-REACTIVE PROTEIN |
	GOOD CHOLESTEROL	BAD CHOLESTEROL	IMPLICATED IN HEART DISEASE	IMPLICATED IN HEART DISEASE AND ALZHEIMER'S	IMPLICATED IN HEART DISEASE
Oral estrogen	raises significantly	lowers	raises	lowers	raises
Transdermal estrogen (patches)	raises somewhat	lowers	no change	lowers	no change
Raloxifene (Evista)	no change	lowers	no change	lowers	no change or lowers

and stroke, although the topic remains controversial since researchers don't know yet whether homocysteine actually plays a role in causing cardiovascular disease or is just a marker for it. High homocysteine levels may also be associated with Alzheimer's disease. Measuring homocysteine levels to assess cardiac risk is relatively new, so the exact normal range has not yet been established.

Estrogen is linked with lower homocysteine levels in the blood. Premenopausal women, women using oral contraceptives, and pregnant women all have lower blood homocysteine than men and postmenopausal women—except those taking estrogen replacement therapy.

▶ What are triglycerides, and what effect does estrogen have on them?

Triglycerides are the body's storage form for fat. Most triglycerides are found stored in body fat tissue, but some circulate in the blood, fueling your muscles. After you've finished eating, when triglycerides are on their way from your intestines to your body fat for storage, your blood levels of triglycerides are elevated. High levels of triglycerides are associated with increased risk for heart disease.

Oral estrogen therapy is known to raise triglyceride levels, but transdermal estrogen does not.

▶ What is C-reactive protein? What effect does estrogen have on it?

C-reactive protein (CRP) is a protein produced by the liver that plays a role in inflammation. It is thought to be an important marker for cardiac disease. Oral estrogen therapy raises C-reactive protein, but transdermal estrogen does not.

▶ What effect does estrogen have on blood vessels?

It is well known that elevated blood pressure contributes to heart disease and stroke. Many women, both premenopausal and postmenopausal, have angina (chest pain caused by reduced blood flow to the heart muscle) even though their arteries are not clogged and narrowed with fatty deposits. Instead, the reduction of blood flow seems to come from spasm or constriction of the blood vessels.

Researchers have shown that estrogen relaxes and dilates both the peripheral circulation (the blood vessels in your arms, legs, trunk, and the rest of your body) and the coronary arteries that bring oxygen to the heart muscle. A small amount of estrogen will significantly vasodilate the constricted area, just as nitroglycerin does.

> Cheryl D., who is sixty-five, had angina even though her angiogram showed that her blood vessels have no plaque. Her cardiologist, one of my colleagues, took Cheryl's blood estrogen level and found it to be extremely low. He suggested that Cheryl try low-dose estrogen to reduce the risk of spasm in her blood vessels (coupled with occasional use of progesterone, of course, since she has not had a hysterectomy).

Blood estrogen levels fluctuate significantly during the normal menstrual cycle, and episodes of angina occur in many premenopausal women when their estrogen levels are lowest, just before their period begins. Incidentally, women who have cyclic migraine headaches classically experience them at the same time of the month. When these women with angina are checked by cardiac catheterization, it turns out that their blood vessels are not narrowed by plaque; they are constricted by spasm. They do not have obstructive disease; they have unusual responses to their own blood hormone levels. It is possible that there are many more women than men with angina because men do not have these odd responses to estrogen levels.

▶ *Do women who have had their ovaries removed have a higher rate of heart disease?*

When women go through menopause the ordinary way, whereby estrogen declines gradually over a period of years, their risk of heart attack increases gradually. If they have their ovaries removed surgically as part of a hysterectomy procedure and their estrogen declines swiftly, their risk rises quickly. If they take estrogen, however, their risk returns to normal.

▶ *What effect does menopause have on breast tissue?*

Breast tissue is very responsive to estrogen as well as to other hormones. When estrogen levels fall off, the amount of glandular tissue in your breasts decreases. For most women this means a change in the contour of the breast, which tends to sag with age, and some very old women have flat breasts. Many women notice a decrease in breast size, but some notice an increase in breast size as they age, perhaps because body fat tends to gather around the middle section of the body. Women who have had tender and lumpy breasts during the premenopausal years may notice an improvement in these conditions.

▶ *What is the effect of menopause on bone?*

Menopause is not helpful to your bones. Both men and women lose bone as they age, but women are at increased risk for osteoporosis, a disease of bone loss, because at menopause they lose the protective effect of estrogen. To understand this, you must understand something about bone.

Although we think of bone as stable, it is in fact constantly changing. Bone is made of a framework or matrix of organic molecules; crystals of calcium are deposited on this framework, giving it strength and rigidity. Everyone is aware that broken bone heals, that the broken area knits together in a process known as remodeling. But even bone that has not been injured is constantly being remodeled—broken down or resorbed and built up again.

While the scientific picture is complex, basically certain bone cells called osteoclasts break down bone, while other specialized cells called osteoblasts constantly build it up again. If the two activities, osteoclastic breaking down and osteoblastic building up, are balanced, then the amount of bone remains constant. If osteoblastic activity dominates, as it does during adolescence, then bone mass increases. If osteoclastic activity gets the upper hand, as it does after about the midthirties, then bone mass gradually decreases. Peak bone mass is attained somewhere between the ages of thirty and thirty-five, after which it declines gradually.

Estrogen plays a role in keeping this constant construction and destruction of bone in balance. It seems to act on parathyroid hormone, a hormone that increases osteoclastic activity, speeding the breakdown of bone. Estrogen prohibits some of the effects of parathyroid hormone. Without estrogen, bone is resorbed, or broken down, faster than osteoblastic activity can rebuild, and so bone mass decreases.

It is in the first few years after menopause that the rate of bone loss rises dramatically. Researchers believe that a kind of bone thermostat is reset during this period, that eventually the body senses the increased rate of bone loss and resets the thermostat downward to compensate. For this reason, women who are considering hormone therapy at least partially for bone benefits should begin it within four years of menopause, when the thermostat is getting reset.

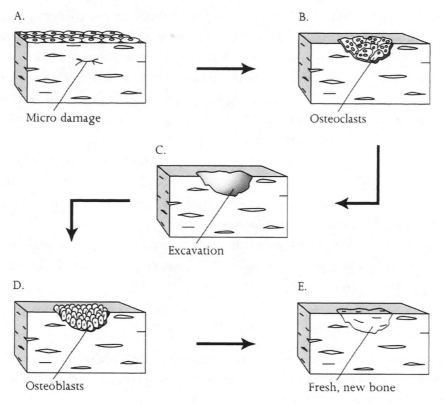

A.

Micro damage

B.

Osteoclasts

C.

Excavation

D.

Osteoblasts

E.

Fresh, new bone

FIGURE 7. The bone remodeling cycle. All bone is constantly being broken down and rebuilt (remodeled). Osteoclasts are the cells that break it down; osteoblasts rebuild it.

▶ *What is osteoporosis?*

It is a disease of bone in which bone mass decreases and the bones lose their calcium, becoming weak and prone to fracture. The name quite accurately describes the condition, porous bones. The little old lady with a dowager's hump suffers from osteoporosis. So does the woman who falls and breaks her hip or blunts her fall with her hand and breaks her wrist.

▶ *Does menopause have any effect on dental health?*

Some researchers believe that tooth loss and periodontal disease increase at the time of menopause and that these problems are related to the same kind of accelerated bone loss that can lead to osteoporosis. If that is the case, then hormone therapy is helpful because estrogen helps you to absorb calcium, which is good for the bones in which your teeth are implanted as well as for the bones in the rest of your body. One of my patients, a dentist and mother of two, believes in the importance of HRT for the maintenance of bone, and of course she believes in adequate calcium intake; I have found her in my waiting room reading a cookbook with high-calcium recipes. There is also evidence that periodontal disease increases the risk of heart attack. Newer theories suggest that people with periodontal disease have a higher inflammatory response to heart attack, which leads to increased plaque and hardening of the arteries, which in turn leads to higher risk for future heart attacks. As risk factors for hardening of the arteries, dental disease and obesity appear to be about equal. Taking good care of your teeth benefits your appearance and your life expectancy by lowering your risk for heart attack.

Because tooth loss and periodontal disease do increase with age, it is especially important to incorporate good dental hygiene into your daily routine. Daily flossing and fastidious brushing are essential.

▶ *What effect does menopause have on the vagina?*

The vagina, which is richly endowed with estrogen receptors, is definitely affected by declining estrogen levels. With menopause the vaginal lining thins, and gradually the whole vagina becomes shorter and narrower.

Among the most common symptoms mentioned by perimenopausal and postmenopausal women are vaginal dryness, irritation or itching, and discomfort with intercourse (technically known as dyspareunia). Some women bleed during or after intercourse. Sometimes this is the first symptom that a woman notices as she approaches menopause: her periods have not changed noticeably, nor is she having hot flashes, but discomfort with intercourse caused by vaginal dryness is beginning to be a problem.

Dryness and the subsequent irritation make these tissues vulnerable to infection. Perimenopausal and menopausal women often have vaginal infections, which may be caused by bacteria or by yeast.

▶ *What effect does menopause have on the bladder?*

One of the most frequently overlooked actions of estrogen is its effect on the bladder. Though it may be well known that many older women have urological problems—urinary tract infections, feelings of urinary urgency, incontinence, and other urinary tract dysfunction—few women realize that these difficulties are often related to estrogen deprivation.

The root of the problem starts before we are born, as the tissues of the human embryo—not yet even at the fetal state—begin to specialize. The same tissue that specializes to form the vagina also forms the bladder. Not surprisingly, this tissue has many estrogen receptors.

So when estrogen is absent, the changes that take place in the vagina also take place in the bladder and other structures of the urinary tract. Just as the walls of the vagina thin out after menopause, the walls of the bladder undergo similar changes. When estrogen is not present, the muscles that support the bladder sag and the bladder loses its muscle tone.

▶ Is incontinence a common menopausal problem?

Incontinence, which is the involuntary loss or leakage of urine, is a common and distressing problem among women, especially as they get older. Surveys show that as many as 16 percent of young women occasionally have incontinence, and perhaps half of women of menopausal age.

There are several reasons why incontinence is more a female problem than a male problem. First, lack of estrogen after menopause means a loss of muscle tone in the structures supporting the bladder. Second, the female urethra is relatively short and has less total muscle with which to control urine flow. Third, the stresses and strains of vaginal delivery during childbearing often weaken or stretch the tissues supporting the bladder.

Stress incontinence, the most familiar variety of incontinence, is loss of small or moderate amounts of urine because of increased pressure in the abdomen—the kind of pressure created by laughing, coughing, or sneezing. Jumping or running can also bring it on, and it is particularly common in women who have had several children. The causes are usually anatomical, that is, loss of muscle tone created by the stress of childbirth or by a decrease in estrogen. This form of incontinence is the most common in menopausal women. Cigarette smoking, which can cause earlier menopause as well as smoker's cough, can be a contributory factor.

Another kind of incontinence, urge incontinence, is discussed in Chapter 12.

▶ What is the effect of menopause on skin?

As we grow older, our skin ages along with the rest of us, becoming less elastic, less firm; it also becomes thinner, drier, and more sensitive to the sun. Are these changes caused or hastened by loss of estrogen? The data here are ambiguous. Researchers have tried to find some relation between estrogen and "youthful skin," which is after all a subjective assessment. A few papers have suggested that estrogen may protect skin from the effects of aging, but at present there is no solid, incontrovertible evidence.

▶ Does menopause cause weight gain?

One concern of many women as they enter perimenopause is weight gain. Patients come to my office complaining that already they have gained five or ten pounds; they wonder what is happening physiologically or hormonally that is making them put on the extra weight, especially since they feel they have not particularly changed either their eating habits or their activity level. At times this concern can escalate to levels of extreme anxiety.

> Recently a patient called me four times in one day. It seems that in reading on her own she had discovered that some psychiatrists were experimenting with two amphetamine-type drugs that, when used in conjunction with each other, produced dramatic weight loss. The woman was very eager to try the drugs and kept phoning me back to see whether I had called the pharmacist yet to fill a prescription.
>
> To her it was an emergency weight-loss issue. She weighed 144 pounds, which in a person of normal height is not a tragedy. But she felt that she had to take these medications because she had ten or fifteen extra pounds that she simply had to shed.
>
> Now I have never considered losing ten or fifteen pounds a medical emergency. But I did call the pharmacy, because I wanted to talk to the pharmacist about the medications. He was busy and said he would return my call later. At five o'clock the patient called back, wondering whether the pharmacist had returned my call. This woman will probably have a very difficult time psychologically when she finds it easier to gain weight as she gets older.

Although I cannot believe that the need to shed ten or fifteen pounds is a medical emergency, I do understand why many women feel anxiety about their weight at this time in their life. We live in a society that says you can't be too rich or too thin or too young. Maybe there is no way you can improve your financial status, and you certainly can't reverse the clock and get younger, but you do have control over your weight.

The scientific community used to believe that menopause itself did not have any specific relation to weight gain, that extra pounds were simply the result of a woman's metabolic clock slowing down as she aged, or perhaps of her becoming less active physically. Becoming sedentary leads to a gradual loss of muscle mass, as muscle turns to fat (witness the aging former football player), which requires fewer calories to maintain. Thus you will gain weight even if you are eating the same amount you did when you were more muscular. Conversely, the more muscular you are, the more calories you burn, just sitting still.

Yet there is evidence that perimenopausal women do experience some weight gain that may be strictly related to menopause and that may be physiological. A study at the Massachusetts Institute of Technology followed a group of perimenopausal women who continued the eating and exercise habits that they had previously established in their daily lives. During the period they were studied (about two years) the women gained an average of five to eight pounds. This gain was independent of whether they started estrogen replacement therapy. It was not the gradual weight gain that both men and women experience as they age and their basal metabolism rates fall.

The good news associated with this bad news is that the weight gain tends to stabilize. The increase does not usually go beyond the initial five to eight pounds, so any further increase is probably not related to menopause. Some of my patients find this information comforting. These are apt to be women who have been making legitimate efforts to keep down their body weight, and while they aren't happy about the five pounds they have added, they aren't frantic either. So when I tell them that yes, most women put on five pounds perimenopausally, they feel better. If they are already running twenty miles a week and eating a normal diet, perhaps the five pounds are not disastrous.

If you think you have gained weight because you are taking hormone therapy (though there is no scientific evidence to support this theory), it is perfectly all right to stop taking estrogen for a while and see whether the weight comes off more readily. I have a number of patients who have tried this and found that HRT was not the culprit.

▶ *Could weight gain at menopause be caused by thyroid problems?*

This is possible but not likely. Many people in our society tend to look for a quick fix to their problems; they hope to take this pill or that pill and suddenly become slender and gorgeous. Patients frequently want me to check their thyroid function, and in some cases this request is justified. I do perhaps a hundred thyroid tests a year and find one or two people who are truly hypothyroid. It is one of the few times when I can call someone on the phone and say, "You have a disease," and she'll be thrilled; she can take a magic pill and feel better.

> Rebecca K. is a patient whom I have known for about eighteen years, since I was an intern, and she has been putting on weight steadily over the whole period. Rebecca is now perimenopausal and has been having problems with heavy blood flow; she has a fibroid uterus, and she has been feeling tired and sluggish. She said to me, "Listen, I swear that I am not really changing my diet pattern, I am not really changing my exercise pattern." She is still having periods, and they are not too erratic, so she is not fully into the menopausal process.
>
> We were considering managing her periods, maybe putting her on progesterone to control her heavy flow, something she has taken well in the past when she needed it. Suddenly I thought, "Let's get a set of thyroid function tests," because fatigue, tiredness, weight gain, and heavy periods can all be symptoms of thyroid dysfunction. Sure enough, she turned out to be one of the very few women I turn up each year with thyroid dysfunction. So she can go on thyroid replacement therapy, which is easy—a pill a day.
>
> We will need to get some blood tests to make sure that her thyroid levels are just where they should be. Her periods should get lighter. She should lose weight maintaining the same diet. And she should achieve a sense of well-being.

Occasionally at this time of life you do have to think about hypothyroidism, but it is confusing because some of its symptoms are similar to the signs of approaching menopause. One difference, however, is that thyroid dysfunction is not like menopause with a waxing and waning, waxing and waning. Thyroid function tends to go down and stay down. For this reason, the American College of Physicians recommends a baseline thyroid test at age fifty, even for people who have no symptoms.

Hypothyroidism can be a significant problem. Thyroid replacement therapy is not to be taken lightly, nor is it purely cosmetic, to be used for weight control. It is a serious metabolic issue, and physicians don't just experiment with thyroid medication. Giving estrogen and giving thyroid are very different matters; you can give somebody estrogen for a month or two, but you can't give someone thyroid extract for just a couple of months.

It is also important to realize that if you have normal thyroid function, you can take all the thyroid pills in the world and you will not get thin. Thyroid medication you don't need may make your heart beat a little faster; it may make you sweat; it may even make you have a fever. But it will not make you thin.

▶ *Does menopause have any effect on allergies?*

Although no significant scientific studies have documented a relation between menopause and allergies, many of my patients tell me that their response to allergens has changed at menopause. Some women note an improvement in long-standing allergy problems, whereas others notice a distinct increase in the severity of their symptoms. It is well known that stress and fatigue contribute to allergies, and insofar as menopause is a time of stress and a time when many women feel fatigued because they have difficulty sleeping, those factors can exacerbate their allergic symptoms.

6 Menopause and Your Mind

MEDICAL science knows a great deal about the effects of menopause and falling estrogen levels on your body. The effects of menopause on your mind and on your mental health are less well understood. These are complex and involve the interaction of physical, biochemical, and even social factors.

Although not many women come into my office every week and say with elation, "Hurrah, I think I'm menopausal," many women feel very positive about menopause. Some of their reasons are physical. There are women who are relieved not to have to worry about birth control. There are women who have elected for religious or other reasons not to use birth control and no longer have to worry about getting pregnant. There are women who strongly dislike menstruating, perhaps because their periods are miserably uncomfortable or perhaps because they just don't like having them. There are women who are debilitated by endometriosis, for whom hormonal therapy has not worked, who don't want surgical intervention, for whom menopause is a great relief.

There are women who have large fibroids or fibroids that bleed, and for them menopause is a positive event because they will no longer bleed, their fibroids will probably shrink, and life will be easier. Women who have undergone surgical menopause because of total hysterectomy often feel grateful that the health problems that made them seek surgery are over.

There are also women for whom menopause is a positive event for other reasons. For many, menopause symbolizes the end of the time when they are bound to family concerns, at least as primary caretaker of their children, and they feel liberated to pursue their own interests and activities. For these women, menopause often brings a sense of selfhood and freedom from binding obligations.

Other women speak of a freedom from the expectations of others. Women are perhaps more strongly than men the creatures of other people's expectations. If we have always been "good girls," we may feel the need to conform less strongly at age forty-five or fifty than we did when we were twenty or thirty. We may have found that living up to the standard expectations of what women "ought" to be has not yielded the rewards we were led to expect. And the overt recognition of middle age that menopause forces on us gives us a chance to reevaluate what we want and how we want to act.

Even though many women feel positive about menopause, there are many myths and (one hesitates to say) "old wives' tales" to the contrary. One persistent and unfortunate myth is that menopause hits with a full barrage of distressing emotional signs: mood swings, irritability, anxiety and panic attacks, and serious depression. The myth of menopausal depression is so strong and so enduring that a large percentage of women who are not yet perimenopausal believe that when they do approach menopause they will become depressed. My own practice bears out not the prevalence of menopausal depression but the level of concern. Every week several people come to me, worried about their mental status—not because they are in fact depressed or anxious but because they have heard that they will be.

In fact, most women do not get seriously depressed as they pass through menopause, although they may notice various emotional changes, which for a relative few include depression or anxiety or even both together. Although statistical studies have long shown that women are at least twice as likely as men to become depressed (or to seek help for it), recent epidemiological studies have suggested that women are no more depressed during their forties and fifties than they are at any other time in life. There is no increase in the number of women hospitalized for mental illness during these years, nor do suicide rates, generally taken as an index of severe depression, rise for women during these decades. As a group, women are much more likely to be depressed in their twenties and thirties, when the life stresses they face are entirely different. You can be comforted, then, that at least statistically you are not automatically doomed to depression or anxiety at menopause.

One reason for the persistence of the myth of inevitable depression is cultural. In the United States today, as the media will readily tell you, youth is in, experience is out. Young is beautiful, old is ugly. Our culture is full of unpleasant stereotypes of the menopausal woman, from the wrinkled, humpbacked crone with a disposition like Snow White's wicked stepmother to the impossible mother-in-law like Wilma Flintstone's mother, Pearl, to the gray-haired airhead, Edith Bunker, made famous by Jean Stapleton.

Nor has science, at least in the past, done women any favors. Around the turn of the century, physicians described a syndrome that they called involutional melancholia. "Involution" means shrinkage or biological deterioration, so involutional melancholia meant depression that occurred at the time of menopause and was caused by menopause. Although the phrase was quickly picked up to describe what was thought to be a common phenomenon, in recent years both the idea and the terminology have been rejected.

A second and equally destructive menopausal myth, one that should wane as science probes the mysteries of endocrinology, is the notion that the symptoms of menopause are "all in your mind." That is, if you are suffering from heavy-duty hot flashes, or if you are miserable because of lack of sleep, it is because you are basically a neurotic complainer. If you were more stoic and heroic, you would either smile at these inconveniences or perhaps you would not even notice them. I was particularly distressed in the spring of 2003 when the *New York Times* ran an editorial saying that all menopausal symptoms were a figment of women's imaginations and a ploy of the drug companies promoting hormone therapy.

Armed with what we know today about how the body works, we can say, yes, to a certain extent your flushes and sleep disturbances and other menopausal symptoms are all in your head. But, as we have seen, they originate in your hypothalamus and your pituitary gland, not in your attitude.

▶ *Is there such a thing as menopausal depression?*

Right now no one really knows. Even though involutional melancholia is no longer accepted as a recognized disease by the psychiatric community and even though, statistically, women are no more likely to become depressed in their fifties than they are in their thirties, the fact remains that many women do report symptoms of serious depression at menopause. Although the final answers are not yet in, many physicians believe that this depression is in some way caused by changes in hormonal levels. Studies undertaken by the National Institute of Mental Health have shown that some women fail to respond to antidepressant medications unless they have some estrogen on board.

▶ *What other kinds of emotional and psychological symptoms do women notice at menopause?*

Although some fortunate women have no menopausal distress, psychological or physical, many individuals do notice emotional discomforts around the time of menopause. These include irritability, tearfulness that is not caused by a sad event, excessive worry, anxiety, diminished energy, problems in concentrating, feelings of low self-esteem, and loss of memory. Some women even find themselves craving certain foods, such as those classic offenders chocolate and potato chips. If some of these symptoms sound like PMS, they are indeed similar. Many women develop PMS-type symptoms in their early forties and then just continue with them into menopause. These women have not had PMS at all earlier in their lives, but they start showing up at their gynecologist's office describing classic symptoms: premenstrual irritability, bloating, malaise, lack of concentration.

> Lois G. is forty-eight and the mother of four children, the youngest of whom is fourteen. Most of her life she was easygoing and even-tempered. She had never had any PMS-type symptoms until after her youngest child was born, but during the past ten years she has had migraine headaches and mood swings, both of which intensified as time went by. We tried all sorts of nonhormonal medications for the migraines, but nothing worked. Finally I persuaded her to try estrogen. After a couple of weeks she said that she felt better than she had in about thirteen years—no headaches, no mood swings, no irritability. After a year or two, when she is through this difficult perimenopausal period, she plans to taper off the estrogen.

▶ *How can I differentiate between symptoms caused by PMS and symptoms caused by approaching menopause if I'm still having regular periods?*

Unfortunately no simple test will say that *these* behavioral changes are caused by PMS and that *those* are caused by the approach of menopause. My approach in this situation is to use techniques of PMS management, including SSRI therapy (Prozac and its relatives).

If these do not relieve the discomfort, my next line of attack is estrogen therapy. Ultimately, many women do respond to estrogen as if they were menopausal, even though their ovaries are still making some estrogen and they are still having regular periods.

▶ What causes emotional changes around the time of menopause?

Again, no one knows. Yet although we lack definitive answers, we are not lacking in theories. One hypothesis is that stressful events in life bring on the emotional changes surrounding menopause. A second theory is that changes in hormonal levels are the culprit. Finally, some observers believe that declining estrogen levels bring about sleeplessness and that sleep problems in turn cause depression and other psychological symptoms. All these formulations have something to recommend them, and all may play a part in a woman's emotional perspective at menopause. It is difficult to separate the strands of the tangle.

▶ Are there particular stresses during the menopausal years?

When I look at my patients as a group, I see very clearly that many women's lives change drastically when they are in their late forties and early fifties. Their children are leaving home, going off to college, dating people (whom their mothers may or may not like), getting married, and having children of their own. Many women who thought they were through raising a family find that they have inherited a whole new set of responsibilities as their children call on them to raise the next generation. Many of my patients tell me that grandmothering, the kind you can go home from when you've had enough, is wonderful. But returning to primary motherhood is another story altogether.

At the other end of the spectrum, elderly people are living well into their eighties, and many of my patients who are dealing with their grandchildren are also dealing with aging parents. Often these parents are becoming infirm or incompetent. They need someone to manage their taxes and sometimes even their checkbooks. Sometimes health issues are involved: finding a nursing home, seeing that someone comes in regularly to help with medications, or other care. In some cases, women in midlife must actually provide this care for their aging parents. Often they have to cope with financial issues, not only managing money but finding enough of it to cover necessities.

Personal issues, such as household management and transportation, also arise. Women, who as a group have been designated society's caregivers, sometimes have to deal not only with their own parents but also with their in-laws. You may have a warm relationship with your husband's parents, but the burden of caring both for them and for your own parents can be heavy and easy to resent.

Sometimes while juggling the demands of parents and children, these same women are trying to go back to school, preparing to reenter the work force or reenter it in a different capacity.

Many a woman in her late forties or early fifties is the victim of her husband's midlife crisis. These seem to be prime years for divorce as men cling to the illusion of their own youthfulness, often in the company of younger women. The male midlife crisis has been quite thoroughly explored in the media, though the midlife crisis in women is more or less terra incognita.

The generation of women who are currently in their fifties often find themselves facing new and different expectations. A middle-class young woman in the 1950s assumed that she would find herself a man, get married, raise his children, support his career, and nurture and share his interests. She was expected to put aside any ambitions for herself or fulfill them in the time she had left over from her responsibilities to husband and family; but she would eventually reap the benefits of her husband's financial success and shine in his reflected glory.

For better or for worse, those days are gone. The dramatic rise in the divorce rate, the convictions of the women's movement, and the changes in our national economy have virtually demolished that set of expectations. The woman in her fifties who has more or less lived by these standards finds herself having to cope with a world that expects different things of her. She may want to enter the working world but may feel that thirty years of housework is a formidable obstacle.

Even women who have worked throughout their adult lives face significant changes. Some of the women I see express the same kinds of dissatisfaction that men seem to experience at midlife. They question the choices they have made. Finding themselves at the zenith of their careers, they wonder whether it is in fact where they want to be. Was the game worth the candle? And where do they go from here?

Now, any one of these factors can be stressful. And all of them together would put a crimp in even the happiest outlook. So there are significant and stressful changes that come into focus around the time of menopause.

▶ *Do cultural factors influence a woman's outlook at menopause?*

Even if you do not have to take care of your sick mother-in-law or your grandchildren or strain your own pocketbook to help your adult children financially or go job hunting when you have worked in your home for the past thirty years, as an older woman you will experience cultural stress. Because women are not accorded a place of esteem and respect in our society, their status sinks as they age. As a nation we are devotees of youth, especially in women. Whereas the silver-haired male may be admired for his power or his financial prowess or even his wisdom, the silver-haired woman—no matter how competent or successful or knowledgeable—is less highly valued. Women who did not feel the brunt of discrimination while in their twenties and thirties—protected perhaps by their youth and physical attractiveness or perhaps because they were not yet near whatever glass ceiling exists in their profession—may begin to feel it more acutely as they age.

Among the women I see are any number of vibrant, handsome, intelligent, athletic, talented, and able women who are considered over the hill because they are over age fifty. Other cultures are kinder to aging women. Marcha Flint, an anthropologist who is a former president of the North American Menopause Society, has performed cross-cultural studies in societies where older women are valued and has come up with some interesting observations. She points out that although all women have declining estrogen levels in their forties and fifties and presumably experience the same physical symptoms, women's perceptions of what they physically feel at menopause seem to be culturally influenced, and their symptoms conform in some ways to cultural expectations. For example, a group of Rajput women in India whom Flint studied had no symptoms whatsoever, nor did Mayan women of the Yucatán Peninsula. Nor did a group of Navajo women studied by the anthropologist Ann Wright; in the Navajo language there is no word for menopause.

Other researchers have pointed out that in many cultures the status of women changes at menopause, and that when it changes for the better, women understandably experience menopause as a positive event. Among the Meo people of Thailand, for example, another group studied by Flint, the condition of menopause is honored. A menopausal woman throws a big party at which she announces that she is no longer of childbearing age and that, having attained this status, she deserves new, heightened respect. Pauline Bart, whose pioneering *Women in a Sexist Society* was published in 1971, pointed out that women in cultures where age is revered, or at least respected, suffer fewer symptoms of menopause than women in cultures where age is denigrated.

▶ *What is the role of sleeplessness in menopausal emotional changes?*

It is evident that sleeplessness can cause emotional changes, including irritability and depression and loss of a general feeling of well-being. Sleep researchers have shown that

REM sleep, the part of the sleep cycle in which dreaming occurs, is important to the feeling of well-being and to the rejuvenation that comes from a good night's sleep. It is also known that women with lower than usual blood levels of estrogen have less REM sleep, even though they may not actually be sleep deprived. Whether sleep deprivation is caused by hot flashes or hormonal changes or just plain stress, it still can interfere with your emotional health.

If you solve the problems of sleep deprivation and your emotional state does not improve, then you will know that other factors are contributing. Improving the quality and the amount of your sleep will not solve the difficulties caused by your family, your marriage, or your inability to get a job that pays a reasonable wage. Nor will it alter depression that is caused by your brain chemistry.

▶ *Do the mood swings, irritability, and other psychological symptoms of menopause go away by themselves over time?*

Although real clinical depression will probably not go away with the passage of time, menopausal mood swings and irritability generally get better on their own.

▶ *What are the symptoms of clinical depression?*

Probably everyone feels dejected and downhearted from time to time, and probably everyone responds with feelings of sadness to life's unhappy events. But depression as a clinical disease has a group of specific symptoms beyond these normal melancholy feelings. The classic symptoms include sleep disturbances, especially difficulty in falling asleep and early morning awakening; these are different from the typical sleep problems of perimenopause, which involve waking up in the wee hours with or without night sweats. The perimenopausal woman finds herself staring at the ceiling at something like one in the morning, while the depressed person wakes at four or five in the morning.

Change in appetite is another classic symptom, as is significant gain or loss of weight. A major change in libido, usually decreased interest in sex, is another warning sign. A depressed person usually experiences feelings of guilt and worthlessness, which may culminate in suicidal feelings. When someone comes to my office complaining of depression and admits to suicidal thoughts, I always ask whether she has made a plan for ending her life. Does she know how she would kill herself? If her vague musings on the subject of suicide have coalesced into a plan for action, I believe that her situation is dangerous and I take immediate action—which on one occasion involved driving someone to the hospital for emergency therapy.

Some women who suffer emotional problems at menopause are afflicted by bipolar disorder, which is characterized by depression but also by periods of mania. During these emotional highs, women may become completely sleepless, spend money recklessly, and experience increased sexual appetite.

▶ Is there a chemical or organic component to postmenopausal depression?

Organic depressions are negative states of mind that arise within an individual because of his or her brain chemistry. An old joke tells of two children, an optimist and a pessimist, confronted with a room full of horse manure. The huge heap simply makes the pessimistic child more depressed. But the optimist is delighted; with all that manure lying around, she knows that there has got to be a pony somewhere. The optimist has a brain chemistry that makes her organically cheerful. The pessimist, for reasons that are not yet understood, unfortunately has a brain chemistry that makes her baseline outlook on life less than positive.

Now, you could argue that the depressed child had good reason to be discouraged and pessimistic when faced with a roomful of manure. This is what is known as exogenous depression; it is caused by events outside oneself. A woman who feels terrible because her son is marrying someone she feels is unreliable and dishonest, or whose mother-in-law with Alzheimer's is moving into her household, unquestionably suffers from exogenous depression.

But there are entities known as organic or endogenous depressions. They are caused by events inside oneself, changes in the brain chemistry. They can happen at any time, and they can come and go; they can be triggered by stressful events. People can get depressed in their twenties or their thirties or their forties. Or they can become depressed when their hormone levels start changing dramatically. Or they can get depressed as they age. Bipolar depression certainly has a genetic component that is independent of external events, and many people who have bipolar disorder have relatives—parents or grandparents—who have had the same disease.

Brain chemistry can be altered, as many menstruating women know, by changes in hormone levels. The depression, listlessness, and irritability that many women experience just before the onset of their periods are caused by the sudden drop in hormones that occurs at this time. Because the years surrounding menopause are marked by wide fluctuations in estrogen and progesterone levels, it is not surprising that mood swings similar to premenstrual fluctuations do occur.

Other accompaniments of aging, factors that are not necessarily mediated by the change in sex hormone levels, can cause alterations in mood. For example, as we get older the secretion of melatonin decreases. Melatonin is a chemical, a sort of natural sleep drug, produced in the brain by the pineal gland—a gland that people used to think was useless (though René Descartes thought it was the home of the soul). The symptoms of fatigue and disorientation during jet lag may be attributable to changes in melatonin level. Because the brain produces less melatonin as we age, we no longer sleep as well as we used to.

Changes in mood can also be caused by certain diseases, among them chronic fatigue syndrome, Epstein-Barr virus, and Lyme disease. Unfortunately, these diseases are frequently often used as smoke screens to avoid facing up to depression. I have had patients attribute a perpetually depressed outlook to fibromyalgia, a disease that causes generalized muscle pain, a sort of "ache all over" feeling. Because mental illness is such a stigma in this society (a worse stigma even than menopause), some people will indulge in a lot of fancy footwork to avoid acknowledging their mental state.

Often women will report to me that they have chronic fatigue syndrome, which is one of today's catchall terms for diseases that diagnosticians and clinicians have trouble pinpointing. Chronic fatigue syndrome is a real disease, it does exist, but it is probably overdiagnosed. Fibromyalgia, which some researchers believe is a less serious cousin of lupus, and Epstein-Barr virus are also real diseases, but are probably also overdiagnosed. Even Lyme disease, which is currently on the upswing and a hot media topic in southern New England where I live, sometimes gets blamed for my patients' depression.

The advantage to confronting depression is that in most cases it is treatable. A colleague at the University of Connecticut, an expert on chronic fatigue syndrome, tells his patients that no, they really do not want to have chronic fatigue syndrome; there are no effective treatments for it. But if they are clinically depressed, however unfashionable that may be, drugs are available that can really help. Other approaches, such as biofeedback therapy and self-hypnosis, can alleviate depression. Between effective psychotherapy and appropriate medical drug therapy, most depressed people can feel much better.

The analogy with diabetes is helpful. Although people may resent having diabetes and wish not to have it, they are not ashamed of being diabetic in the way they are ashamed of being depressed. Yet diabetes is a chemical imbalance that affects millions of people worldwide. When the doctor tells diabetics to take insulin, in general they take it.

In general they don't feel stigmatized by doing so, and fortunately, most diabetics don't believe that by right thinking they can cure their insulin deficiencies.

Many people have an organic chemical depression, which is a real disease, for which we fortunately have effective medicine. If you have a chemical imbalance, then you treat a chemical imbalance. It is not your fault that you have baseline organic depression. You will not feel better by calling it PMS or fibromyalgia or Epstein-Barr virus and trying a lot of different approaches that don't work. But you will feel better if you take the appropriate antidepressant and follow a carefully managed regimen.

▶ *What is the relationship between estrogen or progesterone and mood?*

Although the exact relation between sex hormones and mood is still ambiguous, some facts are beginning to emerge. Estrogen does have a positive effect on mood in some people, though neither the mechanism nor the reason behind it is understood. David Keefe, a researcher at Brown University trained in both psychiatry and gynecology, believes that certain depressive symptoms are triggered by changes in hormone levels, rather than an absolute low level or an absolute high level of estrogen or progesterone. This theory might explain why women taking exogenous estrogen, and thereby keeping their estrogen levels fairly stable, tend to be a little less depressed than women whose estrogen levels are less stable. Keefe has concluded that the same kind of fluctuation in estrogen levels triggers the emotional swings of PMS.

▶ *How can one tell whether depression is caused by hormones, "brain chemistry," or external events?*

The answer is that you can't always distinguish the cause of depression. Sometimes a patient says, "You know, I have gained (or lost) a lot of weight. I am tired all the time. I am not sleeping well at night. I have no interest in activities any more and I am bored with my life." These are pretty standard symptoms of depression, but we need to decide whether this depression is environmental or caused by brain chemistry or brought on by menopause.

I think the only way to rule out menopause as a factor is to try hormonal replacement, if only briefly. If the rapidly changing hormone levels that are characteristic of menopause are at the root of the problem, then estrogen replacement therapy should help. Occasionally the additional administration of testosterone will help enhance mood and give a sense of well-being.

► *Do men experience depression and mood changes related to sex hormone changes?*

Probably they do. However, the production of testosterone in men decreases very gradually over a long period; because men experience no sudden swings in hormonal level, their moods are probably less drastically affected. Another reason for the apparent stability in their moods as they age is that men in our society are trained not to exhibit their feelings outwardly. If their hormones affect their moods, they are less likely to show it.

► *What are the remedies for menopausal anxiety, depression, and mood swings?*

There are several lines of approach, which include hormonal and nonhormonal therapies. If your emotional symptoms are mild and transient, commonsense approaches are in order. Exercise has well-known, positive effects on mood. Support groups, such as Prime Plus/Red Hot Mamas, bring comfort and relief to many women. If you know that what you are going through emotionally is not unique to you, that you are not alone, you may find yourself better able to cope. Education is a valuable tool that can give women higher self-esteem and enable them to communicate more fully with their caregivers.

If your symptoms are more severe and do not respond to these measures, there are other approaches. Among them are antidepressant drugs and hormone therapy, and occasionally testosterone. Estrogen has a well-documented positive effect on mood in women with low levels of this hormone; and HRT relieves mood swings, depression, and anxiety for many women who are perimenopausal, menopausal, and even older.

Annette L., now about eighty-one years old, was depressed for years. She had been to her doctor. She had tried the usual antidepressants but remained down and depressed. When she was about seventy-five, her son, who had worked with me for quite a while, persuaded her to come to my office. We talked about estrogen, and although she is a conservative French Canadian, she agreed to try it. After she started the estrogen replacement therapy, she really took off. She has become a demon housekeeper, filled with energy and a true zest for life. Looking back on her life, she recognized that she had been depressed for almost thirty years.

▶ *How long do I have to take HRT to find out whether it helps my mood swings and psychological outlook?*

Within one or two months you will know whether hormonal replacement is helping. Once you have started taking estrogen, blood tests can measure the amount of estrogen in your blood. If you continue to feel depressed and the hormonal replacement therapy does not help, you will know that your depression is not caused by lack of estrogen. I have treated many women who feel much better with estrogen, whose moods really change, and it is clear that the hormonal swings of menopause were making them feel psychologically miserable.

▶ *How do you determine the correct dosage of estrogen to help with these psychological symptoms?*

In this as in other areas, I am a sort of biotitrater. If someone comes to me with mood swings or what seems to be hormonally mediated depression, I begin by prescribing a small amount of estrogen. If she feels better but maybe not perfect, I try a little more. Some doctors would take blood estradiol levels, but I don't believe that these are entirely helpful. If my patient with the mood swings feels a little better when her blood estradiol level is 75, would she feel a lot better at 175? I don't know. So I tend to juggle dosages according to their results.

The menopause expert Leon Speroff of the University of Oregon Medical School notes that levels above 200 pg/ml probably will not further alleviate symptoms that are caused by menopause. So if someone has a blood estradiol level somewhere around 200 and still feels bad, it is important to pay attention to nonmenopausal causes of her distress. If she finds out after a month or so that the estrogen doesn't make her feel any different than she did before, we need to try to find out what is causing her depressed feelings. If the root of the problem is organic depression or external events, I refer her to someone in the health care profession who can help with biofeedback technique or psychotherapy.

▶ *Can antidepressant drugs help in depressions that are caused by external events?*

Fortunately, the answer is yes. No one knows exactly by what pathways the brain interacts with the external world. But many people who have very good reasons to feel depressed find help with antidepressant drugs. The drugs obviously cannot resolve the troubling situations, but they can help people cope with them.

▶ *What kinds of drugs are used to treat depression?*

Among the advances in medicine in the almost three decades since I was in medical school has been the development of a whole new range of psychogenic drugs, drugs that affect a person's state of mind. Thirty years ago the only available antidepressants were tricyclics, among which were Elavil (amitriptyline) and Tofranil (imipramine). Modern derivatives of these early tricyclics have been developed and include drugs such as desipramine.

These drugs, which work at the level of the neurotransmitter in the brain, are effective and still do the job for many people. In recent years they have been successfully used in treating fibromyalgia and chronic fatigue syndrome. They seem to alleviate muscle pain and also help insomnia, whether caused by menopausal symptoms or something else.

Tricyclics, which increase the levels of neurotransmitters in the brain, do have bothersome side effects. They cause dry mouth and sometimes constipation. Some people gain weight on them, though when people are depressed they tend to gain weight anyhow because they exercise less. A more serious side effect, especially when people overdose on tricyclics, is cardiac arrhythmia (abnormal heart rhythm).

At the end of the 1980s we saw the emergence of Prozac, another kind of antidepressant, and its relatives. Zoloft is a newer medication similar to Prozac, and today drugs that are derivatives of Zoloft, and hence grandchildren of Prozac, are coming on the market. Prozac is a very effective antidepressant and helpful in many situations (including PMS, which is felt to be a separate entity, different from regular depression). Prozac and its descendants are serotonin reuptake inhibitors (SSRIs), which means that they increase the levels of serotonin in the brain. And although all the functions of serotonin are not understood, it seems to be important in controlling mood.

▶ *Is Prozac dangerous?*

Prozac's poor reputation has two principal causes. First, it is overprescribed, like many other psychogenic drugs: there is no question that many people are taking it who should not be. Yet a great many depressed people probably should be taking it who are not, for it is a very effective antidepressant and really does make many people feel better.

Second, Prozac has gotten a very bad press because a number of people who were taking it have committed suicide. And a few people taking it have committed murder. Recognizing this, you have to recognize also the diseases you are treating. Would these people have committed suicide or murder if they were not taking Prozac? Was it the Prozac that caused the violence? These are people who were seriously depressed or had serious mental illness. Blaming the Prozac is like accusing an anticancer drug of killing a cancer patient.

▶ *Can my gynecologist prescribe antidepressants if my depression is caused by menopause?*

Because mental illness carries such a burden of shame in this country, many people feel embarrassed to see a psychiatrist. For this reason, my gynecological patients sometimes want me to prescribe their antidepressants and oversee their therapy. Although some of my colleagues feel comfortable doing this, most of the time I do not. A psychiatrist whose specialty training includes experience with mind-altering and mood-altering drugs has greater competence in this area than I do. Furthermore, many patients will do better with a combination of psychotherapy and medication. A specialist can best judge what psychotherapy is needed. I do feel comfortable prescribing estrogen replacement therapy. Because I am experienced in observing its effects and side effects, I feel competent to oversee therapy, adjusting dosages and dealing with occasional small glitches.

▶ *Are there herbal products that will help with depression or anxiety?*

In Europe, St. John's wort is used widely as an antidepressant, and there are data backing up its effectiveness although no one knows exactly how it works. People who are taking MAO (monoamine oxidase) inhibitors should not use St. John's wort; nor should people who are already taking SSRIs take St. John's wort as well. People who have used St. John's wort for an extended time or at high dosages have sometimes reported an inflammation of their skin or mucus membranes when exposed to direct sunlight. Because the dosages of herbal products are not standardized, ask your pharmacist or someone well informed about alternative medicine to suggest a reliable brand.

Many people have tried Valerian root as an anti-anxiety agent. Like St. John's wort, it is not regulated in the United States and may come in variable doses of whose strength you are not aware. Because it can have dangerous side effects, including congestive heart failure, it is not recommended as a sedative for long-term therapy.

▶ *Is there such a thing as postmenopausal zest?*

Many years ago the anthropologist Margaret Mead coined the term "postmenopausal zest" (PMZ)—a sort of positive PMS—to describe the surge of physical and psychological energy that certain women feel after menopause. There is no scientific explanation, no hormonal or endocrinological evidence, to suggest why women should feel this way.

Does everyone experience it? No, I don't think so. But many women feel very positive about menopause. For many, it releases energies that have been bound up in other things; these women say things to me that suggest that at menopause they are happy to be finished with the part of their life they have lived. They feel that they have succeeded, that they have done well, that they are getting on with their lives.

Some feminist psychologists believe that PMZ is sort of a large-scale equivalent of the positive energy that many women feel after their menstrual periods. If you take as your baseline mood or attitude the kinds of feelings that you have before your period—those sometimes blue or blah or negative emotional states—then what you feel after your period is a kind of high, a sort of postmenstrual zest. Similarly, what you may feel after the hormonal ups and downs of the perimenopausal period can be thought of as a kind of postmenopausal zest.

7 Coping with the Symptoms

IF you are bleeding heavily and irregularly, or suffering the discomfort of hot flushes that drench you with sweat at the most inappropriate moments, or you are becoming irritable and hard to get along with because you haven't had a good night's sleep, or your mood is swinging back and forth like Tarzan on a vine, plenty of help is available. Medical science and feminine experience have developed the tools for dealing with most of these symptoms in the majority of women. And for many of these annoyances, you can find therapies that fit your own pattern of health care preferences.

Some of the available therapies are nonhormonal. Others involve the use of hormones—estrogen, progesterone, and sometimes testosterone—either alone or in combination. Some have been scientifically proven in controlled clinical tests; others seem to help women with their symptoms, though no one knows quite why. No one treatment may be absolutely perfect for you, relieving your own symptoms and at the same time fitting your pattern of expectations and tolerances. If you do not want or cannot use hormonal treatments, you still have options; but you may have to work harder to achieve your desired goal. The choice of whether to use long-term estrogen replacement therapy, which is a very effective way to alleviate common menopausal symptoms, is a controversial issue and merits its own chapter.

Even before the Women's Health Initiative released its results, women had many reasons for not wanting to use hormone therapy. Some women found taking pills regularly to be psychologically uncomfortable. Others preferred not to have the menstrual periods that come along with the progesterone part of the therapy. A few women could not take HRT because some other medical condition counterindicated it. Since the WHI, many women simply feel too anxious about hormone therapy to try it.

But declining to take hormone therapy doesn't mean that you can't do anything to control perimenopausal and menopausal symptoms. The alternative therapies range from vitamins to herbal remedies to other nonhormonal medications. Some hormonal regimens are short term and directed at specific problems. The old standbys, exercise and dietary change, can go a long way toward relieving many discomforts.

HEAVY PERIODS

Many women are content to live with heavier periods during their perimenopausal years once they know that these periods are not abnormal or dangerous. Women who find the heavy periods distressing or disruptive, or those who bleed heavily enough to lower their hematocrit or interfere with their daily routine, have the option of either hormonal or nonhormonal therapy. There are basically two avenues of treatment: replacing the iron that is lost during heavy periods, and controlling the heavy flow so that the iron loss does not have a chance to occur.

Nonhormonal therapies begin with iron replacement. If you are in danger of becoming anemic because of blood loss during heavy periods, but you do not want to try hormonal therapy to regulate the flow, you must maintain your blood count by taking supplementary iron. You can get additional iron through your diet and through iron pills.

Iron is available in tablets. You can start with 325 mg of iron sulfate daily, an amount far higher than that recommended for pregnant women, and enough in many cases to maintain a hematocrit of 38 to 40. If you choose this route, you should have your physician check your hematocrit after a month or two just to make sure that it is within the acceptable range. If your hematocrit is still low, you'll probably need more iron; most women can't absorb much more than three 325-mg iron sulfate tablets daily, which should be taken spread out throughout the day, not all at once.

To maximize the amount of iron absorbed, you should take it on an empty stomach, an hour before a meal or several hours afterward. Taking this much iron every day is not difficult or seriously inconvenient, though some women do not tolerate it well and become constipated. Constipation in general seems to be more of a problem for women than for men, and one that increases with age for a number of reasons, including decreased physical activity. Sensible measures to counter constipation include drinking plenty of fluids, getting a lot of exercise, and eating foods that are rich in fiber. If you find that supplementary iron tablets upset your stomach, you might try taking the pills with food.

Because of these side effects, some women prefer not to take iron supplements and wish to obtain the required iron through dietary sources. Although a woman who is not afflicted with heavy bleeding should have no trouble getting enough iron in her diet, a woman who is trying to maintain her hematocrit by increasing her dietary iron does have to pay careful attention to what she eats.

Many foods contain iron, but not all iron is absorbed equally. There are two kinds of iron, heme iron and nonheme iron. Heme iron, which makes up about 40 percent of the iron in animal tissues, is more easily absorbed by the body and is found in meat (particularly liver and red meat) and to a lesser extent in fish. Nonheme iron, the other form found in animal tissues as well as in dairy products, eggs, certain vegetables, grains, and fruits, is less readily absorbed by the body. Nonheme iron is also used to enrich flour and cereals. "Total" cereal, for example, has 15 to 18 mg of iron per serving. As people eat less and less red meat, it becomes increasingly difficult to get enough iron through diet alone if you have to increase your intake to maintain your hematocrit.

For menopausal women and adult men, the requirement is 10 mg daily. For menstruating women, the requirement is 15 mg. The level previously was set at 18 mg daily, but in 1989 a committee of the National Academy of Sciences lowered the requirement—in part because women were having difficulty achieving the 18-mg level and in part because the lower requirement was deemed sufficient.

The body absorbs about 30 percent of the heme iron from meat or fish, in contrast to only about 5 percent of the nonheme iron content of fruits, vegetables, grains, and eggs. Cooked broccoli, for example, contains 1.8 mg of iron per cup, so six cups of cooked broccoli contain 10.8 mg of iron, just about what you need if you are a menopausal woman. But since only 5 percent of the iron you consume with food is actually absorbed, you would have to increase your daily broccoli consumption twentyfold, to a whopping 120 cups of cooked broccoli a day, if you intended to get your recommended daily requirement of iron solely by eating that vegetable. This example is extreme, because probably no woman intends to get her entire iron requirement by eating broccoli, but it does show how attentive you have to be if you do want to get enough iron without eating red meat or taking iron supplements.

As the broccoli example illustrates, foods do have iron content that is not easily absorbed; but there are several tricks for improving absorption. Eating something rich in vitamin C at the time you are eating something rich in iron improves absorption of non-heme iron. If you were to drink a five-ounce glass of orange juice while eating your broccoli, you would absorb three to seven times the amount of iron. Eating a food with heme iron at the same meal you are eating foods rich in nonheme iron (chili beans and meat, for example) makes more of the nonheme iron available to your body. Cooking in non-enameled cast-iron pots also increases the iron content of foods, especially acidic foods.

▶ *Is there a way to keep perimenopausal periods from being so heavy?*

If instead of replacing lost iron, your concern is lessening the heavy flow of your perimenopausal periods, you can look at either surgical or hormonal options.

One long-standing approach to occasional episodes of heavy, uncontrolled bleeding is the D&C (dilatation and curettage), a surgical procedure that involves scraping the lining of the uterus. It can usually be done on an outpatient basis and often helps to control bleeding for up to two or three years. No one knows exactly why.

Newer approaches that often achieve the same results as a D&C make use of ablation techniques to destroy the layer of glandular endometrial tissue that produces the bleeding. The agent that causes the actual destruction may be heat, cold, or even radio waves: for more detail see Chapter 14.

A hormonal treatment that helps many women with uncomfortably heavy bleeding or very frequent menses is the use of progesterone, which can be administered in several ways. Oral contraceptives, which are a combination of estrogen and progesterone, can be used to manage irregular menstrual periods and to lessen heavy flow. The pills work in the same way as they do to prevent conception: they shut down your ovaries altogether and then reprogram the uterus according to the estrogen and progesterone content of the pills. With birth control pills, you can have a period regularly every month and avoid the kind of "Niagara Falls bleeding" that happens to some women when they have periods several months apart.

A second advantage of birth control pills is that they lessen other menopausal symptoms. A perimenopausal woman who is bleeding three times a month, having hot flashes, and feeling truly miserable is likely to do very well on a low-dose birth control pill. It will put her ovaries out of commission and give her the estrogen that her body needs to control both the hot flashes and the frequent periods.

> Marilyn B. is forty-five. She has signs of approaching menopause: a mild and not especially bothersome hot flash now and then, and irregular periods. Her menses are coming further and further apart (three- or four-month intervals) and are very heavy. She wears tampons plus pads, but the frequency with which she must change this protection still keeps her near a bathroom all day long for several days.

Progesterone without estrogen is an important adjunctive therapy for women like Marilyn. By taking progesterone to challenge her uterus every three months, or more frequently if she desires, she can trigger a period that will clean out the endometrium she has built up.

If you are using progesterone to control your period, you can schedule it more or less at your convenience. When you plan your vacation, you can manage your progesterone so that when you arrive in Kenya or Boca Raton or wherever you are going, you probably won't start flooding with a heavy period.

The therapeutic regimen is simple: you take one tablet, usually 10 mg, of medroxyprogesterone each day for ten days. When you withdraw the progesterone, your period will usually arrive within a week of the day you took your last pill. Because progesterone is on board, this period should result in a controlled bleed as opposed to an extravagant flow.

▶ *Can women over forty safely take birth control pills?*

The attitude toward birth control pills has changed dramatically in the past twenty years here in the United States, among both gynecologists and the general public. In years past, the Food and Drug Administration restricted birth control pills to women under age forty (thirty-five if they were smokers), since the pills were associated with a higher incidence of cardiac disease. Then the FDA reviewed all the data on cardiac disease, thrombotic phenomena, and other complications of birth control pills. They discovered that in nonsmokers there is no increased risk at any age. Today most ob-gyns are very comfortable prescribing birth control pills to nonsmoking women over forty.

The story with smokers is very different, however. For them, the risk of cardiac disease associated with birth control pills rises significantly at thirty-five and dramatically at forty. Occasionally I have a patient in her forties who would benefit overwhelmingly from birth control pills, but she smokes. I suggest that she try the pills for perhaps two months to see whether they help her heavy bleeding or her frequent periods. I use the two-month figure to represent an arbitrarily short period, limited enough so that the positive effects of taking the pills will be apparent but the risks will be minimal. I advise her to call me immediately if she feels any uncomfortable side effects or symptoms such as chest or leg pains. And then I suggest that perhaps she will feel so much better being on the birth control pills that she will think seriously about giving up cigarettes.

Clearly, she must be closely supervised, and some physicians will not prescribe birth control pills under any circumstances to a woman who smokes. But because the pills are available by prescription only, it follows that any woman who is taking them has to be under a physician's care and observation.

After the smoker has tried birth control pills for a couple of months, she will have to decide whether to continue them and give up smoking or to give up the pills and continue smoking.

▶ *What therapy is available to reduce clotting?*

If you are one of the women who does not need therapy to control heavy flow but who finds clotting gross and offensive, you can benefit from anticlotting drugs. The most commonly used is Ponstel (generically, it is mefenamic acid), a cousin of Motrin (or ibuprofen). Like all prostaglandin inhibitors, Ponstel can upset your stomach, so always take it with food.

HOT FLASHES

You can do many things to reduce the intensity and frequency of hot flashes or to get rid of them altogether.

The temperature surrounding your body seems to be critical in bringing on hot flashes—so much so, that some women notice that hugging or other skin-to-skin contact with someone will trigger a flush. Try to sleep in a cool room (although battles be-tween bed partners over the thermostat are not uncommon during menopause). Al-though you cannot control the temperature of every room in which you find yourself, you can control what you wear. Dressing for menopause can be like dressing for travel to a country with an unknown climate: think layers. Many women find that fabrics of nat-ural fibers are more comfortable than synthetics.

Some things you can avoid. If you know that alcohol or hot coffee brings on hot flashes, sidestep them. If you notice that eating large meals brings on hot flashes, re-arrange your eating schedule.

Some women find that relaxation techniques, yoga, meditation, or other spiritual ex-ercises help relieve the stress that causes or intensifies hot flashes, and there is scientific evidence that these approaches may work. One study, for example, showed that breathing techniques reduced the frequency of hot flashes.

Beyond these simple, commonsense measures, which may not alleviate all your hot flashes, other steps are possible. Therapy for hot flashes can be directed toward the low-ered estrogen levels that stimulate the activity of the pituitary and the hypothalamus; or it can work to stabilize the blood vessels, whose inconsiderate constriction and dilation cause the flushing and sensations of heat that constitute a hot flash.

▶ How can estrogen help?

Estrogen replacement therapy raises the level of estrogen in the blood so that the pitu-itary and hypothalamus glands do not release the hormone FSH, whose vasodilating action can trigger a hot flash. You can take estrogen alone, estrogen with cyclic proges-terone, or oral contraceptives—which, as we have seen, contain both estrogen and pro-gesterone. Androgens are sometimes effective. Any of these regimens, calibrated for your own body's needs, will in almost every case take care of hot flashes. Nonhormonal ap-proaches include the use of vitamins or drugs that stabilize the blood vessels.

Finding just the right way of controlling hot flashes can be a process of trial and er-ror. Certainly no solution is perfect for everyone, and there may not be an absolutely per-fect answer for you. Still, you and your physician together eventually should find a solu-tion that works for you.

▶ *What other medications for hot flashes are there?*

Medicines that prevent blood vessels from dilating prevent hot flashes for many, but not all, women. A host of these drugs exists, from old standards to more modern medications.

Bellergal

The archetypical drug of this sort is Bellergal S, which has been around for years. It is a combination of several drugs including belladonna, atropine, and barbiturates, and comes in a standard dose. The usual dosage is one to two tablets daily. Bellergal is a prescription medication, but you take it as you need it, that is, when your hot flashes are troublesome. It is not like estrogen, which you take daily to prevent hot flashes, although some people do take Bellergal daily until their hot flashes have disappeared.

Like all other drugs, Bellergal has side effects. The main one is drowsiness; so if you are going to be driving or doing anything where your safety demands alertness, Bellergal may not be appropriate for you. If you can take it at night and not wake with a hangover, then the drowsiness should not be a problem. Many people also experience dry mouth.

Bellergal does not help everyone; among my patients I find about a 50 percent success rate. But if you are really bothered by hot flashes and have decided against hormonal therapy, Bellergal is relatively safe and certainly worth a try.

Beta-Blockers

Other nonhormonal mainstays of hot flash treatment are the beta-blockers, drugs such as propranolol (brand name Inderal) and the newer versions of these drugs that have been developed over the past twenty years. Beta-blockers work on the principle of vascular stability, preventing your blood vessels from going through the massive dilation-constriction-dilation-constriction routine that typifies hot flashes.

In small doses, about 40 to 80 mg of Inderal daily, beta-blockers can work effectively to prevent hot flashes. By comparison, cardiac patients who use a beta-blocker such as Inderal take up to 800 mg daily—ten to twenty times the dosage for preventing hot flashes.

Although beta-blockers work for some women, they are not universally effective. They do have side effects and they are extremely dose dependent, which means that the dosage can differ a lot from one person to another. Some people who are quite sensitive to this kind of drug report that they get depressed from beta-blockers; others report a fatigue or drowsiness that is not the sleepiness people feel when they take such drugs as Demerol, Halcion, or an antihistamine.

A second side effect is that some people, both men and women, find that beta-blockers interfere with sexual function by dulling sexual responsiveness. Men may have difficulty getting or maintaining an erection; women may have difficulty reaching orgasm.

Beta-blockers can also lower blood pressure; people taking them should have their blood pressure checked regularly. (Light-headedness is a symptom that might indicate low blood pressure.)

One of the beneficial effects of beta-blockers is that they tend to make people calmer, to take the edge off stage fright or general nervousness. People who perform in public, everyone from concert violinists to doctors presenting papers at scientific meetings, occasionally take beta-blockers to blunt the physical symptoms of nervousness—the shaking knees or trembling voices that interfere with successful performance.

Clonidine

Another drug that provides vascular stability is clonidine, which is marketed under the name Catapres; it is an antihypertensive drug, used normally to lower blood pressure, but may be useful in suppressing hot flashes. Again, since clonidine lowers blood pressure, you have to be sure that the dosage you are taking doesn't reduce your pressure to the point where you feel faint or dizzy. I cannot say that I have had overwhelming success with clonidine, but if other efforts have failed, it is worth a try.

SSRIs

In recent years, physicians have looked at SSRIs and SNRIs (selective norepinephrine reuptake inhibitors) for relief from hot flashes. The most important SNRI is Effexor (venlafaxine), whose success in suppressing hot flashes has been documented. This approach was pioneered by oncologists for women who had breast cancer and could not take estrogen but were troubled by hot flashes. These medications, which are generally used as antidepressants, do have side effects. Among them are sweating, decreased libido, and weight gain.

Alternative Treatments for Hot Flashes

Since the Women's Health Initiative results have become public, more women are considering alternatives to conventional hormone therapy to relieve menopausal symptoms and possibly to seek long-term benefits. In fact, a study conducted by the North American Menopause Society in 1997 suggested that even before the WHI results were released, more than 30 percent of American women had already tried some form of alternative therapy: acupuncture, natural estrogens, herbal supplements, or plant estrogens (phytoestrogens).

Unfortunately, at present we don't have enough scientific evidence to determine the effectiveness or the safety of many of these therapies. We don't even know whether alternative therapies are as safe as the conventional drugs being used for hormone therapy. Just because something is "natural" doesn't mean that it has no harmful effects: the herbs kava and comfrey, for example, have been linked to serious liver damage.

Many of the few studies of herbal products have fallen short of strict scientific standards. Some have involved only a few women or have involved them for only a short time. As we've seen before, randomized double-blinded, placebo-controlled studies are the gold standard of clinical research. If a study doesn't have a placebo arm—that is, if the women taking black cohosh are not compared to a group of women taking pills with no active ingredients—then its results aren't reliable. All studies on hot flashes show a placebo effect of about 40 percent (that is, the women taking the inactive pills experience a 40 percent reduction in hot flashes), so the vitamin or botanical preparation being tested must show a reduction of significantly more than 40 percent to be considered effective.

We do know that in traditional and folk medicine, plant estrogens have long been used to treat a range of problems involving menstrual disorders as well as the discomforts of menopause. Currently, the National Center for Complementary and Alternative Medicine (NCCAM), an agency of the federal government, is undertaking research on several botanicals that have shown promise for reducing menopausal symptoms. They include dietary soy, dong quai, black cohosh, ginkgo, red clover, and flaxseed.

Although scientific studies suggest that some of these plant estrogens work effectively and many women find that they help, herbal preparations present problems that drugs produced by pharmaceutical companies do not. First, herbal medicines (also known as botanicals) do not come in standardized dosages. When you are taking 0.625 mg of Premarin, you know exactly how much estrogen you are getting. When you drink three cups of ginseng tea, you have no idea how much estrogen you are getting. In fact, a recent study in San Francisco of four hundred ginkgo preparations showed that some of the products contained no ginkgo at all, whereas others as much as five times the amount described on the label. It is a lot easier to overdose on ginkgo, for example, than on Premarin.

A second risk of botanicals is that plant estrogens, like estrogens synthesized in the laboratory or developed from natural animal sources, act on the body in ways other than those primarily intended. Plant estrogens may well help control hot flashes, but they theoretically could cause overgrowth of the uterine lining, just as other estrogens can. If you decide to try plant medicines, you should do so under the guidance of a naturopathic physician, since very few medical physicians know anything about herbal medicines.

Botanicals may also interact with other drugs you are taking, so you should be sure to let your caregiver know what herbal medicines you are taking.

Soy

Among botanical preparations, soy and soy derivatives are the most commonly used for relieving hot flashes. Soy contains phytoestrogens called isoflavones, particularly genistein and daidzein, which have estrogenlike properties. It isn't surprising, then, that Japanese women, whose traditional diet has the world's highest in soy intake, experience very few hot flashes.

Many experts in alternative medicine recommend eating full-soy products as Japanese women do. Unfortunately, soy isn't a staple of the American diet, and many American women find it hard to eat enough whole-plant soy (soy beans, tofu, and soy milk) to reap the benefits of their phytoestrogens. Therefore soy extracts have become available, and most list the isoflavones they contain. The standard dosage recommendation is 45 to 60 mg of isoflavones daily.

The effect of soy on breast tissue is controversial, though most studies have shown that it is either beneficial or neutral. It is certainly true that Japanese women in Japan, who have the world's highest per capita soy consumption, have one of the world's lowest breast cancer rates. Some researchers believe that timing is important: the breast cancer protection comes from eating a high-soy diet during the teen years when breast tissue is actively differentiating. Boosting your soy intake later in life may not provide the same benefits.

Researchers also believe that soy works as a selective estrogen receptor modulator (SERM), acting like estrogen at some tissues but blocking estrogen at others, notably the breast. However, a few in vitro studies of breast cancer tissue exposed to soy do show increased growth of the cancer cells. Basically these studies involved dumping soy extract on breast cancer cells in a petri dish. The soy actively promoted proliferation of the cancer cells; water, used as a standard of comparison, did not. Putting soy into a dish containing cancerous cells, however, is different from eating it, since the soy you eat is metabolized before it contacts breast tissue.

Because of this controversy, I ask my patients who have had breast cancer to talk to their oncologists before trying soy. In fact, oncologists should have the final say over use of any medication, including botanicals, just as obstetricians like to have final clearance on any medication taken by pregnant women.

Because soy contains phytoestrogens, the other potential area of concern is stimulation of endometrial tissue, the lining of the uterus. No experiments have shown that soy does encourage overgrowth of the uterine lining, a precursor of cancer, but if you get irregular bleeding, call your doctor right away.

After reviewing the few controlled experiments suggesting that soy may reduce the risk of heart disease, FDA decided in 1999 to allow a health claim on food labels stating that a daily diet containing 25 gm of soy protein and also low in saturated fat and cholesterol may reduce the risk of heart disease.

Ginseng and Dong Quai

There are several types of ginseng, a plant valued for its roots, which are brewed as tea or swallowed in pill form. Chinese ginseng, the variety known botanically as *Panax ginseng*, is native to Asia and has been valued for its medicinal properties for more than two thousand years, especially by the elderly, who take it to enhance vitality and mental acuity. Also known as Asian ginseng, panax, ren shen, jintsam, ninjin, Japanese ginseng, Oriental ginseng, and Korean red ginseng, it is contained in such products as Ginsana, G115, and Ginsai.

The active ingredients are thought to be substances called ginsenosides or Panaxosides, though the exact mechanism by which they act isn't known. Chinese ginseng may act like estrogen in some circumstances, but the data are inconsistent and there is little scientific evidence to suggest using ginseng for relief of hot flashes and other menopausal symptoms.

This herb is definitely associated with an increased risk of bleeding, so if you are going to have surgery, you should discontinue ginseng (along with all other herbal medications) a week before your operation. Because its estrogenic properties are not understood, you should not take it if you have an estrogen-sensitive disease (for example, some types of breast cancer). Nor should you use it if you take MAO inhibitors, certain drugs given for depression and to relieve vascular headaches. Most people don't suffer side effects from this herb, but those that have been reported are dry mouth, rapid heart beat (tachycardia), nausea, vomiting, diarrhea, insomnia, and nervousness.

Dong quai, whose Latin name is *Angelica sinensis,* has been called the "female gin-seng" because in traditional Asian medicine, it has long been used to treat menstrual problems including PMS and menopausal problems including hot flashes. However, there are very few data in Western literature proving its efficacy.

Black Cohosh

Black cohosh, made from the root of *Cimicifuga racemosa,* is not a phytoestrogen, but it seems to help with hot flashes. Also known as black snakeroot, rattlesnake root, squaw-root, bugbane, and bugwort, it was used by Native Americans for relief of painful men-strual periods, rheumatism, and even sore throat. Lydia Pinkham's Vegetable Com-pound, a popular patent medicine, relied on it as a principal ingredient—along with a high percentage of alcohol. Cohosh has only minimal side effects.

Our scientific knowledge about this plant comes from Germany, where it gained popularity for the treatment of menopausal symptoms. The German scientific literature recommends trying cohosh for six months to see whether it does reduce hot flashes; if it does, then it is not harmful to continue. It is available in the United States as Remifemin and Estroven. The standard dosage is 20 mg twice daily.

Because cohosh is not a phytoestrogen, it has no effects on breast or endometrial tis-sue. Nevertheless, if one of my patients who has had breast cancer wants to take cohosh, I suggest that she talk to her oncologist before trying it. One study of cohosh done at Co-lumbia University with breast cancer patients did show a significant reduction in the severity of hot flashes.

Ginkgo

The leaves and seeds of the ancient Ginkgo tree (*Ginkgo biloba*) are used to make ginkgo extract, which is available as a liquid or in tablets. Alternate names for the product are fossil tree, maidenhair tree, kew tree, bai guo ye, and yinhsing. The medication is believed to help with circulatory disorders, including poor blood circulation to the brain—hence its reputation as an enhancer of short-term memory. No scientific evidence suggests its use for relieving hot flashes. Like ginseng and dong quai, ginkgo use is associated with in-creased risk of bleeding; if you take it, you should stop doing so a week before you have any surgery.

Red Clover

Like soy, red clover *(Trifolium pratense)* contains isoflavones (formononetin and bio-chanin). Little research has been done on red clover yet, but a few studies have suggested that it may be helpful in relieving hot flashes, while others have shown no positive effect. Red clover is available as an extract, under the trade name Promensil.

Flaxseed

The phytoestrogens in flaxseed are lignanes, closely related to a material that forms the woody parts of trees and other plants. The highest amounts are found in the husks of seeds used to produce oils. The whole seed is added to salad or cereal; when ground into meal or flour, flaxseed can be used as a food additive. Again, there have been few studies on flaxseed, but what data we do have suggest that it may have a beneficial effect on hot flashes.

Vitamins

As little as we know about soy, cohosh, and other herbal medicines, we know even less about the effect of vitamins on menopause. Many women find vitamin E works well, both in reducing the intensity of their hot flashes and in easing the sleep disturbances that are secondary to the flashes. Research is beginning to suggest that vitamin E may be useful in other medical conditions, for example in lowering the risk of atherosclerotic heart disease and as an antioxidant in soaking up free radicals and secondarily lowering cancer risk. Since cancer and heart disease are both associated with aging, vitamin E certainly cannot hurt; and it may help.

The dosage generally recommended is 400 to 600 units daily. Skipping a day won't hurt you. If vitamin E helps your hot flashes, they will probably return if you forget to take it, but there is no danger in starting and stopping vitamin therapy. Usually you will notice an improvement in about two weeks.

Some women report anecdotally that vitamins B and C help suppress hot flashes. Although there have been no supporting scientific studies, these vitamins may help and won't hurt if you use them in moderation. Try 500 mg daily of vitamin C and see whether it helps. The standard dosage of B-complex vitamins is contained in one B-50 tablet.

Acupuncture

Right now it is hard to say whether acupuncture reduces hot flashes, but ongoing studies suggest that it may well be helpful.

▶ *Are there women who are resistant to all these therapies and still have hot flashes?*

Almost everyone responds to estrogen, and most women respond to one or more of these other therapies, but a small fraction still report some hot flashes. Since the amount of discomfort experienced with hot flashes is quite subjective, it is hard to know just how uncomfortable these people are. If you are one of these women, it is worthwhile to check your blood levels of FSH and estradiol, because hot flashes can have causes other than lack of estrogen. If your estradiol and FSH levels are premenopausal and should not be giving you hot flashes, then you will know to look for something else.

INSOMNIA

Some old-fashioned commonsense approaches to sleeplessness are good starting points, especially if you prefer not to take hormones. Cut down on caffeine or cut it out altogether, especially later in the day. Alcohol may make you feel sleepy, but it can cause you to wake up in the middle of the night.

Try vigorous exercise during the day and a warm (not hot) bath before bedtime. Drink a glass of warm milk before you go to bed; milk contains tryptophan, an amino acid that has mild sedative properties. (To be honest, I am not sure why people always suggest that the milk be warm, but it certainly is the standard recommendation.) If you practice yoga, you may find that controlled breathing helps you get to sleep or go back to sleep if you have wakened in the middle of the night. Some women find that herbal teas or ginseng promote relaxation. Remember that ginseng has hormonal properties and like other herbal preparations should be used with care because you never know how much (or sometimes what) you are taking.

If these remedies don't work for you, there are other approaches. Because insomnia is often a by-product of hot flashes, the first line of attack is to relieve the hot flashes (by any of the methods we have already discussed). The second is to deal with the sleeplessness as a separate entity.

Remember that hot flashes and the sleeplessness that accompanies them tend to be worse in summer. If you are taking hormone therapy, you may have been completely comfortable with your dosage in January and suddenly find in July that you are awake in the wee hours, awaiting the dawn. You should check with your gynecologist and have your dose adjusted if your symptoms change in this way. Estrogen is also effective in relieving insomnia caused by hormonal changes, even though that insomnia may not be accompanied by hot flashes.

Many women wake up at two in the morning and can't get back to sleep though they don't have hot flashes. And there are women who don't mind the hot flashes but can't live with the insomnia and the fatigue that follows it. Using traditional sleep medications is one obvious approach.

Sleep medicines belong to a variety of chemical families, including benzodiazepines and barbiturates, and almost all of them can be addictive. Some people get habituated to a certain dosage level and have to increase the dose or switch from one medication to another. While most people know that barbiturates (which include phenobarbital, Nembutal, and Seconal) can cause chemical dependencies, benzodiazepines can also be addictive. Valium (diazepam), for example, along with its cousins Xanax (alprazolam), Ativan (lorazepam), and others, is sometimes prescribed as a sedative and sometimes as an antianxiety drug. Although Valium is now recognized as addictive, it is still prescribed too freely in many parts of the country.

Sleep medications can also cause a hangover, making you tired or sluggish the next day, and possibly giving you a headache. If you must be fully alert, for example when driving or negotiating a contract for your company, we have indicated that you should be very cautious about sleep medications. Most physicians do not encourage nightly use of sleeping pills, but they can be used judiciously. Be sure to discuss the subject thoroughly with your physician.

▶ What therapy exists for insomnia and hot flashes together?

Therapy to deal with hot flashes and insomnia can take one of three general directions: it can be directed toward the lowered estrogen levels that stimulate the activity of the pituitary and the hypothalamus; it can work on the sleep centers of the brain; or it can be directed at stabilizing the blood vessels.

Estrogen replacement is the one major therapy for insomnia that also controls hot flashes. To speak simplistically, estrogen tells the brain to go to bed. There is a constant feedback loop between the brain and the ovaries, and the brain continuously responds to the levels of estrogen that it senses being produced. But the brain is "dumb"; if it sees an elevated estrogen level in the blood, it doesn't know whether the estrogen is coming from the ovary or entering the body by mouth and being absorbed by the intestines. It merely recognizes the estrogen and allows the pituitary and hypothalamus to remain quiescent; they are not urged on to greater nocturnal activity. Increased quantities of FSH are not secreted into the bloodstream. Since estrogen replacement short-circuits the whole hypothalamus-pituitary cycle, and FSH with its vasodilating activity is not released into the blood, hormone therapy also controls hot flashes and decreases the component of insomnia caused by the flashes themselves.

Estrogen therapy works very quickly. Women who have been troubled with sleep disturbances and insomnia usually find relief within a week of beginning HRT.

With hormone therapy it is possible to adjust dosages from the outside in much the same way your ovaries do it from the inside when they are functioning at peak levels, say in your twenties and thirties. Some women who are perfectly comfortable with a certain dosage in the winter might start flashing in summer, and it is acceptable to increase the dosage during the hot months. If one of my patients for some reason wants her dosage reduced during the summer, I prefer to wait until autumn; it can be confusing to decide whether a woman is getting more hot flashes because her estrogen dosage is too low or because it's ninety degrees outside and she needs more estrogen anyhow.

BREAST DISCOMFORT

Strictly speaking, breast discomfort is not a perimenopausal problem. Many women have it throughout their reproductive years, but many report that their breasts feel more sensitive as menopause approaches. Although researchers have not discovered the causes of fibrocystic breast condition, as tender, lumpy breasts are called, many doctors have noticed that certain foods can stimulate the breasts and make breast tissue lumpier or more painful. Anything that contains caffeine (coffee, tea, cola, chocolate) can have this effect. Although drinking coffee won't give you breast cancer and there is no association between the amount of caffeine you ingest and your risk of cancer, some women are very sensitive to even small amounts of caffeine. Obviously it makes sense to avoid foods and beverages containing caffeine, if they make you uncomfortable.

A second approach is to take vitamin E and vitamin B6. The standard recommendation is 400 to 800 units of vitamin E a day, and 100 to 200 mg of vitamin B6. The literature contains no conclusive evidence that taking vitamins or cutting out caffeine will improve lumpy or uncomfortable breasts, but many women do notice a distinct improvement. In my experience, about 70 to 90 percent of women are helped by taking vitamin B6 and vitamin E and cutting down on caffeine consumption. Evening Primrose oil, two 500-unit capsules daily, helps many women.

One of my colleagues recommends kelp to her patients with breast discomfort. Available at health food stores, kelp contains iodine, but it is not understood why this treatment should be helpful for breast discomfort.

Testosterone also seems to have a positive effect in reducing breast tenderness. Indeed, young women who have tried reducing caffeine, taking vitamin E and vitamin B6, and so on, often do better on Danocrine, a medication that decreases estrogen production and has some effects similar to those of testosterone.

▶ *Must I give up caffeine if I am not bothered by the lumpiness in my breasts?*

As long as you are not uncomfortable (or nervous and jittery) and the lumpiness does not interfere with self-examination or examination by a doctor, it is not necessary to give up caffeine.

8 The Risks and Benefits of Hormone Therapy

THE biggest issue today for women approaching menopause is whether to use hormone therapy. What are the benefits? What are the risks? What will happen ten or fifteen years down the line if you do elect to use hormone therapy?

Like most important questions, this one does not have a simple answer appropriate for every woman. Women must first decide whether they wish to take hormone therapy at all. If they do decide to do so, then they must decide whether to take it short term to help with the acute symptoms of menopause or long term either for health reasons (to help reduce the risk of certain diseases whose likelihood increases with age) or to improve quality of life (by preventing conditions such as frequent vaginal and urinary tract infections, incontinence, or vaginal changes that can make intercourse painful or impossible).

The question of the risk-benefit relationship, not simple in itself, has been complicated by the conflicting results of recent studies, some of them better designed than others.

LANDMARK STUDIES ON HORMONE THERAPY

The Women's Health Initiative, sponsored by agencies of the federal government, is a fifteen-year project that continues to monitor the health of more than 160,000 women age fifty and older. The study has multiple subsections focusing on such issues as cardiovascular disease, cancer, osteoporosis, and cognitive functioning.

The part of the WHI investigating hormone therapy has two "arms," one for women who used estrogen-plus-progestin and the other for women who used estrogen alone. The estrogen-plus-progestin section involved 16,608 women from age fifty to seventy-nine; the estrogen-only arm has about 10,000 women. The researchers abruptly stopped the estrogen-plus-progestin arm in July 2002, when it appeared that the risks of this kind of hormone therapy outweighed its benefits. Two years later the researchers stopped the estrogen-only arm for similar reasons (see Chapter 1).

The Heart and Estrogen/Progestin Replacement Study (HERS), completed in 1998, under the aegis of the National Institutes of Health, examined the effect of hormone therapy on the cardiovascular health of postmenopausal women who were known to have heart disease. The study found that the use of HRT did not prevent further heart attacks or death from coronary heart disease (CHD), even though LDL (bad) cholesterol was reduced by 11 percent and HDL (good) cholesterol was increased by 10 percent. Women using HRT also had an increased risk of clots in the veins (deep vein thrombosis) and lungs (pulmonary embolism).

An earlier important study was the Postmenopausal Estrogen/Progestin Interventions Trial (PEPI) undertaken by the NIH and completed in 1996. Conducted at seven centers in the United States, the study sought to answer questions about the effect of progestins added to an estrogen replacement regime. The trial tracked 875 postmenopausal women for three years, testing the effects of HRT on certain factors that influence the risk for heart disease and bone mineral density. Early in 1995, the PEPI study reported that estrogen and estrogen with progestin improved some risk factors for heart disease, by raising HDL (good) cholesterol and lowering LDL (bad) cholesterol.

The HERS and PEPI studies and all the arms of the WHI were randomized, double-blinded, placebo-controlled trials that involved many women over relatively long periods of time.

Information from the Nurses' Health Study formed the basis of much medical thinking before the results of the NIH studies became available. In its initial stages, this study, begun in 1976 and continued in 1989, looked at the impact of oral contraceptives on women's health. Although it involved more than 120,000 nurses at the outset and has continued for more than twenty-five years, the Nurses' Study was never intended to be a randomized study; it was and is an observational study. Questionnaires are sent to the nurses at two-year intervals, asking them about their health, their food, exercise, and other daily habits, smoking, menopausal status, and use of hormone therapy. Because it is observational and not randomized, the Nurses' Health Study can be biased: after all, nurses are medically sophisticated and should—theoretically—be more aware of health issues than the general population of women.

Throughout this chapter we discuss the results of these studies as they might affect your thinking about hormonal therapy. To make an intelligent and comfortable decision, you must understand the general risks and benefits of hormone therapy. Then you should consider your medical and family history and your personal risk profile as determined by your lifestyle as well as by your genetic inheritance. Has your mother or your grandmother gotten hunchbacked or significantly shorter as she aged, which suggests that you may be at risk for osteoporosis? Do you have a family history of breast cancer?

Your decision should also reflect your own psychological makeup, your feelings about taking medication either short or long term, and your relative fears about different diseases (for example, cancer and heart disease). If you are one of the numerous women who feel extremely anxious about breast cancer and would blame yourself if you got the disease because you elected to take HRT, then you are probably better off psychologically not taking it. You might also take into account your willingness or unwillingness to put up with the annoyances of continued menstrual periods or the annoyances of menopausal symptoms.

MAKING THE HORMONE THERAPY DECISION: STARTING AND STOPPING

There are several scenarios in which hormone therapy might be a good choice.

Sally N. is fifty, generally healthy, and athletic. She has cycled, run, played golf and tennis, and hiked for recreation all her adult life. Sally has red hair, but not the pale skin that normally goes with it; she has big bones. About fifteen years ago she had a hysterectomy for a precancerous condition, but her ovaries were left intact. She takes care of her health, runs a couple of miles several times a week, and pushes herself to improve her conditioning. She is proud of her energy and the fitness level she has maintained, and in her heart of hearts (like most well-conditioned people) she is a little intolerant of people who cannot push themselves as she can. Sally maintains good dietary habits and has real preferences for healthy foods. She is the kind of person who, without even thinking about it, prefers a couple of slices of seven-grain bread and sprouts to a Big Mac.

Sally drinks very little alcohol and no coffee (because caffeine makes her nervous and edgy), and she prefers herbal tea to nonherbal. She would rather not take medication, if she can avoid it. She has never smoked. Her politics are liberal; she is concerned about world hunger, pollution, women's rights, and other such issues. There is no history of breast cancer or heart disease in her family.

Sally obviously has an enviably healthy lifestyle, and she is fortunate in her genetic endowment. She does not seem to be at risk for osteoporosis, in that she is very active and large boned. Her low alcohol consumption, her status as a nonsmoker, and her general fitness level lower her risk for both osteoporosis and cardiac disease. Her liking for natural foods and a healthy diet, along with her general political outlook, suggest that for psychological reasons Sally might feel uncomfortable with HRT. Her pride in accomplishment and endurance, which are apparent in her level of fitness and conditioning, suggest that Sally is a person who can tolerate discomfort fairly easily. Since she is not at risk for osteoporosis, there is no reason for her to try HRT if she does not feel so inclined.

Priscilla F. is fifty-one, blonde, attractive, and the mother of four. She was twenty-four when her first baby was born, and she breast-fed all four. These days she is slender to the point of being skinny. She is a highly excitable and nervous woman who smokes to calm herself and cannot break the habit. Although Priscilla has plenty of energy, she does not enjoy exercise, saying that she is too nervous even to play tennis. Obviously she doesn't need exercise to help control weight because she tips the scales at about ninety-eight pounds, and although she admits she should exercise for other reasons, she cannot bring herself to do so. Her mother had osteoporosis and in fact died of the complications of a hip fracture. Her family has no history of breast cancer.

Priscilla might consider trying (short-term) hormone therapy. Her fair hair and skin, her smoking and slenderness, and her family history all put her at high risk for osteoporosis. She is a low-risk candidate for breast cancer, in part because of her family history, in part because of her youth at the time her first child was born, in part because of her breast-feeding. Priscilla seems, to some extent, to be the victim of her habits—smoking and low exercise tolerance—so there is little chance that she can change her habits to adjust her risk for osteoporosis. She has no psychological objections to HRT.

If Priscilla begins getting hot flashes and night sweats, it would be reasonable for her to take HRT to control them. When she decides to stop the hormone therapy, she must attend to her bone health, probably taking some bone-building medication.

▶ Which menopausal symptoms eventually go away by themselves?

In general, hot flashes will resolve themselves eventually, but a few women have them throughout their life. Other vasomotor disturbances also will probably disappear in time. Sleeplessness, if caused by vasomotor disturbances, improves with time, although both men and women may have increased trouble sleeping as they age. The acute mood changes and feelings of anxiety or even panic that are brought on by hormonal changes at menopause tend to get better with time, peaking early in perimenopause and then gradually fading away.

▶ Which menopausal symptoms don't go away with time or get worse as time goes on?

Vaginal dryness and atrophic changes get progressively worse with time. Incontinence gradually increases. Bone loss starts when we are in our thirties, apparently accelerates just after menopause, and continues more slowly throughout life. Cardiovascular risk increases gradually with age. Menopausal short-term memory loss and its companion, difficulty in concentrating, probably do not get better spontaneously, though so far the evidence may not be conclusive. One of my patients reported that during her perimenopausal years, she regularly forgot her appointment with her hairdresser; now, ten years past menopause, she is able to show up regularly and on time at the beauty salon.

▶ If I start on HRT, do I have to take it forever?

No, you can stop any time you want. If you are taking hormone therapy to control your hot flashes or your sleeplessness, two symptoms that will probably get better on their own as time passes, then you can stop the HRT for a while and see what happens. If the symptoms return, you can go back to HRT; if they don't, you can assume that you are probably in the clear. But if you have chosen hormone therapy to protect yourself against osteoporosis, you will lose the protection estrogen provides when you stop taking it.

▶ *If I decide to stop HRT, can I stop "cold turkey," all at once?*

Gradual withdrawal by cutting down on your dosage will probably produce fewer symptoms. We know that women who have a sudden menopause—women whose ovaries are removed surgically or shut down in response to chemotherapy—often have severe hot flashes. But many women can just stop their therapy and not be uncomfortable.

HORMONE THERAPY FOR THE SHORT TERM

▶ *Are there short-term risks of HRT?*

Since the publication of the Women's Health Initiative results on hormone therapy, the healthcare professions are reevaluating the risks and benefits of short-term HRT. At present the North American Menopause Society, the American College of Obstetricians and Gynecologists, and the FDA approve of short-term HRT to relieve menopausal symptoms including hot flashes and sleeplessness, using the lowest effective dosage for the shortest period of time.

▶ *If I take HRT for the short-term do my risks revert to normal after I stop?*

According to a study published in 2002 by the National Institute of Child Health and Human Development, breast cancer risk for women who have been taking HRT begins to return to normal within six months after stopping the hormones. Other studies show reversion to normal risk anywhere from six months to five years after stopping hormone therapy.

▶ *What are the short-term benefits of HRT?*

Hormone therapy is the best, most effective way known to medical science to relieve the discomfort of hot flashes and other vasomotor symptoms such as sweating and clamminess, crawly skin, tingling fingers, and palpitations.

Researchers do not yet know exactly what mechanism triggers an individual hot flash. Scientists do have some understanding of the mechanism by which falling estrogen levels at menopause lead to hot flashes and other vasomotor symptoms, but it is still a mystery why 20 percent of American women (all of whom have falling estrogen levels at menopause) never have any menopausal discomfort at all. So although areas of mystery still exist, numerous scientific studies as well as mountains of anecdotal evidence show that HRT does work for practically everyone.

Hormone therapy is also very effective in preventing the sleeplessness and frequent awakening that are among the most distressing symptoms of menopause. Some women say they wake in response to feelings of being overheated or the sweating and cooling of hot flashes; others do not notice hot flashes or heavy perspiration, but they wake anyhow, sometimes several times a night. Even if you are not aware of having a hot flash before you wake, estrogen can still be a big help in giving you a solid night's rest. But if you can't sleep because your children are in trouble or your husband is out of a job or your boss is driving you crazy, then HRT won't help.

Some women notice an improvement in their moods or psychological outlook when they are taking short-term HRT. Since it is certainly possible that sleeplessness and fatigue contribute to mood swings or a negative outlook on life, HRT can certainly help here. There is also some evidence that estrogen in itself has a positive effect on mood, at least in some women; some researchers believe that it is the fluctuations in estrogen levels that account for swings in mood and perhaps by keeping estrogen levels quite stable, hormone therapy can help in this regard. You can try HRT for one or two months to see whether it helps you.

As long as you continue to take it, HRT will have beneficial effects on your vaginal lubrication and the general health of your vaginal tissues, making intercourse more comfortable. Again, as long as you take it, hormone therapy will protect the walls of your bladder, which in the absence of estrogen will thin out and become more prone to infection.

▶ *How long do I have to take HRT before I notice improvement in hot flashes, sleep disturbances, and other vasomotor symptoms?*

Usually women notice that their symptoms are abating within a week or two.

▶ *Will HRT help with short-term memory lapses and lack of concentration during perimenopause?*

Some women say that they are less susceptible to strange memory lapses and lack of concentration when they are on HRT. But these feelings are very subjective, and we all forget things from time to time, especially as we age.

As you may have noticed, mental capacity doesn't decline across the board with age. Your eighty-year-old mother can probably recount incidents of her childhood—and also yours—but she may have difficulty absorbing and recalling new verbal information, for example a set of directions or the names of new acquaintances.

Beginning in the late 1980s, Barbara Sherwin, a psychoendocrinologist at McGill University in Montreal, undertook studies on the relation between memory and estrogen deprivation. She and her coworkers gave several tests of memory and abstract reasoning to women whose ovaries had been removed surgically as part of a hysterectomy. The women were divided into two groups: one received estrogen therapy, the other a placebo. Sherwin discovered that the women who were given estrogen therapy after the operation did better on the tests of short-term memory than did the women who were given a placebo, though long-term memory in the two groups was about equal. Sherwin believes that estrogen's effect on verbal memory may be seen as comparable to its effect on bone density.

▶ *Will HRT help with the mood swings, tearfulness, and irritability of menopause?*

Many women say that hormone therapy helps their psychological outlook, that they are less likely to become grouchy and angry when they are taking estrogen. Irritability and mood swings can be caused by sleeplessness, and insofar as HRT promotes a good night's sleep, it helps with these problems.

HORMONE THERAPY FOR THE LONG TERM

▶ *What are the long-term risks of HRT?*

The Women's Health Initiative study showed slight increases in the risk of breast cancer and cardiovascular disease. Like many studies before it, the WHI trial also showed a significantly increased risk of blood clots in the veins (thromboembolisms); the increase usually quoted for all these studies is in the range of a two- to threefold higher risk, with most of the clotting problems occurring during the first six months of HRT use. In addition, the WHI also showed a slight increased risk for stroke, probably a consequence of estrogen's potential to increase clotting problems. The memory subsection of the study (WHIMS) found that, contrary to earlier findings, estrogen-plus-progestin does not protect women over age 65 from normal decline in cognitive function but instead increases the risk of dementia.

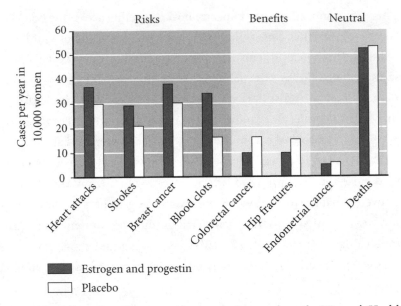

FIGURE 8. Risks and benefits of long-term hormone therapy, from the Women's Health Initiative study. The WHI study showed that women taking HT had higher rates of heart attack, stroke, breast cancer, and blood clots but lower rates of colorectal cancer and hip fractures compared to women taking a placebo. The overall mortality rate, however, was almost identical. Source: Women's Health Initiative, National Heart, Blood, and Lung Institute.

HORMONE THERAPY AND BREAST CANCER

The Women's Health Initiative reported that of the women taking HRT (estrogen-plus-progestin in the form of Prempro), there were 38 new cases of breast cancer per 10,000 women per year. Women not using hormones experienced 30 new cases of breast cancer per 10,000 women per year. That is a difference of 8 cases per 10,000.

The WHI study was not the first to investigate this important issue, as studies for two decades have attempted to determine whether breast cancer risk increases with estrogen use. Early investigations, undertaken during the 1970s and 1980s, produced conflicting results. Some suggested no increased risk, some suggested slightly increased risk, and some suggested slightly decreased risk of breast cancer in women who took HRT.

In 1989 researchers at University Hospital in Uppsala, Sweden, published a large epidemiological study involving 23,244 women that made the front page of the *New York Times*. The research showed that women on long-term HRT (that is, women who had been on HRT for longer than nine years) had a slightly increased risk of breast cancer. Their risk factor was placed at 1.1, which means that if 10 women per 1,000 would get breast cancer without HRT, then of 1,000 women taking HRT for more than ten years, 11 would get breast cancer. The study also showed that women who were taking combined therapy, estrogen plus progestin, had a higher risk than those taking estrogen alone.

Scientists who reviewed the study, however, found several significant differences from the way HRT is prescribed in the United States. First of all, the estrogen used in the Swedish study was primarily estradiol, while in this country the most commonly prescribed estrogen, Premarin, is conjugated equine estrogen (estrogen isolated from the urine of pregnant mares). Second, although the statistics were gathered for a period beginning in 1977, many of the women might have begun taking estrogen well before that. Furthermore, the dosage levels in the European study were much higher than those conventionally used in the United States, as were the recorded blood estrogen levels of the women receiving these dosages.

In 1995 a group of researchers at Harvard University published further statistics from the Nurses' Health Study, incorporating data from 1976 to 1992. These researchers found that women aged fifty-five to fifty-nine who had been taking HRT for five or more years had a 40 percent higher risk of breast cancer than women who had never taken HRT. That

TABLE 3. Results of the Women's Health Initiative Study
(Per 10,000 women each year)

	WITH HRT	WITHOUT HRT
Heart attacks	37	30
Strokes	29	21
Breast cancer	38	30
Blood clots	34	16
Colorectal cancer	10	16
Hip fractures	10	15
Endometrial cancer	5	6
Deaths	52	53

Note: Only 2.5% of the women in the WHI had these negative health events. The study results suggest that during one year, for every 10,000 women taking estrogen plus progestin, we would expect 7 more women with heart attacks, 8 more with breast cancer (and so on), but that the overall number of deaths would be almost equal.

is, if no women in this age group had taken HRT, the expected number of cases of breast cancer for 1,000 women would be about 35. If all the women in the same age group did use HRT for five years or more, then statistically there would be 50 cases of breast cancer. The risk increase was higher in older women, who have a higher incidence of breast cancer under any conditions. In the sixty to sixty-four age group, long-term use of hormones was associated with a 70 percent increased risk. Again, this means that of 100,000 women in that age group, if 100 were expected to get breast cancer without taking hormones, then 170 cases would be expected among women who had taken hormones for five years or longer.

The study further concluded that women who stop taking HRT revert to their original risk category within two years. Use for longer than five years makes no difference in risk; that is, women who take HRT for ten years are not at higher risk than women who take it for five. The addition of progestins does not protect women against breast cancer.

Other researchers, both clinical and epidemiological, questioned the validity of the study on the basis of estrogen's known tendency to speed the growth of some types of breast cancer. In an interview with the *New York Times,* the late Trudy Bush, an epidemiologist at the Johns Hopkins University School of Public Health, pointed out that although estrogen may increase the growth of small tumors that are already present but not yet clinically detectable, it is doubtful that it stimulates the growth of new tumors. If hormone therapy caused a true increase in tumors, she said, doctors would be seeing this increase clinically in their practices. The fact that the incidence of breast cancer does not increase with length of HRT use beyond five years suggested the same thing. This controversy remains unresolved.

Doctor Bush's reasoning would explain the fact that neither the Swedish study nor the Harvard study pointed to an increased rate of mortality, more deaths from breast cancer. Nor did the WHI study find an increased risk of carcinoma in situ, a precursor stage of cancer. If the hormones were truly causing the cancer, we would expect to see increases in precancerous stages as well as full-blown cancer. And yet, HRT does make breast tissue denser and therefore makes mammograms somewhat harder to read. This, though, is not new information: radiologists have known this for years.

Perhaps the explanation of my colleague Dr. Isaac Schiff, faculty member of Harvard Medical School, best summarizes the risks of hormone therapy and breast cancer. He explains that if you are a fifty-five-year-old women who does not take HRT, your chances of getting breast cancer in the next year are one in four hundred. If you take Prempro, the form of estrogen-plus-progestin used in the WHI study, your risk after about six years of use rises to one in three hundred.

▶ Does HRT cause fibrocystic breast changes?

Because one of the side effects of HRT can be breast tenderness, HRT may in some cases make fibrocystic breasts more tender.

HORMONE THERAPY AND ENDOMETRIAL CANCER

If you have a uterus (that is, if you have not had a hysterectomy) and you take estrogen without taking progesterone, then you do increase your risk for cancer of the lining of the uterus. The longer you take the ERT, the more your risk rises.

If you take progesterone along with the estrogen, however, either cyclically or as continuous therapy, you do not increase your risk for endometrial cancer, as several scientific studies have shown.

Estrogen causes the lining of the uterus to grow. During your premenopausal years, you shed this lining every month during your menstrual cycle. After menopause, unless you take and withdraw progesterone to mimic the menstrual cycle or limit its growth with a continuous small dose of progesterone, the endometrium just grows and grows, sometimes leading to a condition called hyperplasia.

Hyperplasia is not uterine cancer, but it can precede uterine cancer. Still, even with unopposed estrogen, the risk of endometrial cancer is quite low. Not only is the risk statistically small, but uterine cancer associated with ERT is, as cancers go, easily treated. It is usually what is called "well differentiated," which means that the cancerous cells don't look much different from the normal cells lining the uterus. There may be more of them (hyperplasia), but to use the pathologist's term, they don't look "nasty."

Second, uterine cancer associated with ERT is usually diagnosed early, because its first symptom in most women is bleeding at an abnormal time. Women bleed; they go to their gynecologist; and they get diagnosed early. Treatment is usually by hysterectomy, which for women beyond their reproductive years is not a tragic event.

A fascinating study about twenty years ago investigated women with endometrial cancer. It compared women who had very early, noninvasive stages of endometrial cancer with women who did not have cancer. The two groups were matched by age and comparable medical histories. It turned out that essentially the women with the cancer had a better survival rate than the control group. Why? What the study showed is that the factors that put you at risk for endometrial cancer—obesity, hypertension, and diabetes—also put you at risk for other, potentially more serious problems. The reason that obese women are at high risk for endometrial carcinoma is that fat tissue converts adrenal-gland hormones to estrogen. Heavy women are walking around with a lot more than one tablet of Premarin a day in their bloodstreams; they have their own estrogen factories, which are constantly stimulating the uterus.

Fat women are also at high risk for other disorders, especially diabetes and high blood pressure. What probably happens is that women who have early, well-differentiated tumors of the endometrium go to their doctors because of their bleeding, and their other risk factors are taken care of. Their blood pressure will probably be checked. If their blood sugar is out of control from their diabetes, it will be taken care of. If they are obese, they will probably be reprimanded and perhaps they will take off a few pounds.

CARDIOVASCULAR HEALTH: HEART ATTACKS AND STROKE

A few years ago, medical practitioners were confident that hormone therapy protected postmenopausal women against cardiovascular disease. Several studies had shown that postmenopausal women on HRT had better cardiovascular health than women who did not take estrogen. One of the most important of these was the Nurses' Health Study, whose results seemed to provide solid evidence to support the cardiovascular benefits of HRT. Statistical results, first published in 1989 and based on the first ten years of data, showed that the 48,470 postmenopausal women who were taking HRT had significantly fewer heart attacks than the women who were not. Furthermore, the PEPI study suggested that women on HRT had better cholesterol levels—higher HDL and lower LDL—than women not taking hormones.

The Women's Health Initiative study, however, contradicted these findings. It found that in one year for every 10,000 women taking estrogen plus progestin, 37 women would have heart attacks compared to 30 women not taking the hormones, an excess of 7 women per 10,000.

It offered similar statistics on strokes. Although studies before the WHI had shown neutral results—HRT did not significantly either increase or decrease risk—data from the WHI suggested that HRT slightly increased risk for stroke. The WHI rates projected that for 10,000 women over a one-year period, we would expect to see 29 strokes in women taking HRT compared to 21 in women taking a placebo. The excess risk of stroke due to the hormones was 8 strokes for every 10,000 women over one year; it is likely that the increase is due to the clotting problems associated with HRT. The increased risk of stroke for women taking estrogen only (with no added progestin) seems to be similar.

▶ *How could the WHI data be so different from earlier studies of cardiovascular disease and HRT?*

When the WHI data came out, many health care professionals expressed concern about the group of women enrolled in the studies. The average starting woman taking part in the WHI had been menopausal for eighteen years. The study's designers had deliberately chosen women who had "outgrown" their hot flashes because they did not want participants to know whether they were taking a placebo or estrogen and the presence or absence of flashes would be a giveaway. The women in the WHI trial did not have diagnosed coronary artery disease, as did the women in the HERS study, but they did have many risk factors. As a group, they were seriously overweight, with an average body mass index (BMI) of 28.5: by this standard a woman who is five feet, five inches tall would weigh about 171 pounds. (People of normal weight have a BMI between 18.5 and 25.9.) Thirty-five percent of the women had high blood pressure, and half were current or former smokers. (The average starting age of those in the HERS study was sixty-seven, so these women, too, were well past menopause when they started taking estrogen.)

Critics of the study pointed out that although women in this group did not have established coronary artery disease, they were very likely to have plaque in their coronary arteries because of these risk factors. There is a big difference between taking estrogen at the time you are going through menopause (which is called "primary prevention") and taking it many years thereafter when you may have developed cardiac disease. No one nowadays recommends estrogen for the prevention of heart disease, but if you have been taking it in the recommended manner, you should not worry about increasing your heart disease risk.

For these reasons, discussions at the 2003 meeting of the North American Menopause Society emphasized the importance of timing in the use of HRT. Beginning hormone therapy around the time of menopause seems to be far different in terms of cardiovascular risk than beginning many years later.

HORMONE THERAPY AND BLOOD CLOTS

It has long been known that estrogen, even in the small amounts used for hormone therapy, does double or triple the risk of blood clots (thromboembolisms), but unless you have a history of clotting problems (for example, thrombophlebitis), HRT is not dangerous to you. Women with varicose veins can use it. Hormone therapy is generally safer than oral contraceptives because it contains quite small amounts of a type of estrogen that is different from the kind used in birth control pills.

In the years after "the pill" was introduced, evidence mounted that the estrogen in oral contraceptives encouraged blood clots, heart attacks, and strokes. Although there were several brands of oral contraceptives with different combinations of estrogen and progesterone, all contained high doses of synthetic estrogen, which lowered the anticlotting factors in the blood and therefore made clots more likely. But times have changed and so has the pill. In the early 1960s, when the pill was first introduced, oral contraceptives contained what would now be considered huge doses of hormones, sometimes up to three times the amount in today's low-dose oral contraceptives. Even today's contraceptive pills contain about six times the amount of estrogen per day in the standard HRT dosage prescribed for postmenopausal women.

Birth control pills contain synthetic estrogen, whereas the estrogen in HRT is "natural," which means that it is identical or very similar in its chemical structure to estrogen produced in nature. The estrogen in Premarin, for example, is isolated from the urine of pregnant mares. The estrogen in Estrace is also "natural" estrogen. Though manufactured in the laboratory, it is still a kind of estrogen called 17-beta estradiol, which is made by the ovaries of female mammals.

If you choose the estrogen patch, the estrogen is absorbed directly into the bloodstream, bypassing the liver. For many years physicians had supposed that this route of delivery lowered the risk of clotting, but only recently was this suspicion confirmed when a well-designed clinical study from France showed that transdermal estrogen doesn't raise the risk of clotting at all.

HORMONE THERAPY AND MENTAL FUNCTION

Dementia is rarely a disease of the early postmenopausal years, though it occurs all too commonly in later life. My experience in medical practice suggests that Alzheimer's disease, which afflicts women one and a half to three times as often as men, is the only illness as frightening as breast cancer. You can be reassured that the fuzzy thinking, memory lapses, and decline in cognitive powers that many women feel around the time of menopause do not usually signal the beginning of serious dementia.

For years it had been thought that HRT might help ward off Alzheimer's disease or other forms of dementia that occur with age. Research on laboratory animals and a few small observational studies of women on HRT suggested that taking hormones does have preventative advantages. We know that there are estrogen receptors in the brain and that blood flow to the brain is intensified when estrogen levels are high.

One complaint about the early prospective studies was that women on hormonal therapy tend to be well educated and well off, and they are likely to keep mentally active—to work in intellectually demanding jobs and in their leisure time to take part in book clubs, play bridge, do crossword puzzles, read the newspaper, and volunteer in community organizations. All these activities demand mental activity and are thought to help prevent dementia.

One of the goals of the Women's Health Initiative, then, was to assess the effect of HRT on dementia. In 2003, the researchers reported that over a five-year period the risk of dementia for women over age sixty-five who took estrogen-plus-progestin therapy was twice the risk for comparable women who did not use hormones. That is, of 10,000 women taking HRT, 45 women per year would be diagnosed with dementia, while 22 women not taking HRT would be so diagnosed. The authors of the study were quick to point out that although the increased risk was significant when applied to large numbers of women, it was relatively small when applied to any individual woman, a difference of 23 cases per 10,000 women per year. The cognitive risks to younger women are still unknown, as are the risks to women taking estrogen only.

Critics of the WHI results pointed out that all the women in the study had been postmenopausal for many years (they ranged from sixty-five to eighty years old) before they started taking the hormones. Some researchers believe that HRT might help protect the brain if it is begun around the time of menopause when estrogen levels are plummeting but that by the time women are sixty-five, the damage is done. Future research should look at this issue.

The WHI dementia study suggested that the biggest increased risk of dementia is from vascular dementia (caused by clogged blood vessels in the brain), which is consistent with the cardiovascular data: starting HRT when you are more than a decade past menopause is not good for blood vessels. No one is suggesting that you take estrogen to prevent dementia, but it does not seem that taking estrogen around the time of menopause will increase your risk of dementia later.

HORMONE THERAPY AND OVERALL MORTALITY

The Women's Health Initiative study showed that the rates of mortality (for all causes) were almost equal in the estrogen-plus-progestin group and the placebo group. That is, about the same number of women died per year from each group.

▶ *What are the long-term benefits of HRT?*

Used long term, HRT has benefits that can affect the quality of your life and can lower your risks for osteoporosis and colon cancer. In the long term as well as the short term, HRT can greatly lessen those degenerative or atrophic changes to the vagina and urinary tract that can make sex uncomfortable and lead to urinary incontinence and frequent vaginal or urinary tract infections.

A host of other benefits, some cosmetic, have been reported anecdotally but not scientifically proved. Among them are improvement in mood or outlook, better skin, and an improved sex life.

HORMONE THERAPY AND OSTEOPOROSIS

The Women's Health Initiative reported that per 10,000 women per year, there would be 10 hip fractures for women using estrogen-plus-progestin, compared with 15 for women not using hormones. According to statistics developed by a team of epidemiologists, if you are a fifty-year-old white woman not taking HRT, the relative risk of sometime in your life having a hip fracture (generally taken to mean your risk for osteoporosis) is 36.2 percent. In other words, of any 1,000 white women who are now fifty years old, 362 will at some time fracture a hip. The risk is lower for black women.

HORMONE THERAPY AND COLORECTAL CANCER

The Women's Health Initiative reported that per 10,000 women per year, we could expect 10 new cases of colorectal cancer for women using estrogen plus progestin, compared with 16 for women not using hormones. Colorectal cancer afflicts men and women more or less equally, and its incidence does increase with age; most people diagnosed with this disease are older than fifty, though younger people, even teenagers, do sometimes have it. Colorectal cancer is the third most common cancer in men and in women and the second leading cause of cancer-related death in the United States. Hormone therapy slightly lowers your risk for this disease but is not recommended by the FDA or any other group for prevention.

OTHER POSSIBLE BENEFITS

▶ *Will HRT keep my skin youthful?*

Is it loss of estrogen or just the process of aging that makes skin lose its youthful elasticity and smoothness? No one knows for sure, and we lack incontrovertible data that estrogen will protect your skin as it will protect your bones. Although nothing known to modern science will make seventy-year-old skin look like twenty-year-old skin, estrogen does seem to have positive effects. The informal observation that plump middle-aged women often have more youthful skin than slender middle-aged women supports this belief. After all, plumper women make more estrogen because their fat manufactures it.

Some researchers also believe that estrogen improves skin tone, perhaps by causing water retention or by stimulating the production of subcutaneous fat or by causing collagen to be built up in layers beneath the skin. Well-designed experiments have shown that the skin of women taking HRT is thicker than the skin of women not getting estrogen replacement.

On an anecdotal level, many of the women I talk to say that taking estrogen has helped their skin. They notice that their skin retains moisture better and feels less itchy and less irritated. A few say that estrogen makes their skin oily, so that in one respect they feel like teenagers again. I even have one patient who complains of getting pimples from her estrogen. She is a slender little woman and is worried about osteoporosis. When we measure levels of estradiol in her blood, we find that at an estradiol of 50, which is low-normal for a menstruating woman, she gets pimples. We have tried different sorts of estrogen preparations, but they all seem to affect her the same way. Her reaction is rare, however.

Is "youthful" skin in itself a reason to choose HRT? Certainly after the results of the WHI study, HRT is not recommended for cosmetic reasons. Nevertheless many people—women and men both—elect to undergo painful and sometimes risky surgical procedures in the interests of their physical appearance. Botox, for example, is neither inexpensive nor risk free, but the product is so widely used that it has become a household name.

▶ *Does estrogen cream rubbed into the skin convey any benefits?*

Because the skin is bound to absorb some of the estrogen in the cream, the risks and benefits will be those of HRT taken orally. But remember that estrogen taken by any route carries with it the danger of causing excessive growth of the uterine lining. And if you are rubbing estrogen cream into your skin, you cannot be sure exactly how much estrogen is reaching your uterine lining.

▶ Will HRT prevent hair loss?

One of the unpleasant facts of growing older is thinning hair—on the head, in the pubic area, under the arms, and elsewhere on the body. No one knows with certainty whether this is strictly a menopausal problem, that is, caused by decreased production of estrogen, or whether it is caused by aging and just happens to become noticeable at about the time of menopause.

Hormone therapy will not keep your hair from graying, and it probably will not prevent it from gradually thinning, though some women tell me that their hair seems to thicken up a little when they start HRT. Nor will HRT necessarily improve the texture of your hair, which may have changed for the worse as you have grown older.

▶ Will HRT prevent unwanted facial hair?

Although hormone therapy will not keep your hair as thick as it was when you were twenty-one, it may help with that other menopausal hair problem, unwanted facial hair. Since the ovaries continue to produce androgens (hormones associated with male characteristics) even after their production of estrogen has dropped off, the premenopausal balance between these hormones changes. There is no circulating estrogen to block the action of the androgens, and many women notice that their hair tends to grow in a more masculine pattern after menopause. This can mean increased facial hair and changes in the texture of this hair, which typically becomes darker and coarser. The HRT may help reverse this process, but its benefits will continue only as long as you take it.

▶ Will HRT prevent weight gain?

Unfortunately, no. Nor will it prevent the redistribution of fat on the body, which tends, as we get older, to rush to the area between our thighs and shoulders.

Some evidence suggests that on a cyclic basis estrogen does influence weight. Very few women are the same weight all through the month, as their hormone cycle changes the amount of fluid their bodies retain. The same is true of women whom I put on HRT; they often report a weight gain of two to three pounds of retained water, which they generally maintain as long as they are taking estrogen. Although we say "never say never" in medicine, it is possible, but highly unlikely, that a person will gain fifteen to twenty pounds from estrogen alone.

Sometimes a patient will call me and say, "Look, I started HRT and I have gained ten pounds, and I really think that it is that darned estrogen." So I suggest that she stop the estrogen for a couple of months and see whether the unwanted pounds melt away. (Contrary to popular opinion, it is not dangerous to go on and off estrogen, though you may notice some symptoms.) Generally I get a phone call about two months later. The ten pounds have not miraculously disappeared, and the patient would like to go back on estrogen again.

Occasional women lose dramatic amounts of weight when they go on estrogen therapy. These are usually people who felt awful, who weren't sleeping at night, and who didn't have the energy to exercise, so it is very possible that they just stayed home and did a little extra eating. When these women found new energy because they were sleeping better, they began running around again and started burning their calories better.

Of course you can certainly diet while you are on estrogen. There is no reason to say, "Well, I might as well not diet because I am on HRT and it is causing me to gain weight." That's equivalent to saying, "Well, I am on birth control pills, so I will gain weight and therefore I might just as well not diet." You can diet any time you want to diet.

▶ Will HRT give me contraceptive protection?

In the doses normally given, hormone therapy will not give you contraceptive protection. If you take low-dose birth control pills as a form of HRT during your perimenopausal years, then of course you will be protected against unwanted pregnancy.

▶ Will HRT increase my fertility?

No, it will not. Nor will it postpone the time when your natural menopause will occur.

9 A Practical Guide
to Hormone Therapy

IF you do decide to use hormone therapy, you have many choices. Physicians have different attitudes about when to start therapy, what kinds of routines or schedules to establish, and whether to use pills, patches, or some other route of delivery. You may have your own preferences, finding that patches work better for you than pills or that one progestin gives you side effects while another doesn't. In most cases you can tailor the regimen to your own needs.

STARTING AND STOPPING HORMONE THERAPY

▶ *Who cannot take HRT?*

There are a few conditions under which it is unwise to take HRT, even for a short time. If you have active thrombophlebitis (that is, an inflammation of the veins involving a blood clot) or active gallbladder disease or active breast cancer, you are not a candidate for estrogen therapy.

You should discuss certain other conditions with your caregiver if you are interested in taking hormone therapy, though these conditions will not necessarily rule it out. If you have a history of clotting problems or a family history of breast or uterine cancer, you should certainly alert your caregiver. If you have had impaired liver function (that is, a history of hepatitis) or have had gallbladder disease, you may still be a candidate for a variant of HRT.

▶ Can I take HRT if I have fibroids?

If you have fibroids, you can still take HRT. Since fibroids are estrogen sensitive, however, your caregiver will need to follow you carefully to see that the estrogen therapy does not cause them to grow.

▶ Can I take HRT if my blood pressure is high?

High blood pressure was long thought to be a reason for not taking HRT. Recent research, however, actually seems to show some beneficial effects of estrogen on the walls of the blood vessels, so current thinking among many physicians is that hormone therapy can possibly help women with elevated blood pressure. For a small percentage of women, however, blood pressure goes up on estrogen therapy. The impact of HRT on blood pressure is lower, however, with the transdermal skin patch than it is with oral estrogen.

▶ What about HRT for women with fibrocystic breasts?

There is no reason, in terms of health risk, why women with fibrocystic breasts should not take hormone therapy. But for some of these women HRT may introduce discomfort.

Probably half the women I see as patients have fibrocystic breasts; it is a common condition. When menopause comes along, most women who were bothered by fibrocystic breast discomfort begin to feel better. Their breasts are no longer affected by the estrogen-progesterone cycle, so they have less lumpiness and less tenderness. If we reintroduce estrogen with HRT, many of these women feel some discomfort again, though usually not as much as when they were having periods (because the dosage of estrogen in hormone therapy is much lower than what the ovaries produce during the reproductive years). Many women can control the discomfort by eliminating caffeine and taking vitamins E and B6, but a very few women cannot tolerate estrogen even in small doses. For these individuals, HRT is probably not a therapy of choice.

Again, you must remember that hormone therapy is an ongoing regimen. You should have a dialogue with your caregiver and know that things may change; the dosage that was appropriate at one point in your life may not be appropriate at all times.

▶ Can women who have not done well on birth control pills take HRT?

For two reasons, many women do well with HRT even if they have had difficulty with birth control pills. First, the dosages in HRT are much smaller, only about one-sixth the amount of hormone in low-dose birth control pills. The amount of estrogen that your body makes during your premenopausal years is somewhere between what you get on HRT and what you get on birth control pills.

A second difference between the two preparations is that birth control pills all use synthetic estrogens, whereas in the United States the estrogens used in HRT are chemically identical to estrogens occurring in nature. So if you have had unpleasant side effects from the synthetic estrogen in birth control pills, your body may respond differently to the naturally occurring estrogen in HRT.

▶ What is the best time to start HRT?

Although the benefits of HRT are clear, the issue of when to start is controversial. Many women begin having menopausal symptoms, especially hot flashes and sleeplessness, long before they stop having periods. These women definitely benefit from taking estrogen and indeed feel better on HRT even though they have not yet reached menopause.

One school of thought, however, holds that women should not take any estrogen until they have had no periods for one year, that is, until they are fully menopausal. The members of this group argue that adding estrogen to what you may still be producing yourself could lead to hyperplasia; because you are probably making less progesterone than formerly, you may not be producing what you need to trigger a menstrual period when you withdraw the progesterone; therefore the uterine lining can continue to build. Physicians who recommend starting HRT before full menopause believe that as long as you achieve a withdrawal bleed at least every two months, hyperplasia is unlikely to be an issue.

Another school believes that women who are still having fairly regular periods should take a small dose of estrogen every day without added progesterone. Since your body is maintaining a schedule of cleanout bleeds, you don't need the progesterone to protect your uterus, and the tiny extra amount of estrogen taken exogenously will not give you hyperplasia.

Yet another group suggests administering some progesterone and synchronizing it with the woman's natural cycle. The approach seems particularly useful for the woman who is having problems with flow. Her heavy bleeding suggests that she is not ovulating properly, that her own ovaries are not making enough progesterone. Giving this woman progesterone roughly day sixteen through day twenty-five of the menstrual cycle, which her ovaries are still more or less orchestrating, often helps to control the bleeding. Some physicians prescribe the progesterone for twelve days, while others give it for ten.

If you are concerned about osteoporosis somewhere down the line, you should begin HRT during the first few years after menopause, because that is the time of most rapid bone loss.

▶ *If I start HRT before I'm completely menopausal, how do I know when I'm going through menopause?*

You will not be able to pinpoint the date of your menopause precisely because you will never know when your last period (regulated by your own hormones) occurred—but you can certainly make some assumptions. Because the average age at menopause in this country is about fifty-one years, you can infer that if you are fifty-five, you have passed through menopause.

If you really are curious to determine your status, you can stop the estrogen for a while (say about four weeks), then have your FSH measured. If you are menopausal, your FSH should be significantly elevated after this time, somewhere over 30.

▶ *What should I do about birth control if I don't know whether I'm menopausal or not?*

For many women the issue is, not simply knowing that menopause occurred at age fifty-one or fifty-two, but dealing with contraception. The old-fashioned attitude is that you should wait a year after your last menstrual period before you stop using contraception. But if you don't have a "last" menstrual period, it is difficult to decide when that year is over. Nevertheless, you can make a pretty good decision based on age: it is extremely unlikely that you will conceive when you are fifty-one or fifty-two.

The problem is similar with women who are on low-dose birth control pills, which some physicians recommend for heavy or irregular perimenopausal bleeding and other symptoms of approaching menopause. If that is your situation, you will not know precisely when you are menopausal and when you should stop the birth control pills and start using HRT instead. What many physicians do is stop the pill, wait four weeks, and do a blood test to check the FSH level. If it is elevated, you can switch over to hormone therapy; if it is not elevated, you can go back on the birth control pills. Obviously the birth control pills will give you contraceptive protection. If you are starting HRT while you are still having periods, let's say when you are forty-six, then you should continue to use some kind of birth control. Your options are condoms, a diaphragm, or an intrauterine device (IUD).

▶ How long do I have to use HRT?

The issue is two pronged: hormone therapy can be used short term for alleviating problems such as hot flushes and sleep disturbances that are associated with the perimenopausal years. Or it can be used long term, which conveys important health benefits but also has potential risks. The benefits have been well defined, but even after the release of the Women's Health Initiative data, the risks are not yet completely understood.

Before the results of the WHI were made public, the average length of treatment in this country was nine months, which means that women were using estrogen to cope with perimenopausal symptoms rather than for its long-term benefits. No increased risk of any disease seems to be associated with short-term estrogen therapy, as long as the woman taking the HRT had no medical reason not to start the therapy in the first place.

▶ What happens if I do stop HRT?

If you decide to stop, you do not have to taper off, since stopping HRT abruptly is not medically dangerous. Hormone therapy is not addictive like nicotine in cigarettes or other addictive substances. But you may be more comfortable if you stop gradually. In general, quitting "cold turkey" does not produce withdrawal symptoms, and most women do not suddenly get depressed or have other symptoms. A few who quit abruptly get significant hot flashes. These flashes usually go away in a few months, but some women find them so uncomfortable that they go back on the HRT.

Of course, if you stop taking estrogen, you will lose its protective benefits. But if you are taking it to maintain strong bones, you will find yourself at age sixty, for example, with more bone than you would have had if you had not been taking HRT since menopause.

ESTROGEN

Most of the estrogen used for HRT in the United States is natural estrogen. Natural estrogens are those found in nature or those made in laboratories whose chemical forms are identical to the estrogens occurring in nature. Among the natural estrogens are conjugated equine estrogens (estrogen isolated from the urine of pregnant mares), 17 beta-estradiol (usually written 17 β-estradiol), estropipate, esterified estrogens, and estradiol valerate.

Synthetic estrogens are estrogens whose action may resemble that of natural estrogens but whose chemical structure is different. Examples of synthetic estrogens are ethinyl estradiol and diethylstilbestrol (DES). These are never found in nature.

▶ *What are the side effects of estrogen?*

Most women tolerate estrogen very well, but 5 to 10 percent do experience side effects. The most common are breast tenderness and fluid retention or bloating—symptoms, incidentally, similar to those that many women feel just before their periods. A few women on HRT feel queasy or slightly nauseated. Too much estrogen may cause these symptoms; changing the dosage usually controls the discomfort.

Some women, especially those who are prone to migraines, find that estrogen brings on headaches. This problem can be hard to solve, because headaches can be caused either by too much estrogen or by too little. I have patients who get headaches from too little estrogen, and when I put them on higher dosages the headaches disappear. I have one patient who gets an occasional hot flash when she takes the usual dosage of estrogen (0.625 mg of Premarin), but when I boost the dosage to 0.9 mg, she gets headaches. Some women who get headaches if they take their HRT orally do not do so if they use the transdermal patch.

Although many women feel that estrogen helps their skin, a few have pigmentation problems: they may develop a darkened area on the face, as some women do during pregnancy. Moles may get darker.

Most of these symptoms are mild and don't mean that you have to give up HRT. Occasionally, however, women are just plain allergic to estrogen and respond to HRT with skin rashes, itching, or other typical allergic symptoms. Sometimes changing the brand of medication will help.

Pills, Patches, and Other Ways of Taking Estrogen

In the United States, estrogen is available in pills, on transdermal patches, in vaginal rings, and in vaginal creams. Pills and patches come as estrogen alone or as estrogen combined with progestin. One brand of vaginal ring comes with estrogen alone in a dose that will help with hot flashes and vasomotor symptoms. For problems with vaginal atrophy, there are estrogen creams, rings, and tablets.

Estrogen Pills

Estrogen is most commonly taken orally, in the form of tablets. The dosages vary from brand to brand, but the usual routine is to take one tablet daily.

Of the pills or tablets, one widely used brand is Premarin, generically known as conjugated equine estrogen. Premarin, derived from the urine of pregnant mares, has been sold since 1941, so most scientific studies on hormone therapy have looked at this brand.

A second widely prescribed brand is Estrace, which is micronized estradiol, a natural estrogen based on plant estrogens but produced in the laboratory. Estradiol is the main form of estrogen produced by the ovary during the reproductive years. Micronizing reduces the estradiol to particles small enough for the digestive system to break them down. Ogen, Ortho-Est, and Estratab are other brands of natural estrogen tablets. In 1999 the FDA approved a new estrogen product, Cenestin, which contains nine synthetic estrogen components chemically derived from plants including soy and yams.

Transdermal Estrogen Patches

Estrogen can also be administered through the skin, by means of a transdermal patch. The original transdermal patch, sold as Estraderm, is a small plastic disk on which estradiol has been dissolved in a jellylike solution contained in a little reservoir on the surface of the patch. You pull off the backing and stick the patch on your skin, usually on your buttocks or abdomen. You should not place the patch on your breasts; because breast tissue is so sensitive to estrogen, it should not be exposed directly to the undiluted dose. The patch remains in place for three or four days. The estrogen is thereby absorbed in a gradual manner through the skin into the bloodstream. In 1995 a new transdermal patch, the matrix patch, was introduced. Marketed under the name Climara, this patch has the estradiol impregnated in the adhesive on the patch instead of being dissolved in a solution on the surface, thus allowing the whole surface of the patch to adhere to the skin. The Climara patch seems to deliver more constant levels of estrogen over its one-week lifetime than did earlier reservoir patches and also seems to stay in place better.

Climara is the only matrix patch that is changed once a week, a real convenience in terms of remembering the correct day. Since its introduction Climara has become available at six dosages levels, ranging from 0.025 mg to 0.10 mg, allowing you to calibrate your dose. For some women, small changes in dosage make a great deal of difference in their response.

Other matrix patches come in the twice-a-week variety, also in various dosage levels, although Alora, approved by the FDA in 1996, comes only in one size, delivering 0.05 mg estrogen daily. The Vivelle patch comes in a very small version, the Vivelle-Dot, about the size of a postage stamp, useful for women whose skin is especially sensitive to adhesives. This patch is also available in variable dosages.

▶ Which is better, patch or pill?

Sometimes people who do poorly on one form of estrogen, say oral Premarin, will do better on another type. If Premarin makes you queasy, you may feel better using transdermal patches, because by this delivery route the estrogen bypasses your digestive tract. If you get headaches from the oral estrogen, you may do better with the patches. Still, some women experience skin irritation from them and find the oral delivery route an improvement. Some data suggest that the matrix patch is less likely to cause skin irritation than reservoir patches.

Advocates of the patch say that patches are better because estrogen that is absorbed gradually across the skin is not metabolized directly, at full strength, by the liver in what is called a first-pass effect. If estrogen can be injurious to the liver, the transdermal route is probably preferable for certain women. Women at risk for gallbladder disease and phlebitis might be better served by the transdermal route. The liver manufactures clotting factors (substances that cause blood to clot). Because high levels of estrogen in the liver increase its production of these clotting factors, oral estrogen is not desirable for people with phlebitis. Oral estrogen also increases triglyceride levels in the blood, while transdermal estrogen does not.

Proponents of oral estrogen point out that by bypassing the liver with the first-pass effect, you get a smaller rise in HDL, your good cholesterol; it is really metabolism of estrogen by the liver that affects the amount of HDL in your bloodstream.

Estrogen for Vaginal Use

Creams: For women who don't need or want full-scale HRT to help with hot flashes and other vasomotor symptoms but do have vaginal atrophy or urinary problems due to declining estrogen levels, estrogen can be applied vaginally, since the body absorbs only a small amount.

Estrogen can be used as a vaginal cream. Premarin and Estrace are available in this form. The cream comes with an applicator, a plastic tube with a plunger (basically the same kind you get with contraceptive foams), which you use to insert the cream into the vagina. Most people devise a regimen that keeps them comfortable and use it perhaps two or three times a week. The cream is best applied at bedtime, because it tends to leak out when you are standing or sitting.

Tablets: Vagifem tablets, estrogen in pill form, are an alternative to vaginal creams. The tablets come in an applicator, which you insert into the vagina; when you press the plunger, a tablet is ejected. As with vaginal creams, Vagifem tablets seem to act locally and not to affect other estrogen-sensitive tissues elsewhere in the body. However, since the bladder sits right over the vagina, some local absorption to the bladder occurs, which can help the bladder. Although the manufacturer's directions suggest that you insert the tablets every night for the first two weeks and twice weekly thereafter, many women don't need such intense therapy. You can regulate your dose, finding a level that relieves your symptoms. You can also alternate creams and tablets.

Rings: A third option for urinary and vaginal problems is Estring, relatively new in the United States though used since the early 1990s in Scandinavia and elsewhere. Estring is a soft silicone ring, something like a small contraceptive diaphragm without the dome, impregnated with estrogen. It is inserted high into the vagina, where neither you nor your sexual partner can feel it. Over a period of three months it releases a constant low dose of estrogen, so you need change it only four times yearly.

Femring, a soft silicone ring impregnated with estrogen, was introduced in 2003. It is similar to Estring except that it is intended for the relief of hot flashes and other vasomotor symptoms as well as vaginal dryness. It remains in place for three months and delivers a systemic level of estrogen similar to the 0.05 mg patch. Women who have not had hysterectomies and who decide on Femring must take progestin to protect against possible uterine cancer, just as they must with an estrogen-only transdermal patch.

Complementary and Alternative Choices

Health food stores carry products advertised for vaginal lubrication, and some women find them helpful. In Europe vaginal soy products are fairly popular. Scientific data on their effectiveness are limited, but these products are not likely to harm you.

Tamoxifen

At least two research teams have looked at using tamoxifen vaginally for relieving atrophic symptoms in women who have had metastatic breast cancer and are advised against using any form of estrogen absorbed into the body. The results look promising. The researchers recommend half a tablet inserted vaginally twice daily. Because tamoxifen is a SERM (see Chapter 10), it works like an estrogen in the vagina but as an estrogen blocker in breast tissue.

▶ What are the pros and cons of vaginal estrogen?

Although small amounts of estrogen do get absorbed through the tissues of the vagina, low-dose vaginal estrogen—whether in the form of cream, pill, or ring—will not protect you from osteoporosis; nor will it relieve your hot flashes. However, because the vagina and bladder are located so close to each other, even low-dose estrogen absorbed through the vagina does affect the urinary tract, and many women find that symptoms of urinary frequency and discomfort improve when they take vaginal estrogen.

Researchers are not in agreement on exactly how much estrogen is absorbed through the vagina, and studies show anything from zero absorption to complete absorption. In general, however, scientists agree that far less estrogen is absorbed from the vaginal cream than from the estrogen taken orally or via the transdermal patch. Less estrogen seems to be absorbed systemically from Vagifem tablets than from creams. With Estring, some estrogen is absorbed systemically during the first twenty-four hours after insertion, but after that initial rise, estrogen levels in the blood fall to the preinsertion level.

If you are worried about breast cancer, yet you still have problems of dryness and vaginal discomfort, this route is a reasonable solution for you. Women who have had chemotherapy for breast cancer that has shut down their ovarian function, either temporarily or permanently, often find vaginal estrogen helpful.

Other Ways to Use Estrogen

Estrogen is also available in injectable form, as estradiol valerate. Before the introduction of the transdermal patch, injectable estrogen was used quite widely for people who did not tolerate oral estrogen well, but nowadays injectable estrogen is used much less frequently, although it is still available. To maintain satisfactory levels you need fairly frequent injections (unlike Depo-Provera, which lasts a long time), and most women are not anxious to have a lot of shots.

In Great Britain, but not in the United States, estrogen is available as an implant, a pellet that a physician places under the skin. The implant slowly releases estrogen over a fairly long period and is replaced at intervals; the procedure is similar to that of Norplant, which is progesterone implanted under the skin for birth control. No particular danger is associated with these implants, and they have been extensively used in England for years. Although many women might find implants a convenient way to take estrogen, there is no apparent impetus toward introducing them in the United States.

Estrogen is now available in products that are applied daily and gradually absorbed through the skin. EstroGel, which dries quickly and without stickiness, is rubbed on one arm from wrist to shoulder. Estrasorb, a lotion containing 17 beta-estradiol (the form in transdermal patches), is rubbed on the thighs and calves. For women with an intact uterus, these products require the counterbalance of progestin to protect the endometrium.

ESTROGEN DOSAGES

▶ *What are the concerns about taking too much estrogen?*

The major concerns are the consequences of increased estrogen levels on the breasts in either promoting or stimulating breast cancer and the side effects of too much estrogen. So far, researchers have not documented the effects of different blood estrogen levels on the breasts and do not know whether the risk of breast cancer is related to dosage. The main side effects of too much estrogen are breast discomfort, bloating, headaches, and queasiness.

▶ *What are the lowest doses of estrogen that will protect me against osteoporosis?*

It used to be thought that 0.625 mg Premarin or 1 mg Estrace were the minimum levels that would protect you against osteoporosis. Although most women are comfortable at up to twice that level, a few experience breast discomfort, bloating, or queasiness. Studies have suggested that dosages half this size are effective: 0.3 mg Premarin, 0.5 mg Estrace, or a patch that delivers .025 mg estrogen. Whereas studies in England have looked at women taking a great deal of calcium as well as the smaller estrogen dosages, studies in the United States generally do not focus on calcium intake, basing their findings only on estrogen intake. Therefore, if you choose a lower estrogen dosage, you should be vigilant about getting enough calcium in your diet or in supplements and about following a weight-bearing exercise program.

▶ *How can I lower my dose if I am taking HRT with the patch?*

A few years ago when patches were available in only a few dosages, women could decrease their dose by wearing the patches longer than the manufacturer suggested, for example changing the once-a-week patch every ten days. Several newer estrogen patches come in lower dosages. While Alora comes in no size smaller than 0.05 mg, low-dose Climara, FemPatch, and Vivelle-Dot deliver 0.025 mg daily. A very-low-dose patch, Menostar, prescribed exclusively for osteoporosis prevention, delivers 0.014 mg daily.

▶ *Do these dosages remain stable forever?*

If you find that the dosage of estrogen that formerly worked for you is no longer appropriate, you might have to increase or decrease the amount you are taking. Dosages change for a lot of reasons. Suppose you start taking hormone therapy in your perimenopausal years. As you get further into the menopausal process, you may find that you need to increase your dose to relieve menopausal discomforts because your ovaries are making less estrogen. Some women, in contrast, find that after they have been on estrogen for a while, they can cut back on their dose and taper off.

Many individuals find that in hot weather they need more estrogen. If it's 95 degrees outdoors and you are hot and sweating, and then you start flashing, you might want to take extra estrogen to help regulate your temperature. If you are going on vacation to a tropical climate, you might want to take a slightly higher amount. There is nothing wrong or dangerous about doubling your dose periodically. So just because at this moment you are taking a certain dosage, it doesn't mean that you will be taking that amount forever.

▶ *How do I find the dosage that is right for me?*

Many physicians, myself included, tend to start with the smallest dose of estrogen that will relieve symptoms and use that as a baseline. From that point I continue to be something of an empiricist; if someone starts flashing uncomfortably again, I adjust the dose slightly upward until it relieves the symptoms. If she feels queasy or gets headaches, I lower the dose a little. This is the approach the Women's Health Initiative sanctions: finding the smallest effective dose by means of small accommodations.

Some physicians believe in taking estradiol levels or FSH levels to determine the appropriateness of a given dose, but problems arise in determining what the tests mean. Let's start with the estradiol levels. The Premarin or Estrace that you are taking in your HRT is converted by the body to several kinds of estrogen, estradiol being just one of them. Even 17-beta estradiol (the main ingredient of Estrace) is converted to other forms of estrogen in the blood. So if the lab test measures only the estradiol in your blood, it is ignoring the other estrogens that are present and may be contributing to the total level of estrogen circulating in your blood. Maybe your estradiol level is low, but you are still comfortable. Do you need to change your dose? Probably not.

Or look at the other extreme. An estradiol level of 100 is, by general consensus, an adequate level. But suppose you are still not sleeping. Suppose you are still getting hot flashes. Is there danger in taking larger doses and reaching a blood level of 150? Probably not.

A problem with using laboratory tests for FSH to determine dose level is that even women who are being adequately replaced on HRT will have slightly elevated FSH levels. You may be comfortable, able to sleep, and undisturbed by hot flashes, you may be getting good osteoporosis protection, but your FSH level will still be high. So the FSH test will not tell you that the dosage is appropriate.

As in the rest of life, there are trade-offs. For some people it is hard to find just the right amount of estrogen. One patient whom I see gets occasional, though not frequent, hot flashes when she takes 0.625 mg of Premarin. When I raise her dose to 0.9 mg, the hot flashes go away but she gets headaches.

What should she do? There are no pills that come in dosages between 0.625 and 0.9 mg, but she could alternate a 0.625 one day with a 0.9 the next. She could break a 0.3 mg pill in half and take that plus a 0.625 mg pill. Beyond that, the decision is up to her. Is it worse to get the headache or is it worse to get the hot flash?

▶ *What happens if I forget to take my estrogen pill one day?*

Again, nothing dangerous happens, since going on and off HRT is not hazardous to your health. You might have a hot flash or two as your body reminds you that you have forgotten your pill, or you may find yourself waking up in the middle of the night. Just take another pill the next day.

PROGESTERONE AND PROGESTINS

Unlike estrogen, which generally seems to make people feel better, progestin (synthetic progesterone) can have negative side effects. It can cause headaches. It can cause chest pain if people have reactive, sensitive coronary arteries. It can increase the levels of LDL (bad) cholesterol in the blood. It can make women irritable, so that they feel very much the way they do just before their menstrual periods.

And when you take progesterone, as you should in order to protect your endometrium from hyperplasia, you will have to decide whether to take it cyclically—in which case you will probably have bleeding when you stop taking it—or daily—in which case you may have considerable spotting or bleeding during the first six months of therapy.

Because of its side effects and because the results of the Women's Health Initiative have suggested that progestin, or at least medroxyprogesterone (the kind used in Provera) may be implicated in stimulating breast cancer, new forms of progestin have been devised, as have new routes for delivering it and new regimens for taking it. Natural progesterone has also become available commercially.

▶ *What are the side effects of progestins?*

If you have your uterus, you will probably be taking progestin along with your HRT. Unfortunately, many women find that progestin gives them the kind of emotional outlook that they used to experience premenopausally, including irritability, jumpiness, anxiety, and mild depression. Others report bloating and breast tenderness. Some women report headaches. These side effects seem to be milder in women taking low-dose daily progestins and in women taking cyclic natural progesterone. Cyclic progestins such as Provera seem to give slightly more severe side effects than either cyclic natural progesterone or progestins taken every day.

FORMS AND DOSAGES OF PROGESTERONE

Pills and Tablets

Most commonly, progesterone by itself is delivered as a pill or tablet. Like estrogen, progesterone is available in natural and in synthetic forms (progestins). Most of the progesterone used in this country for hormone therapy is synthetic.

The progestin most frequently prescribed is medroxyprogesterone, which comes under several brand names: Provera, Cycrin, and Amen. Many physicians try to start with the lowest effective dose, which has been revised downward over the years. In the 1970s, the standard dosage was 10 mg of medroxyprogesterone, but in recent years research has confirmed that 5 mg of progesterone taken cyclically for twelve days of the month will give virtually the same protection of the endometrium with fewer side effects. Although you may get slightly better protection with 10 mg for the same time frame, the higher dosage may not be worth the side effects.

Although continuing research seems to confirm that 5 mg is the smallest amount (assuming standard estrogen dosages) that prevents hyperplasia when you take the progesterone cyclically, you can use a smaller daily dosage if you elect to take your progesterone continuously, every day throughout the month. The dose usually recommended for continuous progesterone is 2.5 mg. Furthermore, since the WHI recommendations suggest using the least effective amount of progestin, you can use the smallest possible cyclical dosage and then leave longer intervals between the cycles.

A newer form of progestin called norethindrone seems to cause fewer side effects, particularly less breakthrough bleeding, when used on a daily regimen. It may also have more bone-protective effects than medroxyprogesterone. Norethindrone is the progestin used in Aygestin, which comes only in 5 mg tablets. The tablets are scored, so you can cut them in half to get a 2.5 mg dose.

Progesterone is also available in combination with estrogen in a single pill. Wyeth-Ayerst markets the combined estrogen-progestin as Premphase for cyclical use and Prempro for daily use. Premphase contains 0.625 mg conjugated equine estrogen (the kind used in Premarin) plus 5 mg of medroxyprogesterone (the kind used in Provera) taken on the second fourteen days of the cycle. Prempro comes in two strengths: a low-dose version with 0.45 mg estrogen and 1.5 mg progestin (28 percent less estrogen and 40 percent less progestin than the current standard dose, which has 0.625 mg estrogen and 2.5 mg progestin).

PremPro and Premphase come in packs of twenty-eight color-coded pills. The

Prempro pills (the same type of pill for each of the twenty-eight days) are salmon colored in the higher-dose version and purple in the low-dose version. The first fourteen of the Premphase pills, which contain estrogen only, are red; the second fourteen pills contain both estrogen and progestin.

FemHRT and Activella are combination pills that contain norethindrone instead of medroxyprogesterone; they are formulated in doses equivalent to 1 mg of estradiol. These brands are associated with a much lower rate of breakthrough bleeding than Prempro.

Natural progesterone is also available commercially in pill form. Oral natural progesterone must be micronized, that is, broken down into tiny particles, so that can be absorbed by the digestive tract. For many years natural progesterone was not available because the micronization process was difficult for commercial manufacturers. Before 1998, when Solvay Pharmaceuticals introduced the product commercially as Prometrium, oral natural progesterone could be purchased only from compounding pharmacies, who made up the pills on an individual basis. The progesterone in Prometrium is derived from yams and is dissolved in a peanut oil base when it is put into capsules, so people with peanut allergies should never use this drug.

If you do have a peanut allergy and want oral natural progesterone, you can still get it from a compounding pharmacy. If there isn't one in your town, you can try the Women's International Pharmacy in Madison, Wisconsin. They seem to be able to formulate reliable doses and will send medications through the mail. They have a Web site at www.womensinternational.com and a toll-free phone line at 800.279.5708. Natural progesterone is a bit more expensive than synthetic progesterone.

Some naturopaths recommend natural progesterone processed from yams and available as a cream. It is well absorbed through the skin, but the amount absorbed varies from woman to woman and the preparations themselves are not usually standardized. This means that you do not always know exactly how much you are getting. Another product, wild yam cream, contains an unprocessed precursor of progesterone; your body cannot use it as progesterone, because humans lack the necessary enzyme to metabolize it. The compound in progesterone cream has already been processed so that it is available to your body.

In addition to reducing side effects for some women, natural progesterone may have less negative effect on breast tissue than a synthetic formulation. This is only a supposition, however: we don't have any scientific data to support this hypothesis. Nevertheless, many women and their caregivers are currently choosing natural progesterone for HRT.

Patches

Progesterone is available combined with estrogen in transdermal patch form, notably the Combipatch, whose hormones are based on plant sources. The patches, changed twice a week, come in two sizes, a smaller patch that delivers 0.05 mg of estradiol and 0.14 mg of progestin (norethindrone) per day and a larger patch delivering 0.05 mg of estradiol and 0.25 mg of norethindrone daily. If you need more estrogen and want it in patch form, you will have to add either a Climara or a Vivelle patch.

The Climara Pro patch, introduced in 2003, combines estradiol and levonorgestrel, a newer form of progesterone. Climara Pro has several advantages. Levonorgestrel, which has been used for many years in oral contraceptives, does not seem to produce many negative side effects Moreover, the patch, which delivers 0.015 mg of levonorgestrel and 0.045 mg of estradiol per day, needs to be changed only once a week, a real convenience.

Unfortunately, we do not yet have the technology to deliver natural progesterone in patch form.

Other Ways to Use Progesterone

Because progesterone can be absorbed through the tissues of the vagina, there is a vaginal option for women who cannot tolerate oral progesterone in any form. Vaginal micronized natural progesterone came on the market primarily to help women suffering from infertility caused by low progesterone during early pregnancy; these women used the hormone vaginally to boost its levels within the uterus. Vaginal progesterone was first sold as Crinone gel and later as Prochieve.

The Mirena intrauterine system, originally intended for birth control, is a progestin-coated plastic device placed in the uterus. The progestin, in this case a low dose of levonorgestrel, is gradually absorbed from the device directly into the endometrium. Using Mirena to prevent hyperplasia is an off-label use—that is, the FDA approved the device for a different purpose. A smaller version for postmenopausal women is being developed but is not yet on the market. Like any IUD, Mirena must be inserted by your healthcare provider, but once in place it can remain for five years.

▶ *What can I do if I am someone who does not tolerate progesterone well?*

The many forms in which progesterone is available suggest some strategies you can try if progesterone gives you unpleasant side effects but you need it to prevent hyperplasia. First, you try using the minimal dose. Instead of the old-style 10 mg of Provera for twelve days of every month, try half the dosage and you may feel better. This is also a good idea in view of the WHI's "less is better" philosophy.

Second, try a different progestin—maybe you will feel better with norethindrone instead of medroxyprogesterone. Among the available brands containing norethindrone are Aygestin and Micronor, which are just as effective as Provera, Amen, or Cycrin (all of which have medroxyprogesterone) in preventing hyperplasia.

If you are uncomfortable with all progestins, maybe natural progesterone will work better for you, as it does for many women. You can try Prometrium as long as you aren't allergic to peanuts. The equivalent dose is 200 mg a day for twelve days cyclically. If you do have a peanut allergy, find a compounding pharmacist and have natural progesterone made up for you.

You can also try changing the route of delivery: instead of oral progesterone, try using it vaginally or in a combination patch with estrogen. Talk with your caregiver about trying the Mirena system.

SCHEDULES AND REGIMENS

▶ *On what days of the month do I take estrogen? What are the usual cycles?*

There are two regimens for taking estrogen—continuously or cyclically.

Back in the late 1970s, when doctors started using a cyclical approach, you would take estrogen on days one to twenty-five of each month and add progesterone on days sixteen to twenty-five. For the last five or six days of the month you would take neither. During the week when you were taking neither estrogen nor progesterone, you would have a period. Then, starting the first day of the next month, you would begin the estrogen again. This regimen mimicked the body's action during the normal menstrual cycle.

Yet many women don't feel well on their days without estrogen. Women who have very sensitive coronary artery disease get chest pains; others experience hot flashes and insomnia. So during the past decade many physicians have switched to continuous HRT. You take estrogen continuously, every day of the month, and add progesterone for twelve days of the cycle.

Some women still prefer to have five days off all hormones at the end of the month, often because they get tender breasts and five days without estrogen will relieve the soreness. Certainly skipping these five days causes no health problems. All the same, more women seem comfortable using the estrogen straight through.

▶ What are the usual schedules for adding progesterone?

As we have seen, the major reason for taking progesterone is prevention of hyperplasia. There are several schools of thought about when and how long to take progesterone, but (as with estrogen) the choices are basically between daily progesterone and cyclic progesterone. The notion of cyclic progesterone (estrogen on days one to twenty-five of the menstrual cycle with progesterone added on days sixteen to twenty-five) was inspired by the hormone sequence of the normal menstrual cycle. The ovaries make estrogen almost all the time, but the body makes progesterone only during the second half of the cycle, after ovulation.

Many physicians still use this method, and most suggest using progesterone for twelve days to get full protection of the uterine lining. Some actually recommend progesterone for fourteen days, which perfectly mimics the twenty-eight-day menstrual cycle in which ovulation occurs on the fourteenth day and progesterone is produced for the subsequent fourteen days. As in the normal menstrual cycle, you will get a period when you stop taking the progesterone.

Because many women objected to the periodic bleeding that cyclic progesterone withdrawal causes, physicians began to experiment with different regimens of progesterone usage. What would happen, for example, if a woman took a very small dose of progesterone every day instead of a larger amount for twelve or fourteen days each month? This continuous regimen turned out to be quite effective in preventing cancer of the endometrium; in fact, all the studies done today show basically equivalent protection from the two approaches.

▶ What are the advantages and disadvantages of continuous progesterone?

The main advantage is that you do not get the regular withdrawal bleeds you get with cyclic progesterone. Unfortunately, some women—not all, but a fairly large number—do get erratic spotting, staining, or light flow when they take these small doses of progesterone. The spotting may come on day two of the cycle, or it may come on day sixteen or twenty-five.

Any unpredictable spotting or staining can be worrisome, and many physicians will biopsy women who have begun spotting after taking daily progesterone, just to be sure that nothing is wrong. This staining usually goes away within three months. If it is persistent, it can become a major annoyance.

Women who would prefer a light period at a predictable time to unpredictable spotting and staining probably would do better on cyclic progesterone, but it is an individual decision.

Not long ago, Justine L., who had chosen continuous progesterone, went on vacation to the Caribbean. She had been taking the progesterone for about a year without any spotting or staining, so she felt confident about wearing white linen slacks on the airplane. It was her bad luck that midway through the journey, she began to spot heavily, which spoiled both her pants and her vacation attitude. I got a very angry phone call when she returned, so now I suggest to women who choose continuous progesterone that they stash a minipad in their handbag, just in case.

▶ *How often do I need to have a period to protect my uterus if I choose cyclical progesterone?*

In the past physicians usually recommended withdrawing progesterone (and getting a period) every month. But gradually it became evident to many of us through clinical experience, though there were no scientifically documented and rigorously controlled studies to verify this hypothesis, that taking progesterone every second or third month provides adequate protection. This squares with the guidelines of the Women's Health Initiative, which suggest using the least effective amount of progesterone for the shortest effective time because of concerns about progesterone's action on breast tissue.

So if you are planning a camping trip in the mountains or a vacation to the Virgin Islands or China, or you are going to be involved in some activity where it would seriously inconvenience you to have a period, you can plan your progesterone around your personal schedule.

In general, the older you are, the less important it is to produce a withdrawal bleed each month. If you are in your fifties or sixties, you should withdraw the progesterone at least every third month; if you are in your seventies or eighties, probably every few months is all right. Doctor Philip M. Sarrel, former head of the Menopause Clinic at Yale, has ninety-year-olds on hormone therapy. He withdraws all these elderly women from progesterone on January 1 each year and gives them one period per year. And sometimes they do not get a withdrawal bleed.

PROGESTERONE AND PERIODS

If you are taking cyclic progesterone, you will probably have periods. Even though you are fully menopausal and your own ovaries are not producing enough estrogen for your uterine lining to build up, the estrogen in hormone therapy will stimulate your endometrium. When you take progesterone and then withdraw it at the end of the month, that withdrawal will cause the lining to shed.

A small percentage of women do not bleed when the progesterone is withdrawn. For them the lack of withdrawal bleeding is normal and nothing to worry about.

Women who have been taking progesterone and estrogen for some time after menopause often find that their bleeding becomes progressively lighter. Some skip a period from time to time. Indeed, many women who have been on estrogen with progesterone for a while have almost no bleeding; a few continue to have periods that seem fairly similar to the ones they had when they were younger.

If you have had cramps, even heavy ones, when you were premenopausal, chances are that you will not have them on HRT.

▶ *How long after withdrawal of progesterone will I get my period?*

Usually bleeding occurs right at the end of the progesterone regimen or within three or four days of withdrawing it. If this pattern changes (if, for example, your period comes very much later than expected), you should notify your caregiver.

▶ *If I start bleeding while I am taking progesterone, what should I do?*

As with any unexpected postmenopausal bleeding, you should alert your physician. You should also keep on taking the progesterone. It is the progesterone that protects you against hyperplasia, not the bleeding, so you must keep taking it for the length of time your physician recommends. If you bleed while you are taking progesterone, it is possible that you are not taking enough, so you should also be able to discuss the pattern of bleeding when you talk to your caregiver. When did the bleeding begin, on the fourth day after you started the progesterone or on the tenth? Is there any pattern to the bleeding? For example, have you occasionally started bleeding on day ten after you started the progesterone, whereas this month you suddenly began to bleed on day four?

▶ *If I have been taking cyclic estrogen and progesterone and don't get a period when I stop the progesterone, can it mean that I am pregnant?*

If you have never skipped a period except when you were pregnant, it can be worrisome if suddenly you skip one even after withdrawing progesterone. If your ovaries have shut down and are no longer releasing their monthly follicles, you cannot be pregnant. But if you worry that you started HRT before you were fully menopausal, you can have a blood test to ascertain whether you are pregnant.

▶ *If I'm taking progesterone cyclically to get a withdrawal bleed, do I have to take it every month?*

Because of the present concern that progesterone may be implicated in stimulating breast cancer, many physicians have suggested using progesterone only every two or three months. It is harder to remember to do things at longer intervals, so be sure to mark your calendar. You do have to take progesterone regularly if you choose the cyclical routine, but it doesn't have to be every month.

> Juanita S., fifty-one, a teacher, really needs estrogen. When she doesn't have it, she has debilitating headaches. But she doesn't like taking progesterone at all. Since she calls me every few months with a question about something or other, I always ask her whether she has had her progesterone recently. Usually her answer is no. When I haven't talked to her for about six months, I make it a point to call her and remind her.

▶ *Do I still get the protective action of progesterone, even though I don't have periods when it is withdrawn?*

Yes. Even if you don't get the withdrawal bleed, progesterone is acting to flatten out the lining of the uterus, to control the growth of the endometrium. The situation is similar to that of many women who don't get much of a period on low-dose birth control pills. It's not the period that counts but the progesterone. So even if you stop getting periods when you withdraw the progesterone, you still need to keep taking it.

▶ *What happens if I forget to take a progesterone pill one day?*

Nothing. You might have some bleeding, but continue with your regular progesterone schedule.

▶ *What should I do if I forget to take progesterone altogether for several months?*

Take the progesterone when you remember and continue with your regular schedule through the month. If your flow is very heavy, repeat the progesterone the next month.

THERAPY WITH ESTROGEN ALONE

▶ *Do women who have had hysterectomies need progesterone?*

Because the sole reason for taking progesterone postmenopausally is to protect the uterus, there is no reason whatsoever for anyone who has had a hysterectomy to take it. This is especially true in the light of the WHI results, which suggested that progesterone, at least medroxyprogesterone, the kind used in that study, might be implicated in stimulating breast cancer.

▶ *If I am taking estrogen alone because I can't tolerate any form of progesterone but I haven't had a hysterectomy, are there ways to check for possible excessive growth of the uterine lining?*

First of all, if you experience any bleeding, you should report it to your caregiver right away. Beyond that, many physicians recommend either an annual ultrasound of the pelvis or a yearly routine biopsy for women who are taking estrogen but not countering it with progesterone.

The traditional way of checking for endometrial hyperplasia is with a biopsy, during which a sample of the endometrial tissue is taken for checking. A newer method, which may not be available in smaller population centers, is the use of ultrasound technology, which makes the lining of the uterus visible as a kind of stripe along the muscular inner wall of the uterus. Physicians who have access to the technology are using ultrasound, in part to distinguish those who are bleeding from normal atrophic changes in the uterus from those with hyperplasia. By measuring the width of the endometrial stripe, as it is called in the technological jargon, a doctor can get some information about whether there is hyperplasia. If the endometrial stripe measures 6 mm or less, you can be reason-

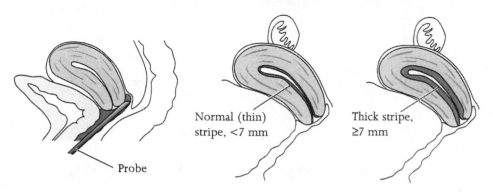

Normal (thin)
stripe, <7 mm

Thick stripe,
≥7 mm

Probe

FIGURE 9. The endometrial stripe. Ultrasound can be used to measure the thickness of the lining of the uterus, which shows up on the scan as a stripe. A thin stripe is rarely associated with precancerous conditions or with cancer itself.

ably sure that there is no hyperplasia. This does not mean that if the stripe is wider than 6 mm, hyperplasia is definitely present, but it does mean that a biopsy may be in order.

▶ *What if I have hyperplasia and still want to continue with HRT?*

If women on estrogen replacement therapy who cannot tolerate progesterone develop hyperplasia, the only alternative to stopping the estrogen is a hysterectomy. This significant decision should be made only after careful thought. Some of my patients feel strongly enough about HRT that they have preferred hysterectomy to withdrawing the therapy.

Grace Q. is fifty-nine. She has significant arthritis but keeps it under control by exercising daily, so she is quite mobile. When she doesn't exercise, she stiffens up and has increased pain. Grace has taken estrogen since menopause and does well on it. However, she cannot tolerate progesterone, which gives her headaches. Without the progesterone she developed endometrial hyperplasia and clearly needed a hysterectomy if she wanted to continue with the estrogen. After some thought, she decided that hysterectomy was her choice. As it turned out, her uterus was quite small, so that she was a good candidate for a laparoscope-assisted hysterectomy. She had the operation and recuperated so quickly that she was back in the gym after only two weeks.

10 Osteoporosis and Heart Health

TWO LONG-TERM ISSUES

OSTEOPOROSIS

Osteoporosis, the progressive loss or softening of bone through time, is one of the risks of aging. Avoiding bone loss is a primary reason why many women have chosen long-term hormone therapy. No one wants to lose height or to be hunched over, but this, after all, may seem to be merely a cosmetic problem. Nor does anyone hope for a broken hip or wrist, yet those injuries may also seem tolerable: lots of people have suffered from broken bones and recovered. Until a blitz of publicity brought osteoporosis to everyone's attention about a decade ago, it was easy to underestimate the seriousness of this disease.

In fact, the consequences of osteoporosis in terms of human suffering are often extremely grave. According to the American Academy of Orthopaedic Surgeons, women have two to three times as many hip fractures as men, with white, postmenopausal women, the highest risk group, having a one in seven chance of hip fracture during a lifetime. The rate of hip fracture increases at age fifty, doubling every five to six years, so that about half the women who live until age ninety have suffered a hip fracture. Of people older than fifty who fracture a hip, 24 percent die of complications in the following year. About half will require canes or walkers when they return home, while 53 percent of hip fracture patients age sixty-five and older are discharged from hospitals to long-term care facilities. A broken hip, then, can permanently alter the shape of your life. Osteoporosis also causes tiny fractures in the spinal column and elsewhere that account for chronic severe backaches and other pain. These microfractures often go undetected.

▶ *Who is at risk for osteoporosis?*

Although bone mass decreases in everyone as the years go by, not all women develop osteoporosis. The factors that increase risk are well known. Some are beyond your control; others can be minimized.

You are at higher risk if you are female. Bone size influences risk: if you are small boned and delicate, you are at higher risk than someone with a large, strapping frame. Small-boned people simply have less bone to lose. If you are slender, you are at greater risk than someone fatter. Although fat is not desirable in many respects, it does protect women from osteoporosis. People think of fat, like bone, as being inert, as just lying around your waist and hips. But fat tissue takes adrenal hormones, particularly one called androstenedione, and converts them into an estrogen called estrone. Although it is not the kind produced by the ovaries, it still retards bone loss. So a slender, small woman who doesn't have much fat does not have as much peripheral conversion from androstenedione to estrone as her fatter friend.

The down side of being fatter is that the same women who are protecting their bones from osteoporosis are significantly increasing their risk for cancer of the uterus. Estrone from their fat factories constantly stimulates the uterus, which can lead to excessive growth of the uterine lining (hyperplasia) and sometimes eventually cancer of the uterus. Obesity is indeed the biggest risk factor for uterine cancer.

Another risk factor for osteoporosis is activity level. If you fail to get adequate weight-bearing exercise, you are at increased risk of osteoporosis. Weight-bearing exercise, such as walking or running, increases bone strength by increasing osteoblastic activity. There is also some indication that bone mass can be improved by strength training, such as weight lifting or working out on exercise machines. The more you exercise, the more bone you build. Some types of exercise, swimming for instance, are great for your cardiovascular system, but because your bones are not bearing weight, they do not help prevent osteoporosis.

Family history affects risk in ways other than by influencing body type. Fair-skinned women of northern European, Chinese, or Japanese ancestry are at higher risk than darker-skinned Mediterranean women. African-American women have a much lower risk of osteoporosis; their hip fracture rates are one-third the rates of white women. Black women in Africa have even lower rates. Some researchers believe that this advantage has to do with absorption of the sun's rays, that darker-skinned people get improved vitamin D action and use calcium better from their diet than light-skinned people.

Calcium intake over your lifetime is another risk factor. If you have had several children, breast-fed them, and never drunk much milk or eaten many dairy products, your bones are probably not rich in calcium even before you reach menopause. If, in contrast, you have maintained your dietary calcium, you probably have not depleted your calcium store. One reason sometimes given for the high risk of Asian women is that their traditional diet is low in calcium.

Smoking and heavy alcohol intake are also harmful to your bones. Smokers are doubly damned: they go through early menopause, and once they are menopausal, smoking destroys their bones much faster than normal aging destroys the bones of nonsmokers. Although scientists believe that nicotine has some effect on bone metabolism, the mechanism is not well understood. Alcoholics have more osteoporosis than people who do not drink heavily, but again the reasons are imperfectly understood. It is possible that part of the cause relates to nutrition: alcoholics tend to drink rather than eat and may not get adequate dietary calcium. Other factors may also be at work.

Some specialists believe that caffeine adversely affects calcium absorption and that coffee drinking increases bone loss. Other studies fail to confirm this.

Bone loss accelerates at menopause, so you are at much greater risk for osteoporosis if you have an early menopause, either naturally or surgically, because you start losing bone rapidly. If, for example, your ovarian function is knocked out by chemotherapy when you are forty, or you simply have an early natural menopause at that age, you will have ten more years of accelerated bone loss than a woman who goes through menopause at age fifty. If several of these risk factors are working against you, you might consider HRT.

▶ Are there tests for osteoporosis?

The best test for diagnosing osteoporosis is a bone-density scan, called a DEXA scan. Ordinary X-rays do not detect bone loss until it has become significant, but more sophisticated diagnostic machines can establish a baseline density and compare it with later measurements, providing a way to monitor bone loss before it becomes dangerous.

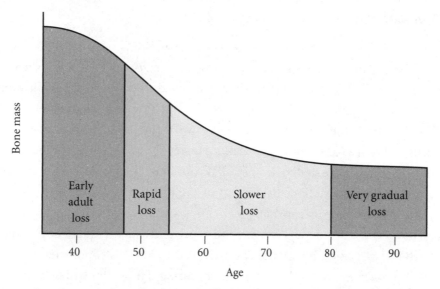

FIGURE 10. Bone loss over time, showing periods of rapid and slow bone loss. Bone loss starts by a woman's midthirties. Without estrogen, it accelerates right after menopause. If you take hormonal therapy and then stop, the rate of loss increases.

The test uses a technique called dual-energy X-ray absorptiometry (DEXA) to measure the amount of bone in your hip and spine, and in some cases your forearm, sites where fractures are likely to occur in people with osteoporosis. The scan works on the principle that the more energy a tissue absorbs, the denser it is. A DEXA scan is performed just like a standard X-ray and involves no discomfort and minimal radiation.

Ultrasound, usually of the heel, is sometimes used as a screening tool. It is less expensive than DEXA scanning but provides less information. If your ultrasound shows osteoporosis, you should then have a DEXA scan so that your bone loss can be accurately measured. A normal ultrasound of your heel, however, is not a guarantee that you don't have osteoporosis.

You may have heard about blood or urine tests for bone loss. Physicians use these tests to measure how well you are responding to bone-loss therapy or to diagnose why some women have excessive bone loss, but the tests are rarely used for screening.

The easiest and least expensive test is your annual height measurement. Many adults will lose an inch or perhaps an inch and a half from their peak height, but if you have lost more than that, your bone density should be evaluated.

▶ *What do the results of my DEXA scan mean?*

Bone density is measured in milligrams of bone per cubic centimeter. DEXA scans compare the density of your bones first with those of a thirty-five-year-old woman whose bone mass is at its peak, and then with age-matched controls, that is, with women of about your age. These comparisons are called "T" and "Z" scores, respectively.

The "T" score is the more important of the two. If your bone density lies within a certain statistical range (one standard deviation) below the bone density of the thirty-five-year-old woman, you are said to be normal. If your bone density is between one and two and a half standard deviations below that of the thirty-five-year-old normal woman, then you are said to have osteopenia, which simply means "insufficient bone," that is, not enough bone. If your score puts you more than two and a half standard deviations below the thirty-five-year-old's norm, then you are said to have osteoporosis, which can be translated "porous bones." If the names are confusing, simply think of bone density as a continuum, with "osteopenia" and "osteoporosis" as stages in bone loss.

The risk of fracture is correlated to the amount of bone loss as calculated in your "T" score. In ballpark figures, people with osteopenia have three times the fracture risk of that thirty-five-year-old woman enjoying peak bone mass; people with osteoporosis have about ten times that risk.

In the past several years many radiologists have added bone density scanning equipment to their facilities, so it has become relatively easy to find a radiologist who can do the procedure. Five years ago there was only one doctor near where I work who had the equipment to do serious bone density studies. Nowadays as the medical profession and the population as a whole have become aware of osteoporosis, there are about eight facilities in my area, some at major hospitals, some in suburban clinics.

▶ *How much do bone density studies cost?*

A DEXA bone density test costs about three hundred dollars. In this day of HMO medicine, many insurance companies are not willing to pay for bone density studies, and paying three hundred dollars for a test that will be repeated in a few years can be hard on your pocketbook, so check with your insurance company to see about your coverage.

▶ Who should be tested?

This is controversial, but most physicians agree that all women should have a test by the time they are sixty-five. In my own practice I recommend bone density studies for women at high risk for osteoporosis. If you do weight-bearing exercise four times a week, get 1,000 mg of calcium every day, take hormone therapy, have no family history of osteoporosis, and are big-boned and dark-skinned, you probably don't need a bone density study, though there is always some minimal risk that you might have osteoporosis.

But if you are blond, slender, and have a family history of osteoporosis, or if you smoke, chances are your doctor will send you for a bone density study. In my own practice I might use the test as a way to encourage you to start appropriate preventive therapy, because I have learned that it is hard to convince people to do something healthy if they don't physically feel ill or uncomfortable.

▶ Can I prevent bone loss by exercising?

Many women wonder whether they should exercise or take either estrogen or some other bone-preserving agent. The answer is that to maximize bone health throughout life, you should do both. There is no question that if you are not taking estrogen postmenopausally, you will lose bone. Exercise helps, but studies have shown that moderate exercise alone, for example brisk walking, will not prevent osteoporosis.

The ideal preventive is a combination of estrogen and exercise, plus adequate calcium and vitamin D intake in your diet. Although estrogen alone may prevent significant postmenopausal bone loss, estrogen or a bone-preserving medication plus exercise may even help you build back bone that has been lost.

▶ Can I prevent bone loss by increasing my intake of calcium?

Studies have shown that you can increase bone mass by exercise at any time during your life, but if you are not taking estrogen, the effect of drinking even a gallon of milk a day is debatable. Remember that women in their thirties and forties should be sure they are getting enough calcium (about 1,000 mg) in their diet, because they still have enough estrogen to absorb it; in terms of building healthy bones, now is better than later. Physicians recommend 1,500 mg of calcium daily for postmenopausal women.

▶ What drugs other than estrogen help prevent osteoporosis?

There are two medical options. One is a class of medications called bisphosphonates; the other is raloxifene, which acts in some ways like hormone therapy.

Bisphosphonates

Two bisphosphonates are available: alendronate, marketed as Fosamax, and risedronate, sold as Actonel. Fosamax was introduced in 1995, replacing its parent compound etidronate (trade name Didronel), a drug used originally for a rare bone affliction called Paget's disease and later for postmenopausal osteoporosis.

Both alendronate and risedronate work by decreasing the resorbtion of bone, by slowing down the destructive action of the osteoclasts (see Chapter 5). Both effectively increase bone mineral density within the first year you use them, and both have been shown to decrease fracture rates.

These drugs don't have many side effects, though some people who take them experience irritation of the stomach or esophagus. To minimize these symptoms, bisphosphonates must be taken first thing in the morning with a full glass of water, while you are sitting upright. You must continue sitting or standing (no lying down again) and then eat breakfast half an hour later. This ensures that the medication goes straight down your esophagus and gets absorbed as quickly as possible from your stomach. Most people don't have difficulty following these instructions, but some elderly folks find them hard to remember. Back in the 1990s, when bisphosphonates had to be taken daily, this regimen could be annoying, but now that bisphosphonates are available in weekly dosages, it is not so difficult to follow the directions.

Raloxifene

Raloxifene, introduced in 1998 as Evista, provides the bone-enhancing benefits of estrogen without increasing cancer risks. Raloxifene belongs to a new category of drugs called selective estrogen receptor modulators (SERMs). Evista is easy to take—one smallish pill daily, with or without food. It doesn't irritate your stomach or esophagus.

How SERMS Work

Estrogen, a hormone produced mainly by the ovaries, travels through the body by circulating in the blood. When the estrogen in the blood encounters cells that have appropriate estrogen receptors, it binds to those cells. Researchers use the metaphors of a lock and key or pieces of a jigsaw puzzle to explain the relation between the receptor and the molecule that binds to it. Once attached to a target cell, the hormone makes that cell do something—produce a chemical that will stimulate growth, for example. There are cells with estrogen receptors in the uterus, breasts, and vagina, as you would expect, but also in such unlikely organs as the brain and heart, and, in men, in the testis and prostate. Thus estrogen has far-reaching effects throughout the body.

SERMs change the behavior of the estrogen receptors in specific tissues. They can act as estrogen "turn ons," activating the cell, or they can act as estrogen blockers, preventing estrogen from binding and doing its work. SERMs can block the action of estrogen in one tissue but mimic its action in another. Thus estrogen may bind to the receptors in the brain, for example, but not to those in the uterus. In this characteristic lies the vast therapeutic potential of SERMs.

Tamoxifen, a drug used since the 1970s to treat breast cancer, is a SERM. Women whose cancerous tumors were estrogen-receptor positive, that is, stimulated to grow by the action of estrogen, take tamoxifen because it works at the level of the breast tissue to block the action of estrogen. Because some 75 to 80 percent of breast cancer tumors in postmenopausal women are estrogen-receptor positive, many older women are being treated long term with tamoxifen.

Because tamoxifen therapy originally lasted many years, doctors and researchers began to worry that women taking this estrogen blocker might develop osteoporosis. When tests were done, however, it turned out that the women taking tamoxifen, instead of losing bone density, were in fact building bone. Nor did their cardiovascular risks seem to increase. These observations suggested that tamoxifen acted as an estrogen blocker on breast tissue but not on bone and blood vessels.

All of this made tamoxifen seem like the perfect drug, but there was one catch. Tamoxifen stimulates uterine tissue and raises the risk of endometrial cancer. A fairly small percentage of the women taking it developed uterine polyps, a worrisome finding, because hundreds of thousands of women undergo long-term tamoxifen therapy.

Researchers then went back to the drawing board and looked at a drug called raloxifene, which had been discovered at about the same time as tamoxifen and is closely related to it. They wondered whether raloxifene would act differently from tamoxifen, would bind to different tissues. Experiments showed that raloxifene blocks estrogen's action on the breasts but mimics its bone-enhancing action. It also seems to offer cardiovascular protection but does not stimulate the endometrial lining. Consequently the FDA has approved raloxifene for use in menopausal women.

Three large-scale studies—the American, European, and international studies—examined the effects of raloxifene on bone density. The international study traced bone loss in women who had undergone hysterectomy, whereas the American and European studies focused on women who had not. The women chosen for the studies were at least two years postmenopausal; none were experiencing hot flashes or other perimenopausal symptoms; none had osteoporosis. The researchers followed the women for two years, doing bone-density studies at regular intervals. In each study, a control group took a placebo and an experimental group took raloxifene. Both groups took calcium supplements. All three studies showed that the placebo group lost bone during the two years, while the women taking raloxifene actually increased their bone mass. The studies were extended another year, with the same results: the group treated with raloxifene continued to gain bone mass, while the placebo group continued to lose it.

▶ Is raloxifene a good choice for me?

If you are not experiencing severe menopausal symptoms (hot flashes, sleeplessness, mood swings, vaginal dryness) but are at risk for osteoporosis and don't want to take estrogen, raloxifene might be right for you.

> Françoise Z. is sixty-two, small, slender, and fair-skinned. Although she is physically active, she is not keen on drinking milk or taking calcium supplements. Her daughter Joanne is a gynecological endocrinologist, the kind of person who is likely to think about osteoporosis with some frequency. When Françoise went through menopause at fifty-two, Joanne sent her to have a bone density test, which showed bone loss.
>
> Joanne put her mother on ERT, which Françoise disliked because it gave her breast discomfort that made her miserable. This year her mammogram showed a breast cyst, and when the radiologist asked for repeat pictures, Françoise announced that she had had enough and was not going to take ERT any more. Because Françoise wasn't having mood swings, sleeplessness, hot flashes, or other symptoms that needed relief, but did need bone protection, Evista worked out well for her.
>
> Wendy L., now forty-nine, had a complete hysterectomy twenty years ago because of severe endometriosis. This early removal of her ovaries puts her at risk

for osteoporosis, but when she tried estrogen, she became bloated and uncomfortable. We tried diuretics to reduce her swelling, but they make her lightheaded. Evista was a better choice for her.

Kathy W., who has been postmenopausal for five years, is at least a hundred pounds overweight. Since she was a young woman, she has had breast cysts, which must be drained at fairly frequent intervals. Kathy had hoped that menopause would give her relief from the cysts, since her ovaries would no longer be producing the estrogen that stimulated their growth, but unfortunately the extra fat she carries produces enough peripheral estrogen to make the cysts a continuing problem. Kathy has severe osteoarthritis, and I am concerned the she will develop osteoporosis on top of her arthritis. Evista would conserve her bones, while protecting her breasts from the action of estrogen.

▶ *Does raloxifene protect against breast cancer?*

Because raloxifene is an estrogen-receptor blocker in the breast, it protects breast tissue against the effects of estrogen. Although Evista has been on the market for only a short while, large clinical studies conducted for about three years before it was approved by the FDA showed that it did not increase the risk of breast cancer and might even lower its incidence; the FDA did not approve it as a cancer preventative, however.

More recently, when the protective benefits of raloxifene's cousin tamoxifen became apparent, studies were undertaken to compare the two drugs in terms of breast cancer protection. The most important of these is the STAR (Study of Tamoxifen and Raloxifene) trial, a five-year study involving some nineteen thousand postmenopausal women who are at high risk for breast cancer. Preliminary data suggest that raloxifene, as well as tamoxifen, may very well lower the risk of breast cancer.

This makes good common sense, given raloxifene's function as an estrogen-receptor blocker in breast tissue. About 75 to 80 percent of postmenopausal breast cancers are estrogen-receptor positive, which means that estrogen stimulates these tumors to grow. Evista, however, blocks the receptors and prevents any estrogen, including that made in body fat, from affecting the breasts.

We won't know with certainly until further research has been done whether Evista prevents breast cancer or lowers the risk for it. In the meantime, its estrogen-blocking effects on breast and uterine tissue and its estrogen-protective effects on bone and the cardiovascular system make it the drug of choice for certain women.

About nine years ago, Shirley C. came into the office. She was fifty-two, a capable woman with two children. She doesn't have a lot of formal education, but it was immediately clear that she was an intelligent woman who read a lot. She works on an assembly line in a factory, where her job involves a certain amount of lifting and moving, so that she is quite active physically even though she does not follow a specific exercise program.

Shirley has an unfortunate genetic heritage. Her mother had a mastectomy while still young but died of coronary artery disease at age fifty-five. Her aunt had premenopausal breast cancer. One brother had coronary artery bypass surgery eight months ago; another died in his forties of coronary artery disease. Shirley herself had had a coronary bypass when she was forty-eight.

Her question to me was, which was more important? Her history of coronary artery disease (which HRT was then thought to help)? Or her family's history of breast cancer? We discussed her choices at length and she decided to begin HRT. When the HERS study showed that estrogen provided no benefits for women who already had cardiovascular disease (as Shirley did), she had already been on estrogen for about four years and was doing very well, both cardiovascularly and in terms of breast health. After more discussion we agreed that she would continue.

Then the WHI study came out. Again, we discussed the pros and cons. Shirley decided to stick with the hormone therapy. "No one in my family has ever reached the age of sixty," she said, "and I don't want to rock the boat."

If Shirley had made her first visit to the office today rather than in 1995, I would not have encouraged her to take hormonal therapy long term to prevent further heart disease. But it will be interesting to see what the RUTH (Raloxifene Use for the Heart) and STAR trials show. If they do suggest that Evista has benefits to breast tissue as well as the cardiovascular system, it might be a good choice for Shirley.

As Shirley's decision suggests, another important psychological consideration in a woman's choice are her fears about disease. Many women are concerned about the possibility of getting breast cancer, and realistically, it is a worrisome disease, but in some women this concern reaches the level of phobia. If the studies about breast cancer and HRT unravel you emotionally, then you probably should chose alternative ways of dealing with the discomforts of menopause. Shirley, despite her family history, was not phobic about breast cancer. When we discussed it, she said, "Oh, well, I'll just go out and get a mammogram."

Both heart disease and breast cancer—the two risks in Shirley's genetic heritage—are serious, life-threatening, and life-compromising diseases. Breast cancer also carries a stigma that is independent of its seriousness as a disease. That stigma puts an additional burden on many women who have it and adds to the fear of women who do not.

Although no one goes out and asks for heart disease, it does not have the fearsome reputation that breast cancer does. Nevertheless, heart disease is serious business and can end your life abruptly or compromise your life to the point where you cannot move from your bed without serious pain. Perhaps Americans think of heart disease as a man's disease, although half of the nearly one million people who die yearly of heart attacks are women. In the popular imagery, heart disease has a macho connotation: it fells hard-driving business executives or basketball superstars, not carpool-driving mothers or underpaid officer workers. Furthermore, the heart is a socially acceptable organ, unlike the bowel or the breast. People don't make denigrating jokes about the heart. You can talk publicly about your heart and its infirmities, as you cannot about your colon, vagina, or breast. So, for several reasons, breast cancer carries heavy emotional baggage.

> Sharon G. has high LDL (bad) cholesterol. She dislikes all forms of exercise, even walking. She is also extremely afraid of getting cancer, and every time she comes for a check-up, Sharon is sure that I will find cancer somewhere in her body. Her son, an endocrinologist, encouraged her to take estrogen but Sharon refused, because she was certain that it would give her cancer. Given her fears, taking estrogen would only have made her more phobic than she already is.
>
> Still, her high cholesterol and her inactivity put her at risk for cardiovascular problems. Evista is a good choice for Sharon because it certainly will not increase her cancer risk; if it lowers her LDL, which is now 150, by 10 percent to 135, it might benefit her.

▶ *Can women who have had breast cancer take raloxifene?*

Unfortunately, there have been no studies to assess the impact of Evista on preexisting breast cancer. If women who have had breast cancer are currently taking tamoxifen therapy, they don't need raloxifene because the two drugs are quite similar.

For women who have finished their course of tamoxifen therapy, however, raloxifene makes good common sense, because it will protect them against osteoporosis and perhaps against coronary artery disease while blocking the action of estrogen in the breast. This is a matter to discuss with your oncologist, however. Oncologists will often decide against using raloxifene, which is reasonable conservative practice, because no data establish raloxifene as helpful or even safe in this situation.

▶ Does Evista affect the lining of the uterus?

No, and that is one of its most appealing features. Since Evista does not stimulate the uterine lining, women taking it do not need to take progesterone, which can cause uncomfortable side effects. It might be a good choice for women who cannot tolerate any form of progesterone whatsoever, as well as those women who can't tolerate the menstrual periods elicited by stopping the progesterone each month.

▶ What are the side effects?

Its main disadvantage is that it can contribute to hot flashes. In the studies mentioned earlier, about 24 percent of the women who took raloxifene had hot flashes, while only 19 percent of the placebo group did, a statistically significant 5 percent difference.

Perhaps "suggestibility" contributed to the perception of hot flashes. That is, if you query someone long enough about a symptom, he or she may begin to feel, "Yes, I have that," just as 30 percent of people taking a placebo experience improvement in the symptoms that the "medication" is supposed to cure. The women in the study, none of whom had perimenopausal symptoms at the outset, were questioned repeatedly, at about three-month intervals, about their hot flashes; sooner or later some of them began to remember that they had had a few flashes.

Raloxifene's other side effect is leg cramps, which troubled 6 percent of the women in the study taking the drug and only 2 percent of the placebo group. The researchers studied the women's calcium metabolism, blood flow, and other likely causes of leg cramps but arrived at no satisfactory answer. When the women stopped taking the drug, the cramps disappeared. Neither the leg cramps nor the hot flashes were severe enough to cause women to drop out of the study; only 2 percent of those who signed on quit because of adverse effects of the drug.

Other peri- and postmenopausal symptoms—weight gain, depression, anxiety, mood swings, irritability, decreased libido, vaginal dryness and other urinary tract symptoms—seem unaffected by raloxifene. Unlike estrogen, which has been associated with migraine-type headaches, Evista does not seem to cause headaches. Anecdotal evidence suggests that it may even help with headaches that are associated with estrogen.

▶ *Are there women who should definitely not take raloxifene?*

Unless a year or more has elapsed since your last menstrual period and there is no chance you could become pregnant, you should not even consider this drug because it can cause serious birth defects. If you have had problems with thrombophlebitis (inflammation of a vein, caused by a blood clot) and thromboembolisms (blocking of blood vessels by clots), you should not take it.

Studies published in 1996 showed that estrogen does indeed increase risk for thrombophlebitis and thromboembolisms, although the risk remains small. For women not taking estrogen, the risk of these complications is one in ten thousand; although this rate doubles or triples with estrogen use, the risk remains small, three in ten thousand. Most thrombotic problems with Evista occur during the first few months.

Because Evista is metabolized partly through the liver, it may not be desirable for women with severe liver dysfunction, such as cirrhosis.

Before you try Evista, tell your gynecologist about your other medications. If you are taking coumadin or another anticoagulant, you should be careful about your clotting time, because some drugs can alter the concentration of these blood thinners. If you are taking cholestyramine to lower cholesterol, you probably shouldn't take Evista.

▶ *Since men also lose bone as they age, can they try bone-enhancing drugs?*

Unfortunately, we have no scientific studies that have tested the efficacy or the safety of raloxifene in men. However, bisphosphonates have been used to help men maintain bone mass.

CARDIOVASCULAR HEALTH

▶ *Who is at high risk for heart disease?*

Risk factors for heart disease include age, heredity, diet (high fat, heavy salt consumption), high alcohol consumption (generally defined for women as more than two drinks a day), stress, obesity, and smoking. Some of these factors—diet, smoking, alcohol consumption, obesity—are controllable. Others are not.

The single most lethal controllable factor is smoking. Many women say they continue to smoke in order to keep their weight down. Although obesity is certainly a risk factor for heart disease, smoking is even riskier: according to the American Heart Association and the American Cancer Society, to offset the health benefits of quitting smoking, the average smoker would have to gain seventy-five pounds.

Smoking seems particularly deadly in women because in addition to accelerating the hardening of the arteries, it weakens women's two best defenders against cardiac disease, estrogen and HDL (good) cholesterol.

▶ How important a threat for women is coronary heart disease?

According to epidemiologist Deborah Grady and her colleagues, a fifty-year-old white woman has a 46 percent lifetime probability of getting coronary heart disease, the leading cause of death among postmenopausal women. In a sample of one hundred of these women, then, forty-six of them can be predicted to get coronary heart disease. The average fifty-year-old white woman's chances of dying of this disease are 31 percent. The median age at which women die of coronary heart disease is seventy-four years, which means that half of the women are older and half are younger at the time of death.

▶ Does adding progesterone to HRT have any effect on risk for heart disease?

When American physicians prescribe HRT, they usually prescribe a progestin (synthetic progesterone) as well as estrogen to protect women from uterine cancer. Unfortunately, progestins tend to increase the LDL (bad) cholesterol or decrease the HDL (good) cholesterol levels in blood, so that some of the estrogen's benefit is lost. Many researchers believe that natural progesterone does not have this negative impact, and preliminary data suggest that natural progesterone has almost no adverse effect on blood lipids.

▶ Does HRT raise blood pressure?

It was formerly believed that HRT did raise blood pressure, but more recent research shows that blood pressure generally doesn't change much with estrogen therapy. A small proportion of women taking oral estrogen, however, about one in twenty, responds to HRT with higher blood pressure. Estrogen delivered through the transdermal skin patch is less likely to affect blood pressure.

BOX 2.   Your Risk for Heart Disease (for Women)

Circle the number of points relating to your personal health information in each category. When you have added up your points, compare the total with the guide at the bottom of the page, which suggests your risk for developing heart disease within the next ten years based on your present information. If you are unsure about some of your levels, ask your doctor about getting them checked.

AGE	POINTS	AGE	POINTS
20–34	−7	55–59	8
35–39	−3	60–64	10
40–44	0	65–69	12
45–49	3	70–74	14
50–54	6	75– 79	16

TOTAL CHOLESTEROL	POINTS				
	AGE 20–39	AGE 40–49	AGE 50–59	AGE 60–69	AGE 70–79
<160	0	0	0	0	0
160–199	4	3	2	1	1
200–239	8	6	4	2	1
240–279	11	8	5	3	2
≥280	13	10	7	4	2

	POINTS				
	AGE 20–39	AGE 40–49	AGE 50–59	AGE 60–69	AGE 70–79
Nonsmoker	0	0	0	0	0
Smoker	9	7	4	2	1

HDL (MG/DL)	POINTS	SYSTOLIC BP (MMHG)	IF UNTREATED	IF TREATED
≥60	−1	<120	0	0
50–59	0	120–129	1	3
40–49	1	130–139	2	4
<40	2	140–159	3	5
		≥160	4	6

POINT TOTAL	10-YEAR RISK %	POINT TOTAL	10-YEAR RISK %
<9	<1	17	5
9	1	18	6
10	1	19	8
11	1	20	11
12	1	21	14
13	2	22	17
14	2	23	22
15	3	24	27
16	4	≥25	≥30

Source: *Third Report of the National Cholesterol Education Program (NCEP) Expert Panel on Detection, Evaluation, and Treatment of High Blood Cholesterol in Adults (Adult Treatment Panel III): Executive Summary,* NIH Publication No. 01-3670, May 2001, table B2.

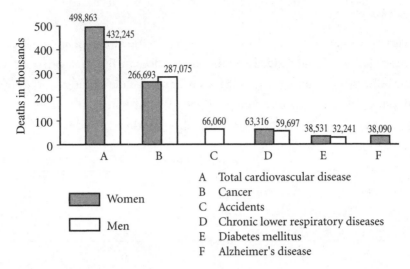

FIGURE 11. Leading causes of death for American men and women, 2001. Contrary to popular belief, more women than men die of cardiovascular disease; more men than women die of cancer. In 2001, 232,000 more women died of cardiovascular disease than of all kinds of cancer combined. Source: American Heart Association, *Heart Disease and Stroke Statistics—2004 Update* (Dallas: American Heart Association, 2003).

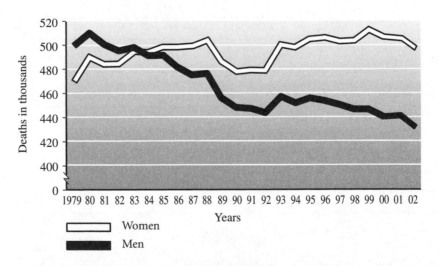

FIGURE 12. Trends in cardiovascular disease mortality for American men and women, 1979–2001. In every year since 1984, cardiovascular disease has killed more women than men, with the "cardiovascular gender gap" rising to almost 67,000 in 2001. Source: American Heart Association, *Heart Disease and Stroke Statistics—2004 Update* (Dallas: American Heart Association, 2003).

▶ *Do any of the medications used for osteoporosis protection also protect against heart disease?*

Bisphosphonates—Fosamax and Actonel—have no known effect on cardiovascular health. With Evista, the picture is less clear. Because Evista came on the market in 1998, we do not have long-term epidemiological data, but we can look at what are called markers of coronary artery disease. Researchers do this by measuring the levels of several components in the blood. The most important, and the most familiar, are LDL (bad) and HDL (good) cholesterol. We know that women taking Evista have about a 10 to 11 percent reduction in LDL; women taking estrogen have about a 12 percent reduction, so Evista and estrogen are virtually equivalent in reducing bad cholesterol. Estrogen, however, raises good cholesterol, whereas Evista does not.

Other components of the blood, called triglycerides, are fatty substances something like cholesterol. With triglycerides, as with LDL, less is better. Beyond that, the role and even the importance of triglycerides in coronary artery disease are controversial. Some cardiologists think that triglycerides influence the risk of coronary artery disease at least as much as cholesterol; others say their influence is negligible. We do know that women taking estrogen in pill form (but not women using the estrogen patch) have elevated triglyceride levels. Evista does not affect triglycerides.

Fibrinogen, which influences clot formation, is another piece in the big puzzle of cardiovascular disease. Scientists generally believe that, as with triglycerides, less fibrinogen is better. Unlike estrogen, Evista lowers fibrinogen and a substance called lipoprotein A, which is similar to fibrinogen.

11 Menopause and Sexuality

ONE of the myths of menopause suggests that a woman's sex life ends when she reaches menopause. As many women at midlife know, this is not true. But if menopause is a time of biological change, then for many women it is a time of sexual change also. Sexuality in middle age, as in other times of life, has physical, emotional, and even social components; so the changes that take place during the years surrounding menopause may be influenced by all these factors.

Physical factors may include changes in the structure and lubrication of the vagina that lead to discomfort or pain during intercourse, diseases (for example, heart disease or high blood pressure), or surgical repairs to correct incontinence, which could make sexual functioning difficult. Emotional factors include a woman's general outlook during menopause and her specific feelings about being menopausal. In the past, when female sexuality was presumed to be bound to reproductive capacity, women were thought to become disinterested in sex when they became menopausal because they were mourning their lost ability to produce babies. Although the close ties between reproductive capacity and sexual pleasure may be extremely meaningful to some women, they certainly are not significant to all women. For many, in fact, the certainty that pregnancy is no longer a risk heightens sexual pleasure.

Self-esteem also affects sexual functioning. A culture that holds that only young women are sexually desirable, or that sex is the exclusive province of the young, may make it hard for an older woman to hold onto her self-esteem and to see herself as desirable. Women who feel unattractive—too fat, too flabby, too saggy—may feel less inclined to sexual activity than women who have higher regard for themselves.

The most important element of sexual activity is a couple's response to their relationship and their ability to communicate within it. If someone comes to me and says that her husband just isn't interested in sex any more or cannot perform, I ask her how she feels about that. Sometimes she is just as glad not to have an active sex life. But if she feels a sense of frustration and loss, then I try to help. As her physician, I want her to be comfortable and happy. I want her to realize that no single standard of sexual activity is acceptable whereas all others are not.

Often patients come to me for reassurance, which is not surprising in a society where sex is emphasized so strongly even though so much ambiguity exists. I cannot emphasize enough the importance of communication in a relationship. If you feel that your libido is diminished and you are worried about it, talk to your partner. If he doesn't have any strong desire for intercourse either, you need not be upset any longer.

Difficulties do arise when one partner's desire is significantly different from the other's. Whether the woman wants sex and the man doesn't or the woman doesn't want sex and the man does, there is a problem. If both partners have active libidos and strong performance abilities and both are happy with that situation, then everything is fine. If neither has strong libido or performance ability and they are equally matched in desire, that's fine, too.

It is also true that many forms of sexual functioning can be satisfying to both partners. As long as they are pleasing to both the man and the woman, oral intercourse and mutual masturbation are healthy forms of sexual activity.

DISCOMFORT DURING INTERCOURSE

▶ *What are the causes of sexual discomfort in postmenopausal women?*

The most common problem reported to me is discomfort during intercourse. The primary reason is that without estrogen the vagina becomes dry, a condition known as atrophic vaginitis, and for many women (but not all) intercourse becomes painful, a condition technically known as dyspareunia. Unlike hot flashes or sleep disturbances, which improve with time, vaginal dryness gets worse the longer a woman is deprived of estrogen.

It makes sense to suppose that the vagina would be sensitive to loss of estrogen, since of all the bodily organs the vagina has perhaps the most estrogen receptors. When a woman's ovaries no longer produce estrogen, the walls of her vagina become thinner. The cells lining the vagina become flatter, less plump, and fewer in number. They produce less lubricant than they did when stimulated by estrogen, and they do not support the vagina as well. Nor are the vaginal walls as elastic and resilient as they were in the presence of estrogen.

An examining physician can see these changes with the aid of a speculum and make a quick assessment of a woman's estrogen status. Fatter women tend to be less afflicted with vaginal dryness than their thinner sisters, because fat produces a kind of estrogen called estrone.

▶ *Does the size of the vagina change after menopause?*

The answer is a qualified yes. Women who remain sexually active tend to remain in better shape, vaginally speaking, than women who do not. The old "use it or lose it" metaphor is appropriate (though not exactly elegant) in this instance.

▶ *Does vaginal atrophy create problems other than uncomfortable intercourse?*

Two problems that sometimes accompany vaginal atrophy are vaginal infections and urinary tract infections. As the walls of the vagina thin out and become dryer, these tissues are more easily injured and irritated and more vulnerable to infection. During your reproductive years the chemical climate of the vagina is slightly acidic, though the degree of acidity fluctuates during the menstrual cycle. This acidic environment discourages the growth of harmful bacteria but encourages the growth of your own vaginal flora, microorganisms that live in the vagina and fight infection. When the vagina becomes more alkaline, as it does when we age, it becomes more hospitable to hostile bacteria and less supportive of helpful ones.

Urinary tract infections occur with some frequency in older women for the same reasons. Just as the walls of the vagina thin out and are less well lubricated after menopause, the walls of the bladder, which also have many estrogen receptors, undergo changes and become more prone to infection. The friction and activity of sexual intercourse can exacerbate the process.

▶ *Does vaginal atrophy have causes other than estrogen depletion?*

Women who have had radiation therapy in the region of their vagina, perhaps for cervical cancer, may have scar tissue in the vagina. In addition to the scar tissue's being less elastic than normal tissue, the vagina itself may have shrunk. Women who have had vaginal repair surgery for a prolapsed uterus, rectocele, or cystocele, may—rarely—end up with a vagina that is too narrow to function comfortably during sex.

▶ *Are vaginal changes reversible?*

Virtually without exception, vaginal changes caused by inactivity, radiation therapy, or surgery are reversible. You can almost always get back into good vaginal shape, just as you can almost always get back into good physical shape generally.

I always tell patients who find intercourse painful after periods of inactivity or for other reasons to come in and talk to me. I have treated a number of women who had not had intercourse for ten years or so and then found a new partner. The first few times such women have intercourse they are going to be uncomfortable, especially if they don't use vaginal lubrication. I encourage those of them who are not on hormone therapy to let me prescribe a vaginal estrogen cream, so that when they do become sexually active again, intercourse will not hurt. In addition to the physical distress, vaginal discomfort is a significant sexual turnoff for both partners.

Some of the women who come into the office are fifteen or twenty years postmenopausal, and their sex lives have gone from satisfactory to nonexistent—because they are uncomfortable. It is understandable that sex would not appeal to them if it is painful, but their husbands or partners are not happy with the situation. If these women are not willing to try systemic HRT, I suggest vaginal estrogen, which can be applied in the form of a cream, ring, or tablet. And I have had husbands write me thank-you notes.

Another possibility is vaginal dilators, which a physician may prescribe to help re-

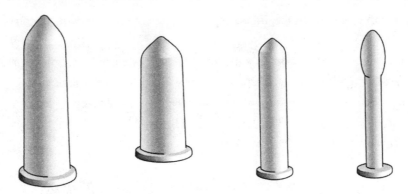

FIGURE 13. Vaginal dilators are rubber cylinders in graduated sizes that can be used to stretch the vagina.

store the vagina to its normal size. Women who have scar tissue in their vagina or who have been sexually inactive for long periods often find them useful. The dilators are little cylinders in graded sizes, which you insert into the vagina with a water-soluble lubricant such as K-Y Lubricating Jelly. Surgical supply companies make them in plastic, rubber, or glass. The smallest ones are narrow, perhaps the width of a couple of pencils. You leave them in for a few minutes each day, gradually increasing the size of the dilator that you insert. With the use of these dilators in combination with vaginal estrogen cream, most women can become functional again.

Some women whose vagina is too tight after surgery need more than dilator therapy. They have to return to surgery to have their vaginal repair relaxed; but this outcome is uncommon.

▶ *Do forms of sexual activity other than intercourse (for example, masturbation) help keep the vagina in good shape?*

The fact that a woman doesn't have a male sexual partner doesn't mean that she must be sexually inactive. Many women who miss sexual activity when they become widowed or divorced turn to masturbation as a source of pleasure or stimulation. This substitute is perfectly all right and certainly contributes to keeping your vagina well lubricated.

Many women do not have sexual partners when they reach menopause. They may be single, widowed, or, more likely, divorced. At this time of life many women, switching their sexual orientation, turn to other women for sexual and psychological closeness. This, too, is a viable solution to sexual loneliness for many older women.

You should feel comfortable discussing these matters with your gynecologist, as should your gynecologist with you. One of the complaints sometimes leveled against male gynecologists, rightly or wrongly, is that many seem to assume that without a male partner a woman cannot be sexually active.

▶ *What therapies are available for postmenopausal vaginal discomfort?*

Although hormonal and nonhormonal therapies are available for most symptoms surrounding menopause, the clear winner as far as vaginal dryness is concerned is estrogen in some form. If you don't wish to take estrogen systemically—via pills or a patch—there are three main approaches to taking it vaginally. Vaginal estrogen creams have been available for some time. These creams stimulate the tissues of the vagina to produce their own lubrication. Very little estrogen is absorbed through the walls of the vagina, and usually the creams make a great deal of difference both in vaginal comfort and in reduction of infections. These products, which come in the same brands as oral estrogen, are available by prescription only.

Two newer contenders in the field, both developed in Scandinavia, are vaginal estrogen tablets and an estogen-impregnated vaginal ring. Vagifem tablets come in boxes of eighteen, each packed in a single-use applicator. You insert the applicator into the vagina as far as it will comfortably go; when you press the plunger, the tablet is ejected and dissolves in the vagina. You can use the tablets as needed, preferably at bedtime. Many women like this product because the tablets are less messy than creams. The manufacturer's directions suggest using a tablet every night for two weeks when you begin the therapy, but most women find relief at lower dosages and end up using a tablet perhaps two or three times a week. If you have dryness around your labia, you may want to alternate the tablets with a vaginal cream.

The other new product is Estring, a soft silicone ring that looks something like a small diaphragm without the cup. You insert it into your vagina and it slowly releases estradiol at a rate of 7.5 μg (micrograms) daily. It can remain in place for three months before it needs changing. Women tell me that neither they nor their partners are aware of the ring during intercourse and that it is perfectly comfortable. The ring is easy to insert and remove, but if you feel uncomfortable doing so, you can either ask your partner or go to your doctor's office, where a nurse practitioner or physician can help you.

There have been no reported cases of toxic shock associated with the Estring, but if you feel anxious about keeping a "foreign object" in your vagina for a long period, you would probably prefer either tablets or creams.

▶ *Will vaginal estrogen keep my vagina in good shape?*

Although systemic estrogen is the best remedy for problems such as hot flashes, sleeplessness, and bone loss, vaginal estrogen is very effective for vaginal dryness. My observations of patients suggest that women who are not using oral estrogen tend to get more vaginitis and more bladder infections if their vagina is dry and atrophic, and I sometimes recommend vaginal estrogen cream for these women also. The cream is not intended as a lubricant for intercourse, because the consistency is not ideal. It is meant to help the cells lining the vaginal walls produce the lubricant that you need to be comfortable during intercourse.

▶ *Can all women with symptoms of vaginal dryness use a vaginal estrogen cream, tablets, or ring?*

These products are safe for virtually anyone because very little estrogen is absorbed into the bloodstream. Vaginal estrogen cream does remain in the vagina for a while (a day or a few days), and during this time the estrogen is absorbed through the vaginal walls, but the amount is much lower than the amount in oral estrogen or skin patches. With Vagifem tablets there seems to be even less absorption than from vaginal creams, and many women find the tablets more convenient and less messy than creams. With Estring, after the first twenty-four hours, almost no estrogen is absorbed. Oncologists sometimes recommend Vagifem and the Estring for women who have cancer and have undergone premature menopause, either through chemotherapy or through surgery.

> Brenda F. is thirty-three and has had breast cancer. Her oncologist has pursued the disease aggressively and prescribed chemotherapy to try to prevent recurrences. Chemotherapy often knocks out normal ovarian function, either temporarily or permanently, and consequently Brenda has undergone a kind of chemical menopause. Her oncologist does not approve of systemic hormone therapy because many breast cancers are stimulated by estrogen. Brenda is young and wants to be sexually active. Estrogen cream can be a big help to her, and her oncologist has no objection to it.

▶ How do I use vaginal estrogen cream?

The same pharmaceutical companies that make oral estrogen make the cream, and it comes in the same brand names (Premarin, Estrace, Ogen, and others). You apply it with an applicator, much like the applicators that accompany birth control creams, and insert it into the vagina two or three times a week at any time convenient for you. Bedtime is usually best, so that the cream doesn't leak out. If your own lubrication is not adequate even with the vaginal estrogen cream, you may also use a lubricant such as K-Y Jelly or the equivalent for intercourse itself.

▶ Can vaginal estrogen cream have any consequences for male sexual partners?

No, it is not dangerous to men even if it remains in your vagina during intercourse. It will not have feminizing effects on him.

▶ Do vaginal estrogen creams have side effects?

I have already suggested that because a small amount of vaginal estrogen cream is absorbed through the walls of the vagina, it can be helpful to women who have frequent bladder infections. It may also aid women with urinary incontinence.

Some women are allergic to certain brands of estrogen creams. The tissues of the vulva and vagina are very sensitive to allergens, and some women experience itching and burning. The cause of the trouble may not be the estrogen itself but the base in which it is dissolved. Since there are several brands, if one does not work, you can try another.

If you have not had intercourse for a long time, putting anything into your vagina may produce discomfort, even something normally nonallergenic such as K-Y Jelly. For women in this situation I sometimes do a little arm-twisting and suggest that they go on oral estrogen for a month to lubricate the vagina and replenish its cells enough so that they can then use topical estrogen cream.

▶ How much does estrogen cream cost?

Like any form of estrogen, these products are expensive. The cream costs something in the neighborhood of $95 a tube. The price differs from brand to brand. The Estring retails for about $135, and Vagifem costs about $75 for eighteen tablets.

▶ *Are there nonhormonal lubricants that can be used for vaginal dryness?*

There are lubricants for intercourse, which are satisfactory for the acute act; but for persistent vaginal dryness and the other complications that sometimes follow it (for example, vaginal infections or bladder infections), estrogen in some form is the best solution.

The products available for lubrication specifically during intercourse include H-R or K-Y Jelly or Lubrin, all of which are water soluble. Another excellent product is Astroglide, made in California. When Astroglide first came out, it was available only in that state and people had to send away for it; now it is widely available. Certain high-quality massage oils can also give short-term pleasure and relief from dryness; these can be purchased over the counter. Although they will not hurt you, Vaseline and other petroleum-based lubricants are less satisfactory because they are sticky and tend to dry the vaginal tissues.

If you don't want to try any form of estrogen, the leading nonhormonal cream for all-day lubrication is called Replens. Although it can be used for intercourse, it is not intended for that purpose. Replens appears to augment surface fluids in the vagina without stimulation by estrogen. You apply it three times a week on a regular basis, not just before intercourse. The manufacturer's literature mentions scientific studies suggesting that the product does increase vaginal lubrication without hormonal therapy.

Many health food stores carry products advertised for vaginal lubrication, and some women find that these work well for them. Although there are no significant data showing that these products work, they do not seem to product unpleasant side effects. In Europe, vaginal soy products are available and quite popular. Again, we don't have data on their effectiveness, but the risk of adverse effects is small.

▶ *If I am on oral HRT and still have lubrication problems, is it all right to use a commercial lubricant?*

Certainly; you can use K-Y Jelly or Astroglide or other products. Many of my patients find this solution satisfactory.

SEXUAL DESIRE AND RESPONSIVENESS

If you notice that you are less interested in sex and less sexually responsive than you used to be, you are not alone. It is a common problem during the peri- and postmenopausal years. No one knows exactly what hormones are responsible for sexual desire, and some researchers believe that libido is wholly brain-driven without hormonal involvement.

Most researchers, however, believe that the hormones estrogen, testosterone, and dehydroepiandrosterone (DHEA) do play a role in this complex response.

▶ *Are there changes in female sexual responsiveness in middle age that are unrelated to vaginal discomfort?*

Some women notice changes about the time of menopause that are not related to vaginal discomfort. They feel fine and sex is comfortable for them physically, but they notice that their sexual desire and their response to sexual stimulation have changed significantly. Perhaps they have less interest in sex, or when they do have sex they find it less enjoyable. They will say that they have no more flushes or other symptoms of menopause, but they have no interest in sex.

Remember that estrogen is a vasodilator. There is strong evidence that estrogen profoundly enhances blood flow to the pelvis as well as to other organs, including the brain. Progesterone, in contrast, may limit pelvic blood flow. Therefore many postmenopausal women who lack estrogen do notice a change in how they feel during sexual activity. This difference may have something to do with their lack of vascular engorgement in the pelvis.

▶ *Can estrogen therapy increase sexual desire?*

When someone comes to me distressed because she has lost her sexual desire, I often suggest a month or two of estrogen alone without progesterone. Such a short regimen is not going to hurt her; the worst that can happen is that it won't help. If it doesn't, she can simply stop taking it. If the ERT does help, she can decide whether she wants to continue with it.

▶ *Does testosterone increase sexual desire in women?*

The role of testosterone in mediating sexual drive in women is one of the controversial topics in gynecology today. Suppose someone comes to the office, concerned about her loss of desire, concerned about her partner and their sex life. She and her partner are getting along well; the cause of her lack of libido probably is not psychological or social. We try hormone therapy, and although it improves her performance a little by making her more comfortable, she really would like to be more sexually interested. At this point I might suggest testosterone.

A lot of libido, however, is emotional, social, psychological—whatever you wish to call it. Testosterone will not solve lack of desire if you are angry at your partner or he is angry at you, or if you feel that you are getting old and unattractive, or if your partner is becoming unattractive to you because he has put on fifty pounds and is out drinking beer with the boys all the time. If your previous basis for communication was limited to your children and they are out of the house now so you and your husband don't talk to each other, if he comes home and reads the paper or turns on the television while you talk to your pals on the telephone, testosterone is not going to help. If, however, the roots of your lack of desire are physiological, or physiological and emotional jointly, then it may well make a difference.

Some researchers, both physicians and psychologists, feel that testosterone increases sexual desire in women and also promotes a sense of well-being. Some studies show that it increases sexual desire, yet other papers in the scientific literature dispute that finding. My feeling is that the majority of practicing gynecologists would say yes, testosterone probably does increase libido. Among my patients who try it, about half say that it makes a big difference for them.

One of the arguments behind the belief that testosterone does not increase libido is that birth control pills lower a woman's testosterone production. A woman who is taking birth control pills has very little testosterone. But most women on the pill still have reasonably normal sex lives. Even though their endogenous testosterone production is low, their libido is intact. The whole issue is murky and complex.

As with the estrogen, I suggest that people give testosterone a three-month trial. If it does not work for you, you can stop taking it.

▶ Will taking testosterone make women masculine?

The first thing I usually hear when I suggest testosterone is something like, "Testosterone, that's the male hormone!" My standard counter is that yes, it is a male hormone, but women make it too—just as estrogen is a female hormone, but men make some also.

The dosages of testosterone that are generally given to improve libido are minuscule. They range from 1.25 to 2.5 mg of methyltestosterone, which really shouldn't masculinize anyone. Testosterone is sometimes prescribed for men, to improve libido or sexual performance, but in far greater doses; if a man were to take only 1.25 to 2.5 mg, he would not notice any change at all.

Most women who take testosterone don't notice any masculinizing effects. However, the symptoms that too much testosterone could cause are facial hair growth, acne, and deepening of the voice. Some women are very sensitive to testosterone and get hair growth rather quickly; for them, the dosage level is crucial. In general, though, if these masculinizing effects take place, they do so slowly and gradually. You won't wake up one morning with a full growth of beard.

On the other hand, many older women get unwanted facial hair even when they are not taking exogenous testosterone. The reason is that our ovaries continue to make small amounts of testosterone even when they are no longer producing estrogen.

▶ Can I take testosterone to enhance desire if I am interested in preserving fertility?

Testosterone is not an appropriate drug for women who are concerned about fertility. Although it may enhance desire, it may also have masculinizing effects on a fetus.

▶ Is testosterone related to anabolic steroids?

Testosterone is a kind of cousin of the anabolic steroids, which some athletes take (illegally) to increase muscle development and athletic performance. The side effects of the two are very different. Testosterone will not give you brain cancer; nor in the dosages we are talking about will it give you the kind of physique we see in muscle-building magazines. In fact, the male athletes who take anabolic steroids turn out to have very low testosterone levels because the steroids block their own production of testosterone. Many athletes who take steroids are sterile, a condition that is sometimes reversible and sometimes not.

▶ Do masculinizing side effects go away when women stop taking testosterone?

Probably in one or two months of testosterone therapy, you will not notice an effect as profound as facial hair. But if you should grow facial hair, it will not disappear spontaneously when you stop the testosterone. New growth of facial hair will stop, however.

▶ Will taking testosterone increase my risk of heart attack?

Although plenty of evidence shows that premenopausal women are less at risk for heart disease than men in the same age group, researchers do not yet know the precise role of testosterone in this statistical picture. In the dosages that we are talking about for libido enhancement, testosterone does not seem to have a significant effect on blood lipids or increase a menopausal woman's chances of having a heart attack.

▶ *In what ways can I take testosterone?*

Like progesterone, pure testosterone does not get well absorbed orally, so several methods have been devised to deliver it. One is a process called methylation, which is similar to the way progesterone is treated so that it can be absorbed. Methyltestosterone does get absorbed from the digestive system, but you cannot take it in high doses because it is toxic to your liver. In addition, the doses that would affect your liver would also give you other unwanted side effects such as facial hair. So methyltestosterone is usually prescribed in tiny doses.

Often testosterone is prescribed in conjunction with estrogen, so estrogen products are manufactured in combination with testosterone. Of the two basic varieties, one is a preparation called Estratest. It has a very small amount of testosterone added to the kind of estrogen used in Premarin. The dosage in Estratest is 1.25 mg of estrogen plus 2.5 mg of methyltestosterone. In another preparation called Estratest HS, the HS stands for half-strength. That is, the estrogen is 0.625 mg with 1.25 mg of methyltestosterone added. This is really the smallest amount that can have any noticeable effect on libido. Its side effects have been well studied, and the company that produces it will be happy to send you literature showing that this minuscule level of testosterone has no significant masculinizing effects and, more important, rarely affects the liver.

Another possibility is testosterone gel, which can be applied to the skin. Although a great deal of the testosterone is not absorbed, enough passes through the skin to help people with libido problems. No liver damage results, first because the cream is rubbed into the skin and thus bypasses the liver, and second because the hormone in these preparations is natural testosterone, not a methylated compound. Topical testosterone applied to the skin can also be used for lichen sclerosus et atrophicus, a vulvar disease. To use it, you dab a little on your skin once a day. You may find this process easier and more pleasant than receiving an injection every four to six weeks. Natural testosterone cream is not readily available commercially, however, so you and your physician may need to search around to find a pharmacist who will make up a testosterone gel in a 1 or 2 percent form.

Androgel is a commercially produced transdermal testosterone gel. It was originally developed for men who do not produce enough of this hormone on their own. Women can use Androgel, but they should apply no more than a quarter of a 2.5-gram packet daily by rubbing it on the skin of the lower abdomen. Testosterone cream or gel should be used daily; these products don't seem to work on an "as-needed" basis, so you can't just use them on Saturday night, for example.

A testosterone patch for women is under development; it will offer lower doses than those available for men.

If these options don't work for you, or you do not want to take methyltestosterone by mouth because you are concerned about liver damage or because you have had hepatitis, injectable testosterone can be used. In some parts of the United States, particularly in the South, it has been popular for years. Men who take testosterone because their own production has decreased get it in shot form. To maintain masculinization, to keep their beard, low voice, and other male characteristics, they would have to take an amount of oral testosterone that could be toxic to the liver. Because the injectable form of testosterone is natural, it does not affect the liver. One disadvantage is that the shots must be taken every four to six weeks.

An anecdote went around a meeting of the North American Menopause Society, a professional organization of physicians and researchers dealing with problems surrounding menopause. A physician forgot to warn some of his patients that he was going on vacation for two weeks. The women who were due for their shots were apparently calling the office to find out when he would return. According to him, or his patients, the testosterone made them feel so good that they missed it when they did not have it.

▶ *Once I start taking testosterone, how long must I continue?*

If you are taking testosterone to enhance libido and it seems to work for you, then you can take it for as long as you want; if it doesn't work for you, you can just stop. I have some patients who vary the routine to suit their needs. If they decide they want more libido, they take their testosterone; when they don't want more libido, they don't take it. So I have some women who take three Premarin and three Estratest tablets a week—that is, three tablets of estrogen alone and three tablets of estrogen-plus-testosterone. In short, they are mixing and matching.

Some sexology experts suggest that you should give these products a three-month trial, since it may take that long to see the full response. If testosterone doesn't work for you during this trial period, continuing its use beyond then probably won't help.

▶ *Does alternative medicine offer approaches to improving libido?*

In recent years attention has been focused on dehydroepiandrosterone, known as DHEA. About forty years ago, Dr. Emile Baulieu, better known for his work on the abortion drug RU 486, began to look at the role of DHEA as an anti-aging hormone. We do know that this hormone is synthesized by the adrenal gland and that its levels in both men and women fall over the course of a lifetime, with significant declines starting as early as the thirties. In the past physicians worried about potential risks associated with DHEA replacement, especially cardiovascular disease and cancer, but these concerns have decreased. Studies on DHEA replacement seem to show increased feelings of well-being and heightened libido.

DHEA blood levels can be measured. If yours are low, you might ask your caregiver about trying DHEA. You can buy it inexpensively as an over-the-counter preparation. Ask your pharmacist, naturopath, or a knowledgeable person in your health food store about locally available brands to find which come from a reliable source. Some practitioners feel that the Schiff brand is reliable. As with all alternative medicines, be sure to tell your caregiver that you are taking DHEA. Remember that because the FDA does not regulate complementary medicines, you cannot be sure of their potency or safety.

Standard replacement doses are 25 to 50 mg daily. As with testosterone, give DHEA a three-month chance to see if it helps you.

There are also some approaches to loss of libido that do not involve medicines. The FDA has approved a device called Eros CSD (clitoral stimulation device), which has a small handheld vacuum device attached to tubing that ends in a cup that fits around the clitoris. The device creates a mini-vacuum at the clitoris, which increases blood flow to the clitoris and vulva and thus enhances sexual responsiveness. It has helped women who have had radical pelvic surgery (for example, for cervical cancer) and whose blood flow to the pelvis in general has been diminished.

The Eros CSD costs several hundred dollars and is available only by prescription. Some insurance companies cover its cost because it is used to treat female sexual dysfunction.

▶ *Is there such a thing as male menopause?*

Yes and no. Men certainly experience physical changes, including changes in hormone production, just as women do. Valid studies show that testosterone production decreases in men over time, but the drop is much more gradual than the profound drop of estrogen production in women during their forties and fifties. Spermatogenesis, the production of sperm, decreases gradually in men. They don't make as many sperm, or as many viable sperm, as they get older; but they do continue to make some sperm into their seventies.

Certainly the physical changes of menopause have social ramifications for women. And to some extent the same is true of men. Both men and women face midlife social changes that may affect their attitudes or their self-image, but in my experience, those that women face are more profound and difficult. Yes, the man's mother is getting older, but usually his wife or sister is taking care of her. Yes, his children are reproducing and occasionally Grandpa takes care of them, but usually the chore is delegated to Grandma. Women face problems relative to rejoining the workforce, but men have been in the workforce for years and found their place in it.

Both men and women feel the pressure to look young and physically attractive, but again the pressure on women seems greater. Men are considered attractive at older ages than women, particularly if they have money or power. Even in the movie star set (a group of people selected in large part because they are more physically attractive than your average Jane or Joe), men have an easier time of it. There is no female counterpart on the screen, for example, of Harrison Ford.

So although we are all aware of the male midlife crisis, which might be the social equivalent of female menopause, in general men have fewer issues to deal with.

▶ *What about male sexuality in midlife?*

Over time, testosterone production decreases in men. This fact may express itself in decreased sexual desire. Men may take more time to achieve an erection and the erection may not be as firm as it used to be. Or men may be slower to ejaculate. These changes may be exacerbated by certain diseases that make it difficult for men to have intercourse as they age: high blood pressure, cardiac disease, angina, diabetes, and prostate problems. Men with any of these diseases can have problems with getting and maintaining erections, that is, the disease itself causes the difficulties. Another contributing factor, however, is the medication given for the disease. Many drugs that block elevated blood pressure can also block sexual performance. In general they do not block desire, but they do block the ability to achieve an erection.

It is difficult to miss the fact that Viagra, a drug that enhances sexual performance but not sexual desire, has changed the playing field for many men. Since "the little blue pill" was introduced in 1998 by Pfizer, more than ten million men have taken it. It has been endorsed by athletes (NASCAR driver Mark Martin and Texas Rangers' first base-man Rafael Palmeiro) and other notables ranging from the respectable Bob Dole to the self-styled sexual celebrity Hugh Hefner. A new anti-impotence drug, Levitra, came out in 2003 and is being promoted by former Chicago Bears coach Mike Ditka. Another Via-gra rival, Cialis, has appeared on the market. Eli Lilly, the manufacturer, asserts that Cialis is effective for thirty-six hours, instead of four or five. In Europe it's called the "weekend drug" since a Friday-night dose will last until Sunday.

▶ What prescription drugs can interfere with sexual performance?

A number of commonly used prescription drugs can inhibit sexual performance, both in men and in women. Among the most common are antihypertensives, that is, drugs that combat high blood pressure. Others are beta-blockers, used in cardiac disease and to treat angina and rhythmic disturbances of the heart, as well as high blood pressure.

Certain drugs prescribed for high blood pressure seem to block orgasmic response in women as well as men. Some women find that their response to sexual stimulation is less-ened or just seems different. This reaction is uncommon but can be troubling.

SSRIs (selective serotonin reuptake inhibitors), often given for depression, can also decrease libido and performance in both men and women. Of course, depression itself can seriously compromise sexual desire. There are ways to get around the problem if the medication and not the depression is responsible. Some SSRIs are worse than others in this respect, so talk to your doctor and see about switching to see whether another SSRI has the same effect. Another option might be Wellbutrin (buproprion), an antidepres-sant but not an SSRI, which does not seem to depress libido. Some doctors may prescribe Wellbutrin along with an SSRI.

▶ What can be done for men whose medications decrease sexual interest or performance?

If you are concerned about the effect of antihypertensive drugs on your partner's sexual performance, you might talk to his internist. Often men are unwilling to call their physi-cian and say, "Look, I can't get an erection on this medication you gave me." Yet a tele-phone call is all that is needed. Dozens of drugs exist for lowering blood pressure. If one causes unwanted side effects, another one may control blood pressure without giving him an erectile problem.

If it is the disease itself and not the medication that causes the trouble, urologists are available who are skilled in the treatment of male dysfunction, and treatments are available ranging from the simple to the complex. Simplest are the oral medications, including Viagra, that help produce an erection. Or chemicals can be injected into the base of the penis with a very small needle, which will cause an erection even if the man's blood supply to the penis is marginal. The man injects himself before intercourse, like a diabetic taking insulin. The nickname for the three drugs (papaverine, phentolamine, and prostaglandins) in this medication is PEP.

In addition to these drugs, there are mechanical options. Implantable pumps can be placed into the penis surgically. They use fluid as a means to pump up the penis.

▶ What about Viagra for women?

Some doctors have tried Viagra with women experimentally, with mixed response. Unless you have cardiac disease, trying it is a reasonable thought, particularly if orgasmic response has been an issue for you.

▶ Will testosterone increase libido in men?

Sometimes patients complain that their husband or partner has a lower libido than they do. The husband is not taking antihypertensives; he has no prostate problem; he can perform just fine—but he has little interest in sex.

This is a question for male urology experts. Certainly there are physicians who prescribe testosterone for men to see whether it enhances their sexual performance. But in the doses that men require, physicians need to address such issues as blood lipid levels.

▶ What about sex after my partner has had a heart attack?

Almost all cardiac rehabilitation programs address this important issue. Occasionally someone with end-stage coronary artery disease probably should not have intercourse, but in general, once a person has recuperated from a heart attack, intercourse is quite all right. You should check with your partner's cardiologist that he has recovered sufficiently and that there is no reason to be afraid of strenuous sexual activity. Remember that Viagra can exacerbate cardiac problems, so men should consult their cardiologists before trying it.

As a gynecologist, I am frequently asked, "Will my husband have another heart attack if he gets sexually aroused?" I cannot answer that question; only the cardiologist who knows the degree of damage caused by the previous heart attack can assess that individual. Usually after a man is fully rehabilitated, there is no reason he can't engage in full sexual activity.

If your husband or partner is not willing to raise the question with his cardiologist, you can certainly call the doctor yourself. Ask how much sexual activity is safe for your husband.

▶ Is sex safe for women who have had heart attacks?

Again, check with your cardiologist. If you are getting on your treadmill and working out, if you are out walking, there is probably no reason not to have sex.

12 Fibroids, Incontinence, Itching, and Other Midlife Annoyances

CERTAIN gynecological discomforts accompany middle age, no matter how healthy your habits, and can be classified as annoyances rather than as life-threatening illnesses. Among these problems are fibroids, incontinence, and vaginal itching. Although your mother may have been forced to put up with some of these difficulties, you may well be spared.

FIBROIDS

Called myomas in medical terminology, fibroids are technically defined as exuberant growths of the smooth muscle wall of the uterus. In this context "exuberant" merely means an excessive growth of basically normal tissue; the tissue grows too much, but there is nothing pathologically wrong with it.

At least one in four women past thirty has fibroids. It is important to emphasize that more than 99 percent of the time they are benign. They are not life threatening, and they won't harm you in any absolute sense. But they can make you bleed and give you pain. They can also cause infertility, which may be of concern to a small proportion of women who are approaching menopause. About 20 to 40 percent of women have fibroids by the time they are menopausal, with black women having a slightly higher frequency than white women.

▶ How big are fibroids?

Fibroids come in sizes ranging from that of a pea to that of a small watermelon, to use common round objects as a basis of comparison. Physicians speak of them in terms of the size of a uterus during pregnancy: the size of a two-month pregnancy (comparable to a tennis ball) or a three-month pregnancy (comparable to a grapefruit). Often fibroids occur in groups, and women who have one fibroid are likely to have several.

▶ Do fibroids grow slowly or quickly?

Fibroids can behave very erratically. Sometimes they appear suddenly, grow gradually to their maximum size, and remain that way forever. Other times they appear, jump to the size of a three-month pregnancy, remain that way for five years, then suddenly change again.

▶ What causes fibroids?

No one knows precisely what triggers the growth of fibroids, though we do know that they are definitely estrogen dependent. Perhaps fluctuation in estrogen levels may play a role in their appearance. Since their growth is related to the presence of estrogen, fibroids tend to shrink or disappear when a woman goes through menopause and her estrogen levels fall.

▶ At what age do women usually develop fibroids?

Fibroids can begin at any age. The youngest woman on whom I ever operated for fibroids was about twenty-three, but she was an exception. From the midtwenties on, the incidence of fibroids increases with age until menopause. Because they are estrogen dependent, fibroids do not ordinarily appear after menopause. Often they appear during the perimenopause, perhaps in response to fluctuating estrogen levels.

Fibroids are so common that it is hard to determine whether there is a familial tendency toward them. There are no other known risk factors, so it is difficult to predict who will get them and who will not.

▶ How can I tell whether I have fibroids?

You can have fibroids without realizing it, because they may not produce symptoms. The symptoms of fibroids are heavy bleeding during periods, pelvic pressure, the need to urinate frequently, backaches, and constipation. But you may have some or all of these symptoms without actually having fibroids since they can be indicative of other conditions.

▶ How can fibroids be diagnosed by a physician?

Your physician can discover fibroids during a bimanual (two-handed) pelvic examination. The physician places two fingers of one hand in the vagina and the other on top of the belly and palpates, or feels, the fibroid. What the physician is actually feeling is, not a lump in the uterus, but a changed contour of the uterus. Mentally the physician will compare the way the uterus feels with the way it would feel if you were pregnant, to get an estimation of size.

Fibroids can also be diagnosed through an ultrasound procedure, which is often used to confirm that what the physician is feeling is indeed the uterus with its fibroids and not a growth on an ovary. More sophisticated methods, such as MRI (magnetic resonance imaging) and CT scanning, can be used to diagnose fibroids, but these tests are more expensive and expose you to more radiation than ultrasound. Ultrasound is preferable and is usually an adequate diagnostic tool.

▶ What symptoms do fibroids cause?

Depending on their size and location, fibroids can cause symptoms varying from none to significant pelvic discomfort, including belly pain or a sense of pressure on the bladder or bowel. Many women who have fibroids feel that they have to go to the bathroom every ten minutes. If the fibroids become sufficiently large and are sitting on the ureters (the tubes that join the kidneys and the bladder), they can exert enough pressure to cause compression of the kidneys or force the urine backward, which can lead to serious problems. If they are pressing on the rectum, they will cause changes in bowel habits, for example constipation or a feeling of fullness.

Fibroids can also cause bleeding, generally in the form of heavier periods; occasionally they cause bleeding between periods. Although many women with fibroids do not experience heavy bleeding, this is the main reason women with fibroids decide to have them removed.

Fibroids can cause backaches, especially during the luteal or second half of the menstrual cycle, when there is increasing edema, or fluid retention, in the pelvis. Occasionally fibroids cause severe pain, classically when they are "degenerating."

I have had patients with fibroids literally the size of small watermelons who were annoyed at me for wanting them to have the fibroids removed. These women felt fine and had no bleeding or other distressing symptoms. I have had other patients with very small fibroids who were extremely uncomfortable.

▶ Where in the uterus do fibroids grow?

Fibroids can be on the inner surface of the uterus, in the middle portion of the uterine wall, or on the outside. Some are a combination of all three. There are names for each lo-

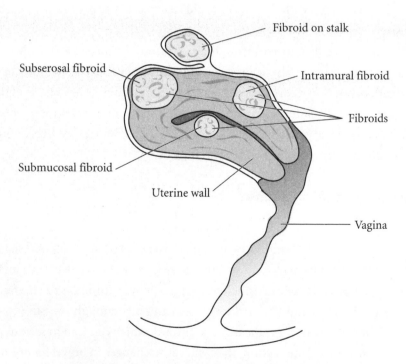

FIGURE 14. Uterine fibroids can occur anywhere in the uterus or may be attached to its surface by a stalk.

cation. The outer part of the uterus is called the serosa; fibroids in this area are called sub-serosal. Those in the uterine wall (*mur* is the Latin word for "wall") are called intramural fibroids. The mucosa is the inner lining of the uterine cavity, and these fibroids are called submucosal fibroids.

If your fibroid is growing off the back wall of your uterus and pressing toward your back, you will probably have a backache. If it is a posterior fibroid pressing on the rectum, you may well experience constipation.

The patients walking around with a baby-watermelon-size object inside, who were angry at me for proposing surgery, have subserosal fibroids. The fibroid is external to the uterine cavity; it is not troublesome; it is just there. Subserosal fibroids are the least symptomatic and they seldom cause bleeding problems because they are outside the main action site of the uterus. Women with erratic bleeding usually have submucosal fibroids, which can cause problems even though they are only a half-inch in diameter.

▶ *Why do fibroids cause heavy periods or other bleeding?*

No one knows exactly. But most people believe that in such a case the fibroid is breaking up the integrity of the uterine lining. Because of this disruption, the bleeding is heavy and erratic.

▶ *What is a degenerating fibroid?*

Basically a fibroid can "degenerate," or collapse on itself, if it has outgrown its blood supply. Like muscle tissue, fibroid tissue needs oxygen. When it fails to get an adequate supply, the fibroid can cause severe ischemic pain. It is the same kind of pain you get when you have uterine cramps, but more severe. Once the fibroid degenerates, the tissue gradually disappears and the pain ceases. The process of degeneration usually lasts for several days, though not for several weeks or months.

Phyllis L., who came to me for her gynecological checkups for a number of years, started experiencing significant abdominal pain rather suddenly when she was in her late forties. She saw her internist, a very good doctor, who thought her problem was appendicitis—but he wasn't sure because her symptoms did not fit those of classic appendicitis.

She went to one of the best surgeons in town, who also thought she had appendicitis, though he agreed that her symptoms were not the ordinary ones.

Her abdominal pain got so bad that she went to the emergency room of the local hospital. Since I was her regular gynecologist, she asked if I could examine her, and I came to the emergency room before her surgery.

There was a lump on the right side of her uterus, without question, and her uterus was tender. The lump was not far from where her appendix would be located. I knew she had a fibroid in that area because I had examined her previously. At this point we did an ultrasound and visualized her fibroid, right where she was feeling the pain. We decided that her problem was a degenerating fibroid and we elected to treat her conservatively and give her pain medication. She stayed in bed for a couple of days and improved. When I reexamined her in my office some time later, the fibroid had disappeared. She has been fine ever since.

The phenomenon of degenerating fibroids is not uncommon in perimenopausal women, but occasionally a fibroid will degenerate during a pregnancy, and again the situation is very uncomfortable. The only therapy during pregnancy is conservative: ride it out with bed rest and pain medication.

▶ What is a prolapsed fibroid?

On rare occasions a fibroid may prolapse, or fall down, into the uterus. Most fibroids are merely little lumps, but sometimes they are on stalks that are called pedicles. If a fibroid on a pedicle prolapses, the uterus may try to expel it; but since the fibroid is attached to the uterine wall, the whole uterus tends to come along with the fibroid. The woman feels contractions like labor; her cervix actually dilates and thins out. The treatment can be either to remove the fibroid from its stalk or to perform a hysterectomy.

▶ Can fibroids become cancerous?

Although it is possible for fibroids to undergo "malignant degeneration," it is extremely rare. The possibility of a fibroid's becoming malignant is so remote that it is not one of the major reasons for hysterectomy. In terms of relative risk, having a fibroid removed because some day in the future it might become cancerous is like refusing to drive a car because some day in the future you might be killed in a crash.

▶ *Do fibroids always lead to hysterectomy?*

Fibroids certainly are the most common indication for hysterectomy in the United States. Just because you have a fibroid, you are not an instant candidate for a hysterectomy, however.

If your doctor discovers that you have a fibroid and it is asymptomatic or not causing significant discomfort, he or she will probably ask you to come back in four to six months to see whether the situation is stable. If the fibroid is not growing or changing, then examinations will probably be scheduled at a wider interval.

▶ *Are there guidelines to how large fibroids should be allowed to grow before removing them?*

A common criterion suggests that the size of a three-month pregnancy (equivalent to a grapefruit) is probably the largest your pelvis can accommodate without danger or discomfort. When a fibroid grows to the size of a four-month pregnancy (a cantaloupe), it may start pressing significantly on other organs. Usually at that point the woman is aware of its presence and may be quite uncomfortable.

Physicians begin to differ in opinion when the mass reaches the size of a grapefruit. My position is that anything larger than a cantaloupe, or four-month pregnancy, should come out. It is difficult to believe that any woman can be comfortable with a mass the size of a five-month pregnancy (or a honeydew melon) in her belly. She may have gotten used to the feeling and be able to put up with it, but it can't be comfortable. The more serious issue is that at this size the mass may well be compromising her ureters, the tubes from the bladder to the kidney.

Opinion on the size fibroid that must be removed surgically varies from gynecologist to gynecologist. Some physicians say you should have a hysterectomy if you have a fibroid the size of a two-month pregnancy; but since there is plenty of space in the pelvis for a mass the size of a tennis ball or even a small grapefruit, you probably don't have to have surgery for a fibroid this size unless you have significant discomfort. If your physician does tell you that you have a mass the size of a two-month pregnancy and that you should have a hysterectomy, it is advisable to get a second opinion. I would like to say that in the area where I practice no unnecessary hysterectomies are performed, but I cannot assert that with total confidence. If size seems to be your doctor's sole criterion for the prospective hysterectomy and you are in doubt, get a second opinion.

Another indication for hysterectomy is rapid growth of the fibroid. If a pelvic examination turns up a mass the size of a two-month pregnancy, and three months later that mass has grown to sixteen-week size, there may be cause for concern. What could be growing in the uterus might be not a benign fibroid but a malignant tumor. Although sarcomas of the uterus are rare, they can occur. The only way to make sure that the mass is benign is to take it out and to examine every bit of it under a microscope.

The other criteria depend on the individual woman, her symptoms, and her response to them. If you are at the point where you can't tolerate the heavy bleeding any longer, or if you have gotten tired of having to urinate every twenty minutes and find that it interferes with your life, then you may elect to have a hysterectomy. If you have a backache that appears at midcycle and continues until your next period, you may well want a hysterectomy to relieve you of the pain. But these decisions are highly individual, and only you can make them.

▶ Will HRT cause fibroids to grow?

No, probably not. Remember that the amount of estrogen you take in hormone therapy is significantly less than what your own ovaries make endogenously during your premenopausal years. If you look at the estradiol levels in normal menstrual women, they range between 50 and 400 pg/ml during the menstrual cycle, which is quite a wide range. In menopausal women on HRT, the range is 50 to 80. So the menopausal woman who is happy walking around all month with an estradiol level of 50 has significantly less estrogen than the premenopausal woman who has a level of 50 for part of the month and a level of 400 for another part of the month.

Most women with fibroids can take HRT, though their physician should watch them to be sure the estrogen is not stimulating the fibroids to new growth. This follow-up is especially important during the first years of estrogen therapy because there is no way of knowing how an individual woman's particular fibroid will respond.

On occasion, however, women with fibroids can't take estrogen because their fibroids are stimulated by even a tiny amount of estrogen.

> Vicki W. is an active and intelligent woman, the owner of a travel agency. She is absolutely miserable without estrogen, in terms of her personality and her mental outlook and her physical comfort. Even my office staff can notice the difference. When she is not taking estrogen, she has been known to call the office, get angry over the telephone, and yell at staff members; the minute she starts taking the estrogen again, she calls back and apologizes.

For psychological reasons Vicki functions much better on estrogen. Unfortunately, she has fibroids. They are fairly small, ten- to twelve-week size at most, and on grounds of size there is no reason at all to take them out. But their location in the uterine wall makes them basically not removable without a hysterectomy.

Vicki is fully menopausal and therefore makes no estrogen on her own. I tried giving her estrogen without progesterone, but she developed hyperplasia; the lining of her uterus built up and built up, so eventually I had to give her progesterone, which makes her bleed.

So the question becomes, which is the worse evil? Should she feel wretched without the estrogen, having hot flashes all the time and feeling angry and upset? Or should she be bleeding heavily? There is no answer. My guess is that eventually she will opt for a hysterectomy. Her travel business takes her into many out-of-the-way spots. In fact, the last time she had a period, she was vacationing in the Virgin Islands. The decision is ultimately hers; she alone must decide that her Jekyll-and-Hyde personality and the discomfort of heavy bleeding disrupt her life so much that she wants to have a hysterectomy and continue her ERT.

▶ *If I have one fibroid, am I at increased risk for developing more?*

Unfortunately, women who have one fibroid are likely to develop others later on. This may be an important consideration if you are thinking about surgery and trying to decide between removal of the fibroid and removal of the entire uterus along with the fibroid.

Medical Treatments for Fibroids

The key decision with fibroids is whether to intervene at all. It may be difficult for Americans, who are used to getting things done, to accept nonintervention, to accept having a fibroid and not trying to make it better, but often this is a wise choice. Biologically speaking, it is a kind of peaceful coexistence. If the fibroid doesn't bother you, if it isn't growing rapidly, and if it is smaller than a grapefruit, then leave it alone.

One of the easiest and least interventionist treatments for fibroids is menopause. Since fibroids flourish and thrive on estrogen, they tend to shrink during the perimenopausal period when the ovaries are producing very little estrogen. Fibroids often disappear after menopause.

Another treatment, which mimics menopause, is the use of GnRH agonists (chemicals that act like GnRH). The GnRH stands for "gonadotropin-releasing hormone," and in the body this hormone is produced in the hypothalamus. During the normal menstrual cycle, gonadotropin-releasing hormone controls the pituitary gland so that it secretes the right amounts of follicle-stimulating hormone (FSH) and luteinizing hormone (LH) at the right time; these hormones in turn contribute to the production of estrogen. Basically, GnRH agonists wipe out your estrogen production, and by depriving fibroids of estrogen you can control their growth. One of the most familiar of these drugs is Lupron, given as a monthly injection and often also used as a medication to control endometriosis. One of the first physicians to use Lupron for fibroids was Andrew Friedman, who showed that within three months, estrogen-deprived fibroids would shrink significantly, often to about half their former size. Unfortunately, when you stop taking the Lupron, your estrogen levels return and the fibroids are apt to grow back to their previous size.

> Anita D., forty-four, came to me with fibroids that had enlarged from the size of a grapefruit to the size of a substantial honeydew in less than a year. She decided to take Lupron to see whether it would control this rapid fibroid growth. After about three months the fibroids regressed, but the minute she stopped taking Lupron, her fibroids began growing again. Within two months they had reached their former size. Her periods once again were miserable, with heavy flooding. Her fibroids were so large that when she walked into the office I could see the change in the size of her abdomen. Eventually she had to have a hysterectomy.

▶ *Can I take Lupron or another GnRH agonist for a long period?*

Lupron has its drawbacks, so you cannot remain on it forever. The first drawback is cost, which as we have seen can be more than five hundred dollars a month. Second, Lupron is like menopause. Because it lowers estrogen levels, it causes all the consequences of menopause. In particular, doctors are concerned about osteoporosis: it has been shown that women who stay on Lupron for more than six months at a stretch begin to encounter bone problems. Women who take Lupron for a shorter time do not seem to have these difficulties. Presumably by taking Lupron you also lose the benefits of estrogen to your cardiovascular system, but it is osteoporosis that has been the concern of researchers.

Because of the adverse effects of Lupron on bone and on cholesterol, some physicians have decided on what is called add-back therapy. That is, they shut down ovarian function and estrogen production with Lupron, then add back a touch of estrogen as if they were giving estrogen replacement therapy. Although this approach preserves bone, it does not give optimal suppression of the fibroid.

For some people Lupron can be a real solution. Recall Cathy H., who found herself bleeding heavily in the supermarket one day during perimenopause. This incident occurred when she was forty-eight or forty-nine; with six months on Lupron, she has done well. Her endogenous estrogen levels declined enough so that her fibroids shrank, even though she still has them. She also still has some menstrual periods, but they are infrequent and not very heavy. The Lupron seems to have seen her through a dangerous time when her estrogen levels were fluctuating rather wildly.

▶ Will taking Lupron postpone menopause?

No. If you take Lupron for six months, it will not delay your menopause for six months.

▶ Will birth control pills help fibroids?

Women with fibroids seem to have very individual responses to birth control pills. Some physicians believe that birth control pills increase fibroid growth; others say their use makes no difference whatsoever to fibroid growth. Some patients who have heavy bleeding seem to do very well on birth control pills, although the pill does not shrink the fibroid. Because birth control pills contain progestin as well as estrogen, the progesterone may help control the stimulation from the estrogen. The bottom line is that we don't know the exact relationship between birth control pills and fibroids. Therefore women with fibroids who take the pill, for whatever reason, need to be monitored.

Nonsurgical Techniques for Treating Fibroids

Uterine artery embolization and cryoablation are two techniques for treating fibroids that, though more invasive than watchful waiting, birth control pills, or Lupron, are less interventional than a hysterectomy or myomectomy, the major surgical techniques.

Uterine artery embolization, a technique developed within the past five years, works by starving fibroids of their blood supply. Performed by an interventional radiologist, this procedure involves guiding a thin tube or catheter into the uterine blood vessels that supply the fibroid and then injecting a "plug" made of a solid alcohol substance into the vessels. The plug causes a blood clot, depriving the fibroid of its nourishment, artificially creating a degenerating fibroid.

This procedure has drawbacks. It is painful. The fibroid shrinks but doesn't disappear altogether. There is a risk of infection. Because it lowers the blood supply to the uterus, uterine artery embolization is not appropriate for women who wish to become pregnant.

> Jane W., age forty, has fibroids that cause her to bleed heavily, so much so that her hematocrit, which should be in the range of 40, is sometimes as low as 20. Her religion prohibits blood transfusions, and because she weighs more than three hundred pounds, surgery would be far too dangerous in any case. Since she is still some distance from menopause, when her fibroids might shrink on their own, she decided that uterine artery embolization would be acceptable to her beliefs and had the procedure successfully. Her bleeding has dramatically diminished and her hematocrit has risen to the mid-30s.

Another relatively new approach involves cryosurgery. The procedure involves inserting a frozen needle into the fibroid and freezing the tissue surrounding the needle, thus killing the fibroid cells. The technique works best for small fibroids; if the growth is large, the frozen needle may have to be inserted again and again.

Myomectomy versus Hysterectomy: The Surgical Options

Several surgical procedures are available for removing fibroids. The most familiar is the hysterectomy. Another procedure is the myomectomy, in which the fibroid is removed but the uterus remains more or less intact. Traditionally, myomectomies are performed with an abdominal incision, but new procedures have been developed using a hysteroscope or a laparoscope. They are appropriate for removing some but not all fibroids. If the fibroids can be removed with the hysteroscope or the laparoscope, there is no prolonged recovery period because there is no major abdominal incision.

▶ *What are the advantages and disadvantages to these different procedures?*

A myomectomy may be done surgically either with an abdominal incision or with a laparoscope, more commonly the former. The surgeries are more or less equivalent in terms of time in the operating room and blood loss. Recovery time after a myomectomy may be somewhat shorter, four weeks rather than six weeks, but it is still significant.

Myomectomies can be more difficult operations than hysterectomies and are often

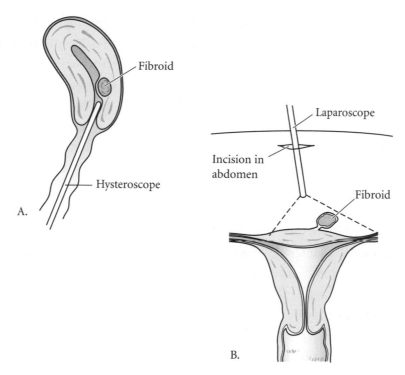

FIGURE 15. Hysteroscopy and laparoscopy. The hysteroscope, inserted through the vagina, is used to remove fibroids from the inner wall of the uterus. The laparoscope, inserted through the abdomen, removes fibroids attached to the outer wall. A, hysteroscopy; B, laparoscopy.

recommended for women who want to preserve their childbearing capability. Although it would seem easier to remove the fibroid than the entire uterus, a myomectomy can become difficult and sometimes involve more blood loss than a hysterectomy, because the fibroid grows into the wall of the uterus and has its own blood supply. In a hysterectomy the surgeon controls the bleeding, clamping off the large vessels to the uterus before beginning to cut. In a myomectomy there is no way to shut down the blood flow to the uterus, because the uterus is being preserved. To remove the fibroid, the surgeon must dig in to the wall of the uterus and peel off the fibroid while the uterus is receiving its full blood supply. The bleeding can be reduced using operative tourniquets or packing towels around the blood vessels to press on them temporarily. These techniques are more or less successful, depending on where the fibroids are located in relation to the uterine blood vessels.

Because a myomectomy can involve significant blood loss, many physicians encourage the patient to have a blood supply available, preferably her own blood.

The other problem with a myomectomy is that the operation often causes adhesions afterward. Adhesions are formations of scar tissue that cause one organ to stick to another; with a myomectomy, the adhesions involve the uterus, which often adheres to the bowel. After the fibroid has been removed, the physician pulls the myometrium (the muscle wall of the uterus) back together and stitches it to stop the bleeding from the blood vessels that once supplied the fibroid. There are different surgical techniques and different coatings that the surgeon puts on the uterus after a myomectomy to minimize the risk, but myomectomy still has the reputation of being an operation that is likely to cause adhesions.

Although a myomectomy is the only surgical choice for a woman interested in preserving childbearing who must have her fibroids removed, the adhesions that may result from this operation can interfere with fertility. Furthermore, women who have had a myomectomy have a significant chance of needing a Caesarean section when they do become pregnant. Scar tissue and a general weakening of the wall of the uterus during the myomectomy may put a woman at risk of a ruptured uterus during labor. The only person who can tell whether a woman who has a myomectomy will need future Caesarean sections is the surgeon who performs the myomectomy. If you are interested in having children and must have a myomectomy, you should realize the possible complications and discuss them with your physician.

> Marlene D. is thirty-eight, recently remarried, and unsure whether she wants more children. She came in with a large fibroid that was sitting right on her bladder, causing pressure and the need for frequent urination. I sent her to a urologist to be sure she did not have any other problems (which she did not), but through the cystoscope the urologist could see the fibroid pressing into her bladder like a little mountain. Because she wanted to preserve her fertility and had no other difficulties, a myomectomy was a good choice for her. Since the operation, her bladder problems have been much better.

▶ Can fibroids be removed with laser surgery?

Yes, there are three tools that can be used for removing the fibroids during a myomectomy: the traditional metal scalpel, an electrified knife or probe called a Bovie cautery, and a laser. Laser surgery has no real advantage over traditional surgery. A laser is a knife—a knife made of a beam of light instead of metal, but a knife nonetheless. Although a laser is a superior tool in many procedures, in a myomectomy it has no advantage over removing the fibroids with electrocauterization or a metal scalpel. But laser surgery gets good press and people are sometimes swayed to want procedures that are new.

INCONTINENCE AND UTERINE PROLAPSE

Among the annoyances of having a middle-aged uterus and pelvis are problems of incontinence, the unwanted leaking of urine. Both the uterus itself and the ligaments that hold it in place are sensitive to estrogen. As estrogen production declines with age, both the uterus and the ligaments atrophy, causing what is known as pelvic relaxation, which means that your pelvic organs are no longer held firmly in place by their ligaments. Unlike most forms of relaxation, pelvic relaxation is not desirable. Women who have gone through term delivery of one or more children almost always have some degree of pelvic relaxation.

The degrees of pelvic relaxation range from very mild to severe. With mild pelvic relaxation, your gynecologist doing a pelvic exam can feel the uterus coming down a little into the vagina. The uterus can slip so far down that it actually protrudes into the vagina toward the perineum, a condition known as uterine prolapse. A cystocele is a slippage or bulging into the vagina of the bladder, which normally sits above the front of the vagina; a rectocele occurs when part of the rectum bulges into the vagina through its weakened back wall.

A common symptom that accompanies pelvic relaxation is stress incontinence, which is loss of urine when the pressure within the abdomen is increased by laughing, sneezing, coughing, or physical exercise such as running or jumping. Many women also experience stress incontinence during pregnancy.

Once the baby has been delivered, the incontinence usually gets better; but it returns with future pregnancies and tends to get more severe with time.

Stress incontinence is a very common problem, and for many older women a serious one. There are women who are afraid to go on vacation because of it or who must curtail certain activities—hiking, camping, sports. We all owe a debt of thanks to the actress June Allyson, star of a groundbreaking series of commercials that brought stress incontinence into the realm of public acceptability. For if people are willing to talk about an issue, some of the stigma disappears.

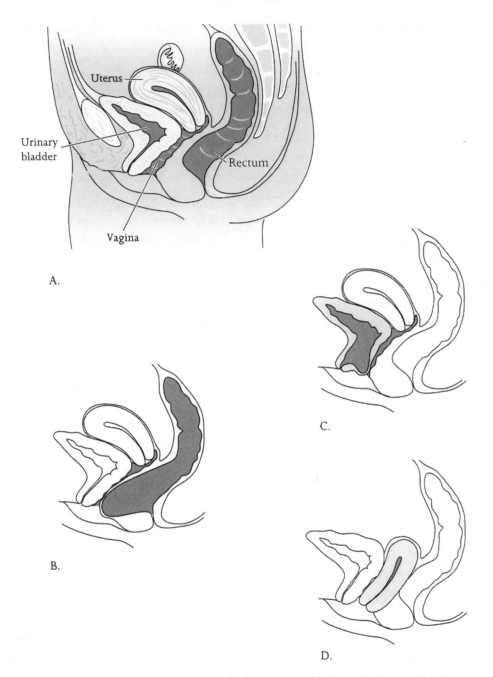

FIGURE 16. Cystocele and rectocele. Weakening of the muscles of the pelvic floor can lead to bulges of the rectum (rectocele) or bladder (cystocele) into the vagina. The entire uterus can also fall (uterine prolapse). Some patients have all three conditions. A, normal anatomy; B, rectocele; C, cystocele; D, uterine prolapse.

▶ Is pelvic relaxation hereditary?

Uterine prolapse and pelvic relaxation seem to have more of a hereditary component than, say, fibroids. When a women tells me that her uterus is prolapsed, she often says that her mother had the same problem. I have one patient whose bladder was repaired when she was only twenty-four years old. Her mother apparently had the same problem, for she had seven children and seven bladder repairs.

▶ What are the symptoms of pelvic relaxation or uterine prolapse?

Symptoms can vary according to the severity of the condition. In its milder forms, when the uterus and bladder have descended only slightly into the vagina, pelvic relaxation can cause back pressure and mild stress incontinence.

If uterine prolapse is severe, the uterus and perhaps the bladder will protrude from the vagina. In some cases of severe prolapse with cystocele, women experience the opposite of stress incontinence: they cannot urinate without manually holding up the bladder. Since the bladder has fallen into the vagina, the urethra is above it; the sac of bladder that remains below the urethra will not contract and empty unless it is pushed up above the urethra. Women with this condition are extremely vulnerable to urinary tract infections.

In addition, women with uterine prolapse and cystocele may feel pressure or fullness between their legs, a sensation described by some as "having my bottom fall out." Many women find the feeling extremely annoying; they cannot stand up comfortably because they experience so much pelvic pressure. Their mobility is decreased because they experience discomfort when they are walking or running, although they do feel better sitting or lying down. Other women with prolapse are less troubled by this sensation.

▶ Can stress incontinence be cured without medication or surgery?

Simple first-line approaches will help many women. If you are overweight and have stress incontinence, you will do yourself a favor by losing the excess poundage. Heavy women have more stress incontinence because they have greater abdominal pressure, caused by the extra fat within the abdomen. If you lose the extra weight, the incontinence may disappear on its own. Second, if you are a smoker and you have chronic smoker's cough, you are doing yourself several disservices. The cough makes a smoker a bad surgical candidate; for even though a urologist may fix your bladder, the constant stress of coughing will undo the best surgery.

All women, fat or thin, smokers or nonsmokers, can benefit from the well-known Kegel exercises, which strengthen the muscles surrounding the urethra and vagina. The easiest way to describe the Kegels is to suggest that the next time you urinate, you stop and start the stream of urine. Of course you can do the exercises when you are not urinating, but the muscles you need to strengthen are the same ones that stop the flow. To do Kegels, contract these muscles and hold while you slowly count to five.

There is no such thing as doing too many Kegels. You can be too thin and you probably can be too rich, but you can never do too many Kegels. If you drive, you might put a sign on your dashboard that says "Kegel." Then at every traffic light, at every tollbooth, in every traffic jam, at every bit of construction on the turnpike, you will be reminded to do your exercises. You can't do much else when you are stuck in traffic, so you may as well make your boredom productive. My experience in clinical practice tells me that Kegels do help many women a great deal.

▶ Does estrogen therapy help with incontinence?

The success of hormone therapy in treating incontinence is controversial in the scientific literature. One researcher, Linda Cardozo, a respected urogynecologist from England, has done controlled studies on women who take and do not take estrogen; her results did not show that HRT helped with incontinence. Nor could she demonstrate that HRT improved the degree of prolapse or lessened the severity of symptoms.

My own experience tells me that HRT does indeed help some women. Women mention it in an offhand way. They notice that they can jog or play tennis without becoming incontinent, though before starting HRT they had more difficulty with this problem. Or they talk about their hot flashes or their concentration, and then mention that, by the way, their urine problem is better. If you do not want to take HRT systemically via pills or patches, you can try topical vaginal estrogen—creams, vaginal tablets, or the Estring—because for this purpose topical therapy is probably just as effective as oral systemic therapy. There are no contraindications for vaginal estrogen cream unless you happen to be allergic to the substance in which the estrogen is dissolved; almost no one is allergic to estrogen. Even most women who have breast cancer can use vaginal estrogen, because so little is absorbed. If your symptoms improve and you don't need an operation, fine. Unlike osteoporosis, in which you can stop bone loss but seldom rebuild bone that has already been lost, changes in urinary control are reversible. Estrogen will improve matters for the seventy-year-old woman just as it will for the fifty-year-old.

▶ Are there medications for stress incontinence?

Although there is nothing currently on the market, Duloxetine, originally developed to treat depression, is scheduled to come out in 2005. It seems to help with stress incontinence by stimulating the nerves that affect the urethral sphincter at the opening of the bladder, causing the sphincter to tighten and thus helping to prevent urine leakage.

▶ Can a pessary help with incontinence?

Another approach to stress incontinence is mechanical. A device called a pessary can be inserted into the vagina to support the uterus and bladder. The most common type of pessary is a rubber or plastic ring designed to raise your pelvic organs, in the way stitches support the bladder if you have a surgical bladder repair. The classic pessary looks rather like a giant diaphragm and is not much harder to put in. (Your gynecologist should be able to show you how.) Other types look like cubes or balloons.

A pessary is inserted temporarily, although it can be used over and over. Some women use it on an as-needed basis, for example when they are going running or participating in a sport; others leave it in longer. For people who are sexually active, it can obviously be a nuisance, but some women just remove the pessary when they have intercourse and put it in again later. In general, pessaries are used by women for whom intercourse is not an issue, especially older women who have uterine prolapse but are not appropriate candidates for surgery. Some younger women who are not ready for bladder repair surgery feel comfortable using one during exercise. Some women don't feel the presence of the pessary at all; other women have reactions ranging from annoyance to discomfort. The pessary may be hard to get in and out, and it may not cure the incontinence. Although pessaries come in different sizes and shapes, some women have such poor pelvic support that they can't keep any pessary in place.

Despite the disadvantages, I frequently suggest to my patients with incontinence or prolapse that they try a pessary. If they like it, they can avoid surgery. If they don't like it, at least they have tried another nonsurgical option.

Remember that a pessary is not a cure; it will not fix your prolapse. For some women it does not work. For others it works so well that surgery is not needed. I estimate that up to half my patients who try a pessary feel comfortable with it, at least on an as-needed basis.

Because pessaries support the prolapsed uterus or bladder whose pressure is contributing to urine leakage, they can help stress incontinence, especially for women who

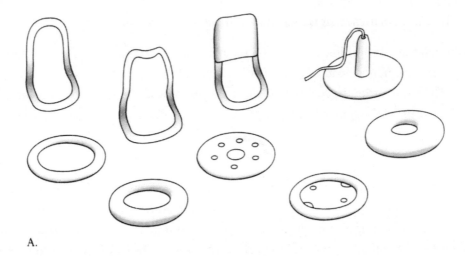

A.

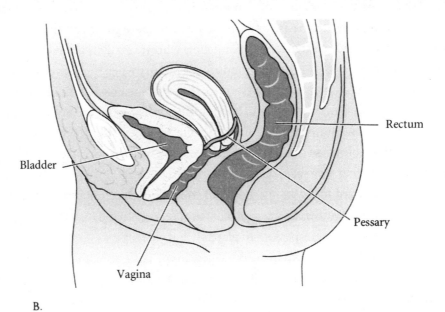

Bladder

Vagina

Rectum

Pessary

B.

FIGURE 17. Pessaries are rubber devices that can help support the uterus, bladder, and rectum. B, a pessary in place.

are weak or in poor health and cannot tolerate surgery. They can also be useful for women who might elect surgery at some later date but would like to put it off to accommodate their schedule.

> Edith L., a tough, smart, healthy sixty-seven-year-old former physical therapist, had a totally prolapsed bladder that made it hard for her to be far from a bathroom for long. Her health was not endangered, but she wanted her bladder fixed. An avid sailor, she also wanted to make a boat trip during the summer. A pessary enabled her to go on the trip and schedule her surgery at a more convenient time.

▶ Is there incontinence not caused by stress?

Urge incontinence, clinically known as detrusor dyssynergia, is named for the detrusor or bladder muscle. Most people are aware of a symptom called spastic colon, also known as irritable bowel, a bowel that contracts too frequently and causes gas and diarrhea. Detrusor dyssynergia is irritable bladder. People who have this symptom feel the need to urinate when their bladder contains only two or three ounces (60 to 90 ml) of urine instead of the usual eight ounces. A urologist or urogynecologist can measure the pressure in the bladder to find out how much urine the bladder contains when the patient feels the urge to urinate. Detrusor dyssynergia is not painful, but it can be embarrassing and inconvenient.

▶ How is irritable bladder treated?

Detrusor dyssynergia is usually treated medically rather than surgically. One do-it-yourself approach is bladder training. If you are in a situation where you are near a toilet all day long, you might want to try it. You begin by urinating every hour on the hour, whether you feel the urge to do so or not. You keep this up for a few days and then start spacing the intervals to an hour and a half, then two hours, then longer. Although you may find it time-consuming and inconvenient to keep up this routine, you may also find it helpful, as some of my patients have reported.

Drugs are also a possibility for treating irritable bladder. The classic medication is Ditropan, a drug that blocks the nerves in the bladder so they do not keep firing off messages that create the urge to urinate. One major side effect of Ditropan is dry mouth, but longer-lasting medications, Ditropan XL and Detrol, have been developed. They cause less dryness and require only one dose a day, instead of the three required by the older form of Ditropan. The newest development is Oxytrol, a transdermal Ditropan patch that you stick on your buttocks or belly and change twice a week. The patch is convenient, delivers a constant low dosage, and has minimal side effects. It is especially useful for problems with nighttime urination.

Some physicians treat detrusor dyssynergia with imipramine and amitriptyline, antidepressants that go by trade names such as Tofranil and Elavil. Some of my patients are offended by the suggestion that they take an antidepressant, feeling that I am suggesting something is wrong with their mental health. But again, the antidepressant has an effect on those nerves in the bladder that keep sending the wrong messages. The antidepressant is prescribed in very low doses, lower amounts than what people with depression usually receive. Interestingly, small children who are nighttime bed wetters are also classically treated with imipramine.

These drugs will not help women who also have stress incontinence or uterine prolapse. If they cough and sneeze or run and jump, they will still be incontinent. Many women have both types of incontinence, and it is important to find out from the patient just when the problem began, how much urine is lost, and so on.

> Monica M. was troubled by the need to urinate frequently and was convinced that she needed surgery. She had never had children, so it was unlikely that she had stress incontinence, which is very uncommon in people who have not been pregnant. When she described her symptoms, it was evident that she had detrusor dyssynergia. She felt that she had to go to the bathroom all the time and that she had to get there in a hurry. She tried Ditropan and it worked well for her.

▶ *Can surgery correct incontinence?*

Surgery is the most aggressive approach to stress incontinence, and most of the time it corrects the problem. Before rushing into it, women should realize that no surgery is 100 percent effective and that all have the potential of coming undone. Just as a face-lift sags with time and increased age, the structures supporting your bladder will do the same. Ten years from now you may need another operation.

Other factors influence the rate of surgical success, such as the difficulty of the operation. Some repairs are relatively simple and some are more complicated. Some approaches, statistically more successful than others, are not performed frequently because they are complex and recuperation is arduous. The operation that is tightest and holds up the urinary tract structures most successfully has a high rate of complications.

▶ *When is surgery a viable option for incontinence and uterine prolapse?*

When you have exhausted the other options and feel that your quality of life is being compromised by incontinence or prolapse, it is time to consider surgery.

Still, I encourage my patients to wait until they have finished their childbearing, because if you have a surgical repair, you may need a Caesarean section to save the repair, and a Caesarean section is a more difficult event than a vaginal delivery. Or if you have a vaginal delivery, you may need another repair operation.

A case in point is the woman mentioned earlier who had seven children and seven bladder repair operations. Unless her symptoms were so severe that she couldn't leave the house (and many women have such symptoms), the operations might have been delayed until later in her life.

Women who seek surgery because of discomfort from a cystocele should realize that any operation to correct the condition may result in some incontinence. If these women have trouble emptying their bladder because the cystocele forms a little reservoir below the urethra that never empties, they may find that they will be able to urinate much more easily; they may even become a little incontinent.

Alice B., an eighty-year-old artist who keeps herself in good shape, had a huge cystocele that she had been controlling with a pessary. After a while the pessary just wasn't working and she found herself really hindered by her cystocele. Although nobody likes operating electively on someone who is seventy-eight or seventy-nine, this woman was a very vigorous person and her life was being seriously compromised. So we fixed her cystocele and she is a new person. She walks around all day in art museums; she stands at her easel and paints for hours; she carries around her large canvases and supplies and has become more active than ever.

Betty H. is about seventy and in terrific shape. Although she has a prolapsed uterus and a cystocele, she generally looks and feels wonderful. One of her hobbies is hiking. Eventually her cystocele began troubling her enough to keep her from doing what she wanted to do. Although her health was never in serious danger because of the prolapse, her activities were curtailed. After her prolapse was repaired, the quality of her life improved dramatically.

Although health is certainly an issue, quality of life is equally important in making the decision to have surgery.

▶ What surgical procedures are available to correct uterine prolapse?

The most commonly performed surgery for this kind of problem is a vaginal hysterectomy with an anterior and a posterior repair. The first question patients ask when I describe the procedure is whether they have to have a hysterectomy; they want to know whether is it possible to leave the uterus in place. The answer is yes, it is possible. The surgeon can use a sling procedure to shorten the ligaments that support the uterus and hoist it back into the pelvis.

But if the uterus is falling into the vagina, why put it back in place, since gravity is going to tend to pull it down again? The ligaments that support the uterus have been badly stretched already, which is why the uterus prolapsed in the first place. So if the uterus is not removed, often the operation must be repeated.

If the woman who needs surgery for her uterine prolapse is premenopausal and is concerned about ovarian function, the ovaries can be, and usually are, left in place. After all, they are not part of the problem.

▶ What are the surgical procedures for cystocele and rectocele?

Often uterine prolapse is accompanied by cystocele or rectocele or both. These are usually injuries associated with childbearing. A cystocele repair, also called an anterior repair, entails taking tucks in the fascia that supports the bladder to shorten and tighten it. Part of the procedure for repairing the cystocele is called a Kelly plication suture. It involves building up the tissue under the urethra, which raises it and thereby helps with incontinence. So there are essentially two components of repairing a cystocele: reducing the size of the cystocele and supporting the urethra.

Many women who have a cystocele also have a rectocele. The surgical repair of this condition involves reinforcing the tissue between the vagina and rectum, rebuilding that wall.

The Kelly plication suture, like many other operations, is named for the surgeon who invented it. John Kelly was chairman of the department of obstetrics and gynecology at the Johns Hopkins University School of Medicine for a number of years at the turn of the twentieth century and invented the Kelly clamp, commonly used by gynecologists in the operating room.

Doctor Kelly also made a significant contribution to literature. One year he asked a fourth-year student to repeat her training in gynecology because she did not seem to be terribly interested and hadn't done a very good job. Although she was almost finished with medical school, she announced that she didn't want to repeat the rotation and would rather just quit and go to Paris. Her name was Gertrude Stein.

▶ *What surgical procedures are used to treat incontinence without cystocele or rectocele?*

Women who have only incontinence, whose bladder or rectum is not bulging into the vagina, are probably better served by a different operation. A number of surgical procedures exist for anatomic stress incontinence, all of which are variations on a theme. They involve attaching the bladder to some other abdominal structure and they differ on what structure to use as support.

One classic operation is the Stamey; another is the Pereira, both named for the surgeons who developed them. Stitches are inserted next to the urethra, and it is attached to some fixed part of the abdominal wall. In these procedures, the stitches go into the rectus fascia, the tight layer that covers the rectus (belly-wall muscles). These operations have become very popular and have more or less replaced the traditional Kelly plication suture because they work better, in general, if incontinence is the primary issue.

A newer procedure developed in Germany makes use of tension-free vaginal tape, called TVT. This procedure is done through the vagina so that it leaves no abdominal scar and can be performed in an outpatient setting. It takes about half an hour and involves placing a tape that is made of a fabric similar to Gore-Tex under the urethra.

Simone B., fifty-three, is the mother of four children, each of whom weighed ten pounds at birth. About three years ago, she found that her bladder problems were so annoying that she had to give up practically all her athletic activities. My colleague Dr. Steve Fleischman, who has done this procedure many times, convinced her and me that a TVT would work wonders for her, and it did. Within a week she was out jogging for the first time in fifteen years.

Another commonly performed surgery is the Marshall Marchetti Krantz procedure and its variations, the most common of which is the Burch. With the Marshall procedure, the stitches are placed into the covering of the pubic bone, the periosteum; in the Burch, the surgeon stitches into some of the other abdominal ligaments.

Although most operations for uterine prolapse, rectocele, and cystocele are performed through the vagina, the Marshall and Burch procedures for incontinence alone are done wholly or partially abdominally. They have a high rate of success, about 90 percent, and success in these terms means complete continence. The 10 percent of patients whose operations are not "successful" do get some degree of relief. Very rarely does a patient experience no relief whatsoever.

Patients should know, however, that any of these procedures for incontinence may fail some years down the road. Although the operations remain successful forever for the majority who have them, a small proportion of women become incontinent again after a number of years.

Patricia G. has a severe eating disorder. A while ago she had a successful Marshall procedure to treat her incontinence. At the time, she was successfully keeping her weight at about 140 pounds. Then she gained about 100 pounds, ballooning to 240. Her Marshall came undone with the extra abdominal pounds, and she is again incontinent. Her urethra was stitched to the covering of her public bone, but the extra weight was too much for three or four stitches to support. Indeed, many gynecologists and urologists will not recommend a Marshall for someone who is seriously overweight.

▶ What can be done if my surgical procedure fails?

The ultimate operation for people whose Stamey or Marshall has failed is the sling procedure. The surgeon takes a strip of tissue and slings it beneath the urethra, then attaches this structure up toward the pubic bone as a permanent support. Many surgeons use the rectus fascia, the very tense, extremely strong tissue that covers the muscles of the abdominal wall, to fashion the sling. Other surgeons use a nonreactive foreign substance such as Gore-Tex to make the sling; tissue from a cadaver is another option. Today researchers are experimenting with injection of collagen around the urethra to make it tighter and build up more resistance within it. Silicone may also be used, but its effects within the body twenty years into the future are not yet known.

▶ *What are the complications of these procedures?*

Any surgery involves the risks of anesthesia and infection. In addition, patients should know in advance that they will have to have a catheter in their bladder for a while after the procedure. Some women experience little discomfort with the catheter; others dislike it intensely. If the patient needs a catheter, she will probably be given preventive antibiotics, since bladder infections can be a complication.

Because the surgery changes your anatomy, obstructing something that was not obstructed previously, you may have difficulty starting to urinate again. Formerly the bladder didn't have to work to empty itself; urine just flowed out, whether you wanted it to or not. Now that the surgeon has introduced an obstruction, the bladder has to work and strengthen itself to force urine out through the urethra.

Many people keep the catheters for three to five days after surgery, while the bladder muscles strengthen. The record among my own patients was three weeks. But nobody is catheterized forever after a Marshall or a Stamey.

One of the major complications of sling procedures, however, is that sometimes these operations hold up the urinary structures too well and people need to catheterize themselves or wear a catheter to start urinating again. On occasion the process can take months. Once in a while a patient will have to go back to the operating room to have the sling loosened a little. So unless you have no control over your bladder at all, a sling operation is not the first option.

▶ *Who performs these operations?*

Usually in the United States, a urologist will do the Stamey and the Pereira, whereas a gynecologist will perform the Marshall. In a Stamey, the physician uses a cystoscope, looking into the bladder five or six times during the procedure in order to place the stitches correctly. Most gynecologists are not trained to use cystoscopes, although some are. Urogynecologists usually perform sling operations.

Sometimes a gynecologist will do a Marshall to treat incontinence, as a kind of bonus along with a hysterectomy that is being performed to treat some other disease. It is becoming rare in the United States to have a Marshall performed independent of a hysterectomy. If you don't need a hysterectomy but need surgical treatment of incontinence, you will probably have a Stamey or one of its cousins or a TVT.

If you are contemplating bladder surgery, you should discuss the procedure with

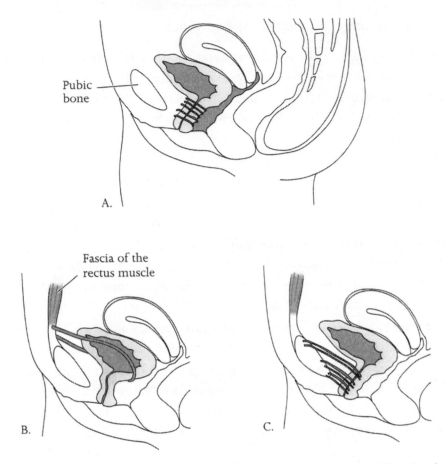

FIGURE 18. Commonly performed surgical procedures for stress incontinence. These involve tucking and tightening sagging tissues and sometimes attaching the bladder to another structure in the abdomen. A, anterior repair; B, urethral sling or TVT. In principle these operations are the same; in both a strip of material is passed under the urethra and attached to the fascia. C, Marshall Marchetti Krantz procedure.

your physician. If your gynecologist thinks you would benefit from a more urological approach, she or he will refer you to an appropriate urologist.

VAGINAL ITCHING

Although there are several causes of vaginal itching, one major culprit is yeast infection. Yeast cells and other microorganisms live in the vagina all the time, normally held in check by its acid environment. When this balance is upset, yeast can become problematic.

▶ *How do I recognize a yeast infection?*

The main symptom is itching. The infection is apt to be odorless, but it sometimes is accompanied by a vaginal discharge, classically described as white and curdy, something like cottage cheese. Some yeast infections have no discharge at all.

▶ *Who is vulnerable to yeast infections?*

Although women of any age may get yeast infections, older women not on hormone therapy are more susceptible to infections of the vagina (vaginitis) and of the vulva (vulvitis). The lower estrogen levels that follow menopause result eventually in thinner vaginal and vulvar tissues, which are prone to invasion and irritation. Women who have diabetes are also at increased risk, as are women who are HIV-positive. I have diagnosed several women with diabetes because they came to me with recurrent yeast infections.

HIV also predisposes women toward yeast infections. Nowadays many people are paranoid about HIV and AIDS. I have had patients come in and say, "I just got my second yeast infection; I must have AIDS." I do HIV tests on women who have recurrent infections just because it is worthwhile to rule out the possibility, but I have never turned up any HIV-positives this way.

Many women who are plagued by yeast infections do not have either HIV or diabetes; they just get recurrent yeast infections.

▶ *Can I lower my risk for yeast infections?*

You can do a few simple things to make yourself a less likely target. First of all, don't sit around in a wet bathing suit or in sweaty exercise clothes. The warm, moist atmosphere offered by these garments is an ideal growing environment for yeast cells.

Next, avoid unnecessary antibiotics. If you don't really need an antibiotic for bronchitis or some other condition, don't take one. While the antibiotics are busy killing off the bacteria that are giving you the bronchitis, they are also killing off your normal intestinal and vaginal flora (the bacteria that normally thrive there). These bacteria could be considered "good-guy bacteria"; they are basically lactobacilli that live in the intestines and vagina and secrete acid to protect the body from excessive growth of yeast. Often if a woman has been on multiple courses of antibiotics, her normal flora will be killed off and her body will be overburdened with yeast.

If you do have to take antibiotics, eat yogurt during the therapy. Buy natural yogurt, which contains live lactobacillus cultures (sometimes this type is more expensive than other yogurts). Or if antibiotic therapy has been lowering your natural vaginal flora and you find yourself susceptible to yeast infections, you can apply plain natural yogurt to the vagina and vulva. To many people this suggestion sounds gross, but it works and it is inexpensive. There are several ways to do this. You can dilute the yogurt and use it as a douche. Or if you have an old applicator for some vaginal medicine, you can fill it with yogurt and apply it that way. Or you can use a yogurt-coated tampon as an applicator. I suggest using the yogurt twice a day for four or five days to see whether you obtain relief.

▶ What is the therapy for vulvitis or vaginitis caused by a yeast infection?

Often vulvitis or vaginitis has two components: the yeast infection itself, and an inflammatory component independent of the yeast and the scratching.

Various antifungal drugs, available over the counter or by prescription, attack the yeast cells. They come as creams or ointments and are applied directly to the infected area. The over-the-counter preparations cost in the range of fifteen to twenty dollars; they are not cheap, but they are less expensive than prescription drugs and they may well work for you. A frequently used brand is Monistat, the commercial name of a drug called miconazole. Another common drug, clotrimazole, is sold commercially as Gyne-Lotrimin and Mycelex. As these preparations are used more and more commonly, certain strains of yeast are becoming resistant; but the significant majority of yeast infections will still yield to these over-the-counter medicines.

Topical antifungals are also available by prescription. They contain slightly different drugs, and fewer strains of yeast are resistant to them because they are less widely used. One commonly used prescription drug is Terazol (terconazole), which is more expensive than the over-the-counter variety, but if your health insurance pays for prescription medications, they will cost you less out of pocket.

Recently many physicians have started to use systemic antifungals similar to the drugs prescribed for AIDS patients who have fungal infections. These drugs are effective. One commonly used antifungal that comes in pill form is Diflucan, the trade name for fluconazole. Members of this family of pharmaceuticals are also used to treat serious systemic yeast infections, including infections of the urinary tract, pneumonia, and certain kinds of meningitis. While therapy for these conditions may last days or weeks, a single small dose of fluconazole will usually cure common everyday yeast infections. One 150-mg pill might be the equivalent of three days of over-the-counter therapy. Diflucan doesn't increase the risk of recurrence, and since most people would rather swallow one pill than use creams or suppositories for a week, it is a useful option. Your symptoms should go away in a few days.

There are also such drugs as oral nystatin, which is not systemic. Oral nystatin is not absorbed into the bloodstream and does not have such side effects as liver toxicity. When you take it, you decrease the load of yeast in your intestine. I sometimes prescribe this drug for people who have increased vulnerability to yeast infections from taking significant amounts of antibiotics. Because nystatin is not absorbed into the bloodstream, it does nothing for your vaginitis or vulvitis per se, but it does decrease your chance of re-infection with your own body yeast.

Because vaginitis or vulvitis may have an inflammatory component, doctors often recommend a topical anti-inflammatory agent if the antifungal therapy alone does not work. The fact that the itching fails to stop when you apply an antifungal cream doesn't mean that yeast didn't start the itching process in the first place. These agents are usually cortisone-like steroids.

▶ *Are there causes of vaginal and vulvar itching other than yeast infections?*

Although vulvar cancer often makes its presence known through unrelieved itching, vaginal and vulvar itching is generally caused by something more benign.

Atrophic changes of the vagina and vulva can cause itching. Postmenopausal women who don't produce their own estrogen often are affected by such changes. Just as the skin of older people often gets irritated and itchy in winter when the air is dryer, these tissues also can become irritated.

Another condition that classically causes itching in the vulvar area, though it can appear anywhere on the body, is called lichen sclerosus et atrophicus, or LS&A for short. It is an inflammation, not an infection. Since LS&A can be difficult to distinguish from vulvar cancer in physical appearance and in symptoms, your physician will probably recommend a biopsy. The tissue affected by LS&A looks whitish, rather than pink like normal vulvar tissue, the white color being caused either by scratching in response to itching or by the disease itself.

The condition is usually treated with topical anti-inflammatory drugs such as steroids. Sometimes LS&A is also treated with testosterone cream applied to the affected area. The amount of testosterone absorbed from the cream is not enough to produce masculinization.

Genital warts, caused by the condyloma virus, can also present with itching or burning. Sometimes, but not always, you can see warts on your skin. Your physician may want to examine you with a colposcope, because the warts have a classic appearance under magnification. A number of specific therapies are used to treat warts, including podophyllin, which comes from an herbal root, and TCA, tricarboxylic acid. Because warts are caused by a viral infection, antibiotics have no effect.

Another disease that can cause vulvar discomfort is something called vestibular vulvitis. Seen more commonly in younger women than in older women, it is a frustrating disease to have and to treat because the physician cannot see much wrong except chronic inflammation. Typically women who have this disease go from doctor to doctor because no one can determine the cause of their discomfort. Even biopsies are of little help.

Vestibular vulvitis can present with itching or with pain. Women sometimes complain of a burning pain, often in a horseshoe-shaped distribution around the bottom part of the opening of the vagina, then reaching back toward the rectum. Usually there is no pain in the rectal area itself. At the present time I have a young woman patient who has vestibular vulvitis periclitorally.

If you do have this problem, find a physician, either a gynecologist or a dermatologist, who is familiar with the disease. Ask your own doctor if he or she knows much about vestibular vulvitis, and if necessary ask for a referral to someone who does.

▶ What is the cause of vestibular vulvitis?

No one knows for certain, but some researchers believe it may be related to previous chronic yeast infections or a chronic infection such as the human papilloma virus or the wart virus. Some women have vestibular vulvitis without any history of these other problems.

▶ How long do these itchy conditions last?

Unfortunately, they can last months or even years, and some older women are significantly troubled by them. Even younger women are occasionally afflicted with vulvar itching. The first line of action is to try a little Monistat or another antifungal medication. If that doesn't relieve your symptoms in a week or two, you should see your doctor. A gynecologist can prescribe medicines that are not available over the counter. If your itching becomes chronic and does not respond to medication, then your gynecologist will have to check on the possibility that you have vulvar cancer.

13 Cancer of the Reproductive Organs

AMERICA is a cancerphobic society; cancer is the one disease that for whatever reason we fear more than any other. One reason I became a gynecologist is that I have a reasonable chance to cure a lot of people. Most gynecological cancers can be detected early and have high cure rates. That alone is sufficient reason for you to continue your gynecological checkups even after menopause.

The most common gynecological cancers are, in order of frequency of occurrence, breast cancer, uterine cancer, cervical cancer, and ovarian cancer. There are also cancers of the vulva, which are very rare, and tumors of the vagina, which are even rarer.

▶ *What can I do to protect myself from cancer in general?*

Cancer is caused both by external factors (chemicals, viruses, radiation) and by internal ones (hormones, immune conditions, and inherited genetic factors), which over time work alone or together to produce cancer. Some of these factors are within your control and some are not. At the risk of boring repetition, the practices that constitute a healthy lifestyle also have cancer-protecting attributes.

The American Cancer Society estimated that in 2003 about 180,000 lives were lost to cancer because of tobacco use, all of these deaths preventable. The most important piece of lifestyle advice concerning cancer prevention is this: don't smoke; don't use chewing tobacco or snuff (probably not a huge temptation for readers of this book, though once when I was in training I almost ordered unnecessary tests on a middle-aged woman patient who spat out a great glob of tobacco juice). Other good advice includes limiting alcohol intake and dietary fat, avoiding exposure to sun, and protecting your skin with sunscreen.

Smoking, as everyone knows, is a prime contributor to lung cancer, oral cancers, and cancer of the bladder, as well as to heart disease. In fact, it seems that smoking contributes indirectly to cancer in many organs of the body—one more reason to stop. Obesity increases risk of breast and uterine cancer. Heavy alcohol consumption is an important factor in liver cancer and cancers of the oral cavity. On the positive side, a lifetime of exercise seems to be a factor that reduces cancer risk. A study of women who had attended the same college found that those who had not actively taken part in athletics developed 86 percent more breast cancer and 153 percent more uterine and cervical cancer than the women who had participated in college sports.

Another way to protect yourself against cancer is to have regular checkups. In Chapter 15 you will find a discussion of physical exams and tests you should be having in addition to your gynecological checkups.

▶ Can I lower my risk of cancer through diet or nutrition?

Many factors contribute to your risk of cancer, and although you cannot assume that you will never get cancer if you follow the dietary guidelines suggested by the American Cancer Society, you can certainly know that you have done what you can, nutritionally speaking, to keep your risk low. Current research suggests that diet plays an important role in establishing your relative risk for cancer.

Keep your weight in the desirable range. People who are 40 percent or more overweight have an increased risk of colon, breast, prostate, gallbladder, ovarian, and uterine cancers.

Eat a diet that includes many different foods. The American Cancer Society recommends the same kind of diet endorsed by the American Nutrition Society, one that includes a variety of fruits and vegetables and high-fiber foods such as whole-grain cereals, breads, and pasta. Studies have shown that eating a lot of vegetables and fresh fruits decreases your risk of cancer of the lung, bladder, rectum, stomach, and esophagus.

Cut down on total fat intake, as a diet high in fat seems to be a factor in the development of breast and colon cancers. High-fiber foods are a healthy substitute for fatty foods. Limit consumption of alcohol if you drink at all. Cancer of the larynx, throat, esophagus, and liver occur more frequently among heavy drinkers, especially those who also smoke cigarettes or chew tobacco.

Don't eat much salt-cured, smoke-cured, or nitrite-cured food, which means cutting down on ham, bacon, and such processed meats as bologna. They seem to contribute to the development of cancer of the stomach and esophagus, diseases that are more prevalent in parts of the world where these foods are a dietary staple.

▶ *Do birth control pills raise my risk for cancer?*

I always find it ironic that when teenagers come in asking for birth control; many of them are reluctant to take the pill because they believe it will give them cancer. On the contrary. No data show that birth control pills increase the risk for any kind of cancer, but reliable studies suggest that birth control pills actually reduce the risk of endometrial cancer and ovarian cancer.

BREAST CANCER

Breast cancer is probably the disease American women fear most. It is not the leading killer of American women—coronary artery disease has that distinction, affecting about 2.5 million and killing 500,000 every year. In 2004 an estimated 215,900 cases of invasive breast cancer will be diagnosed, killing about 40,110 women—less than 10 percent of those who die from coronary artery disease. But breast cancer is the second most lethal cancer for women (after lung cancer, which surged into the lead in 1987) and the most widespread gynecological cancer. Even when it is not lethal, the consequences of this disease—the possible surgical loss of a breast and the physical and psychological aftereffects—are profoundly disturbing to most women.

Breast Cancer Facts and Figures

Breast cancer has been on the rise in the United States since about 1940. Between 1973, when broad surveillance of the disease began, and 1980, the rates of incidence remained constant. During the 1980s, however, frequency of the disease in the general population rose about 4 percent per year and then leveled off at about 101 per 100,000 women during the 1990s. Much of the increase took place among older, postmenopausal women— partly because women are living longer and partly because mortality from other diseases has gone down. In other words, women are living long enough to get breast cancer. Another reason for the apparent higher incidence seems to be the expanded use of mammography, which has led to greater detection of the disease in early stages.

One statistic that has received a lot of attention is that the lifetime risk of getting breast cancer rose from one in nine in the early 1980s to one in eight. The change came about partly because in the early 1990s the National Cancer Institute changed its statistical pool, including cancers diagnosed in women older than eighty-five, a relatively high-risk group, and extending the statistical lifetime to 110 years—an age most people will not reach. The one-in-eight figure is frightening, but it doesn't mean that of any group of twenty-four women chosen at random, three will get breast cancer. It does mean that each baby girl born in America has a one-in-eight chance of getting breast cancer at some point in her life, provided that she lives to be 110.

Risk increases significantly with age. Women between the ages of twenty and twenty-four have a 1 in 2,500 chance of getting breast cancer within the next ten years; women who are sixty have a 1 in 29 risk.

Kinds and Stages of Breast Cancer

To understand breast cancer, you need to know a little about the anatomy of the breast. The working machinery of the breast consists of lobules, the glands where milk is made, and ducts, the passageways through which the milk passes on its way to the nipples. The breast also contains fatty tissue, ligaments to support the ducts and lobules, blood vessels, and lymphatic vessels. The lymphatic vessels are similar to veins, except that they carry lymph instead of blood. Lymph is a clear fluid containing the waste products of tissues along with large numbers of white blood cells that fight infection. Cancer cells can enter the lymph vessels. Most of the lymphatic vessels in the breast lead to lymph nodes in the armpits.

The most common and most worrisome kind of breast cancer is ductal cancer, though the disease can also occur in the lobules. Fortunately, with better technology and more accurate mammograms, we are finding ductal cancer earlier than we did in the past.

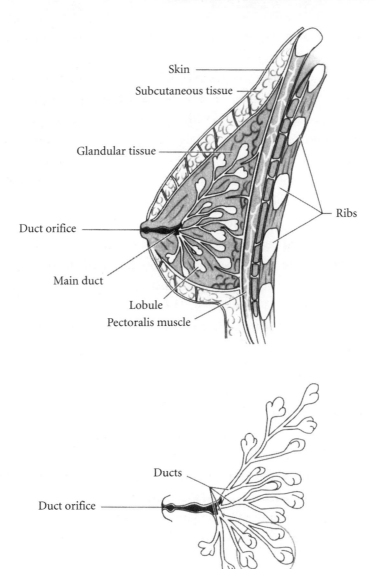

FIGURE 19. A, the structure of the breast; B, one lobe with its ducts and lobules.

▶ *How does breast cancer develop?*

Like other cancers, breast cancer develops through a series of gradual changes that progress from normal breast tissue to full-fledged cancer. The first step is proliferative fibrocystic disease, also called hyperplasia (a word that simply means "overgrowth"). This condition is not cancerous: the cells divide faster than normal cells but are otherwise normal.

The next stage is called atypical hyperplasia. The cells are growing and dividing abnormally fast (hyperplasia), and some of the fast-growing cells have unusual characteristics (atypia). The presence of hyperplasia with atypia is an early warning that the breast is at increased risk for developing cancer, but it is not in itself cancer. Women who have this condition are about four times as likely to get breast cancer as women who do not; they should be vigilant about breast exams and have more frequent mammograms than women less at risk. But most of the time, women with atypical hyperplasia can live normal lives without overwhelming anxiety.

The next development is carcinoma in situ. With this condition, cancerous changes occur within some cells, but these abnormal cells do not invade their neighbors. In the next step, invasive carcinoma occurs. The abnormal cells do invade nearby cells and may also infiltrate blood vessels or lymph nodes. The sequence of changes, from normal to cancerous, is the same whether the cancer is in the ducts or in the lobules, though the prognosis is different.

Ductal Carcinoma

A carcinoma is a cancer that that begins in the lining layer (epithelial cells) of organs. At least 80 percent of cancers and almost all breast cancers are carcinomas. Ductal cancer is the development of malignant cells within the ducts that carry milk.

Another name for ductal carcinoma in situ, sometimes abbreviated DCIS (in which the cancerous changes remain confined to the ductal cells), is intraductal carcinoma. It has a very good prognosis. If the cancer is removed, then the disease is cured. If the cancer has become invasive, the prognosis is more difficult.

Lobular Carcinoma

Lobular carcinoma, which develops in the lobules where milk is produced, has the same two stages as ductal carcinoma: either it is confined to the lobule itself—in situ lobular carcinoma—or it has spread to adjacent blood vessels or cells and become invasive.

If an in situ lobular carcinoma is removed, the disease is cured. No further cancer treatment is needed. However, women who have had in situ lobular carcinoma are at about 33 percent increased risk for developing breast cancer, either in the breast that was previously involved or in the other one. Lobular carcinoma that has invaded nearby cells, blood vessels, or lymphatics must be treated more aggressively.

Inflammatory Carcinoma

Inflammatory carcinoma, the third kind of breast cancer, originates in the lymphatics within the underlying layer of the skin and is quite rare, accounting for only about 1 percent of breast cancers.

Inflammatory carcinoma looks like a hot, red area on the skin of the breast. Often the skin looks textured or pitted, like the skin of an orange. Sometimes the breast develops ridges and small bumps that look like hives. These symptoms are caused by cancer cells blocking lymph vessels or channels in the skin over the breast.

Risk Factors

The highest risk factor is femaleness, the risk of being a woman. Men do develop breast cancer, but with far less frequency. The American Cancer Society's estimates for 2004 are 215,990 new cases of breast cancer in women and 1,450 cases in men.

The second most important risk factor is age, for breast cancer incidence continues to increase with age.

A third risk is family history, especially on the maternal side. It has been standard epidemiology to suggest that if your mother, sister, maternal aunt, or maternal grandmother had breast cancer, your risk of developing it is increased. Having relatives on your father's side who have had breast cancer may also somewhat increase your risk. Newer studies released by the National Institutes of Health de-emphasize the risk of a family history of breast cancer, suggesting that this factor is less important than we formerly thought.

Other factors that increase risk are obesity, delayed childbearing or having no children, early age at the onset of menstruation, and late age at menopause. Women of higher education and socioeconomic status are more at risk for breast cancer than women who are less well educated and less well-to-do. Studies of breast cancer in countries where the traditional diet is lower in fat than in the United States suggest that low fat intake lowers risk of the disease. Some research has suggested that high alcohol intake correlates with increased risk of breast cancer, but the studies are not definitive.

Most of these risk factors are not under your control. You probably will not decide on the age at which you bear your first child in order to minimize your risk for breast cancer. Nor can you control your family history, your gender, or your age. For these reasons the American Cancer Society suggests that your best course of action is screening and early detection.

▶ *How important a risk factor is family history of cancer?*

A couple of studies funded by the National Institutes of Health suggest that family history plays less of a role than we formerly suspected. What seems to be of greatest concern is premenopausal breast cancer. If your mother got breast cancer when she was seventy, that fact has a minimal impact on your statistical chances of getting the disease. If she had breast cancer when she was thirty, that is a different story.

The relatives who are most important to your statistical chances are your mother and sister and your maternal aunt. If your grandmother had cancer, or your cousin six times removed, then your family history is statistically less meaningful than if your mother had the disease.

The actual genetics of this is unclear. Any woman who has a family history of the disease should be aware that she is at higher risk and should be watched more closely.

▶ *Is there a gene for breast cancer?*

In 1994 researchers identified two genes, BRCA1 and BRCA2, whose mutated forms contribute to inherited breast cancer; it is likely in the future that many more contributing genes will be discovered. Every person has two copies of the gene called BRCA1 in the cells of his or her body, one inherited from each parent. Usually both BRCA1 genes function normally, but in some people, one copy carries a mistake, something like misspelling. This alteration can occur at hundreds of different sites along the BRCA1 gene, and some of these changes are associated with increased risk of developing breast and ovarian cancer, as well as cancers of the colon and prostate.

▶ *How do the genes for breast cancer increase risk?*

It is believed that the normal forms of BRCA1 and BRCA2 help to prevent cancer by producing proteins that keep cells from dividing and growing abnormally. However, if a person has inherited a mutated gene from either parent, this cancer-inhibiting protein is less effective, and chances of developing cancer increase.

▶ *How strong is the link between the altered form of BRCA1 and breast cancer itself?*

It is important to emphasize that these genes do not cause breast cancer. That is, if you have inherited one of these mutated forms of the genes, you have an increased susceptibility to breast cancer, but you will not necessarily get it. At present, it is impossible to predict the percentage of women who have inherited one of these genes who will actually develop breast cancer. It is equally impossible to assess any individual woman's risk. The altered gene is not the sole cause of breast cancer, merely a contributing factor.

Only 5 to 10 percent of breast cancer is believed to be inherited, and of these hereditary breast cancers, altered forms of BRCA1 and BRCA2 are associated with only 40 to 50 percent of these cases.

▶ *How common are the genes for breast cancer?*

It is estimated that somewhere between 0.04 and 0.2 percent of women in the general population carry the mutated form of BRCA1; the mutated form of BRCA2 is even less common. The prevalence of BRCA1 and BRCA2 mutations among women of Ashkenazic Jewish descent is estimated somewhere between 1 and 2 percent, depending on whose statistics you accept.

▶ *Can genetic testing determine whether I will get breast cancer?*

Genetic testing, which uses a blood sample to analyze your DNA, can determine whether you have inherited the mutated form of BRCA1 or BRCA2, but it cannot predict whether you will get breast cancer.

Before you decide to have genetic testing, even if you do have a strong family history of breast cancer, it is worth asking yourself what you would do if you discover that you do carry one of the mutated genes. Would you choose, as some women do, to have your breasts surgically removed preventively so that you will not get the disease? Or would you choose to do nothing, but have to live with increased anxiety knowing you were at somewhat higher risk?

Privacy, as with HIV testing, is also a crucial issue. You can't be absolutely certain that your test results will remain private. Suppose your insurance company learns that you carry the mutated form of BRCA1. It is certainly possible, though illegal, that you will be discriminated against because of that knowledge. You may have difficulty getting health insurance or be forced to pay more for your coverage.

▶ *If my mother had breast cancer at a young age, should I have a preventive mastectomy?*

My surgeon colleagues tell me that prophylactic mastectomies—surgical removal of the breasts to prevent the occurrence of breast cancer—are very rare, except in cases where a woman has had cancer in one breast and shows signs of abnormal cell growth in the other. It is also true that about 5 percent of women who do have both breasts removed because of a strong family history of breast cancer still get the disease. Although breast cancer is a worrisome disease, I would certainly urge anyone to get a second opinion and try genetic testing before having a prophylactic mastectomy.

▶ *Am I at high risk if women on the paternal side of my family have had breast cancer?*

Statistics suggest that women with a history of cancer on their father's side are not at such high risk as those with a history on their mother's side. It is possible for the breast cancer gene to be passed on through the father's side, though, as we have seen, only a small proportion of breast cancer seems to be inherited. If you have breasts that are hard to examine—for example, breasts with chronic lumpiness—or if you have had several biopsies, even though they were not premalignant, you should be followed closely.

Part of the reason is your state of mind. If you have a family history of cancer on the paternal side and you worry about increased risk, your doctor should respect your desire to be followed vigilantly.

▶ *Do silicone breast implants increase the risk of cancer?*

No studies have shown that breast implants increase risk. They may, however, compromise the accuracy of mammograms, since they can obscure portions of the breast tissue that need to be examined. The capsule of the implant holds either a silicone gel (no longer on the market, but still present in implants done before 1992) or a saline (saltwater) solution. Over time the capsule can begin to leak. This leakage can appear as a lump in the breast. Even though you suspect that your implant has sprung a leak, you should have the lump evaluated by your doctor. Do not assume that any changes you notice in your breast have been caused by the implants. Women who have implants should be vigilant about breast self-examination and should have yearly mammograms and exams by a physician.

▶ *Should women with silicone breast implants have the implants removed to prevent possible problems later on?*

As the possible drawbacks of silicone breast implants have been broadcast by the media, many women who have gotten them either for cosmetic reasons or for breast reconstruction have started to worry about potential problems. Among the difficulties that women have experienced are pain and lumpiness. Sometimes biopsies have revealed scar tissue around the capsule that surrounds the implant. Other women have reported problems of a systemic nature, symptoms that resemble rheumatoid arthritis, for example (though no scientific studies have demonstrated a relation between arthritic symptoms and breast implants).

If you are not having problems, there is no reason to have the implants removed just because you might have difficulties in the future. If you have lumpiness or breast pain, or symptoms of a vague or systemic nature that you think might be caused by your implants, report them to your primary care physician, who can consider them thoroughly with you and evaluate whether they are related to the implants.

With so much publicity about breast implants, it is easy to acquire tunnel vision and attribute all kinds of symptoms to the implants. The danger is that you might have some other potentially serious condition that you are overlooking because of ascribing your symptoms to the implants.

Prevention

▶ *What can I do to protect myself against breast cancer?*

As we have seen, many of the risk factors involve things you cannot change—your age, your sex, your heredity. Others, like the age at which you marry and have children, depend on many psychological, social, and economic factors. Your best bet is to cut down on the risk factors you can control and to follow the recommended guidelines for early detection.

▶ *Can I reduce my risk of breast cancer by diet?*

Having a diet high in fat may contribute to breast cancer, though the link is far from certain. During the 1980s and 1990s, most nutritionists believed that a high-fat diet was a major culprit in causing breast cancer. This belief rested on international studies that showed women from countries with low per capita fat intake had low rates of breast cancer. Later, more specific studies tended to weaken the link between total dietary fat and breast cancer.

Nevertheless, a high-fat diet is detrimental to your health in other ways. The standard dietary recommendation for general health is to include five servings of fresh fruits and vegetables in your diet every day. The known vitamins and the fiber content in fruits and vegetables are thought to be protective against all kinds of cancer.

The type of fat you eat may be at least as important as the total amount. Monounsaturated fats, including olive oil and canola oil, are sometimes linked to lower risk, whereas polyunsaturated fats such as corn oil and tub margarine, and saturated fats, the kind found in meat, are associated with increased risk. Some studies by European researchers have suggested that women whose diet includes considerable monounsaturated fat (olive oil in particular) have lowered levels of breast cancer.

Although the data are controversial, some researchers believe that lycopene, a natural red pigment found in tomatoes, watermelon, and pink grapefruit, lowers breast cancer risk. It appears that the lycopene in tomatoes becomes more available to your body if the tomatoes are cooked, for example in sauce.

Recently there has been scientific interest in flax seeds. Researchers have experimented with adding ground flax seeds to the diet, though the benefits have not been proven.

Soy products may also have a protective effect. Studies have shown that women from Asian cultures have a much lower incidence of breast cancer than women from Western cultures, but this advantage recedes when Asian women adopt a European or American diet. A timing factor may also be at work: soy may be more helpful during adolescence when breast tissue is actively differentiating.

Oily fish, including salmon, tuna, and bluefish, contain omega-3 fatty acids, which may help in preventing breast cancer. Since omega-3 fatty acids have other benefits, they are certainly worth emphasizing in your diet.

Some researchers believe that folic acid, found in whole grains, fortified cereal products, dried beans, and some leafy vegetables, helps protect against breast cancer. Folic acid also offers cardiovascular protection, so it's a helpful addition to your diet.

▶ *Does exercise have any influence on breast cancer risk?*

This is a relatively new area of research, and more work needs to be done. Some studies, however, show that women who exercise have less breast cancer than women who do not.

This is true both of postmenopausal women and those in the fifteen-to-forty-four age group. Some studies suggest that strenuous exercise in youth has a lifelong protective effect, and though you may be past menopause, you can certainly encourage your daughters to take up the exercise habit. Certainly obesity increases the risk of breast cancer, and exercise is one way to fight off extra weight.

▶ *What about the drug tamoxifen as a cancer preventive?*

If you are at high risk for breast cancer, perhaps through your genetic background, talk to your doctor about taking tamoxifen as a cancer preventive. Tamoxifen, sold under the trade name Novadex, is an antiestrogen drug used for many years to prevent the recurrence of breast cancer in women who had already had the disease. A study in the United States completed in 1998 showed that women at high risk for breast cancer, whatever their age, substantially decreased their chances of getting the disease by taking tamoxifen. In fact, the effectiveness of tamoxifen in preventing breast cancer was so obvious that the study was stopped even before the allotted time period had elapsed. Interestingly, European studies were more ambiguous.

The company that manufactures tamoxifen, AstraZeneca, has promoted a scale for calculating breast cancer risks. Called the Gail Model Risk Assessment Test, it factors in a woman's age, her age when her first child was born, the number of first-degree relatives who have had breast cancer, the number of breast biopsies she has had, and the presence (or absence) of atypical cells in these biopsies.

My own feeling is that every woman considering tamoxifen as a preventive therapy should discuss its pros and cons with her physician. A risk scale is fine, but it should not be used arbitrarily to decide who should use tamoxifen and who should not.

▶ *Does tamoxifen have side effects?*

One side effect is that tamoxifen can put women who are close to menopause into premature menopause. Tamoxifen blocks the action of estrogen, and estrogen is important at many sites in a premenopausal woman's body.

A second side effect is a slightly increased risk of uterine cancer. Women with a strong family history of uterine cancer or other risk factors for this disease must take these risks into consideration before starting tamoxifen. Every woman who takes tamoxifen should have a gynecological exam at least every year and perhaps every six months.

Another risk is the development of deep-vein thrombophlebitis (inflammation of the veins and the formation of blood clots there). These blood clots can move through the circulatory system to the lungs, where they can be life threatening. So if a woman has a tendency to this condition or has had it previously, she should carefully consider whether tamoxifen is right for her.

▶ How long can you take tamoxifen?

The standard recommendation for women who have had breast cancer is five years of therapy. Researchers are currently trying to develop a timetable for preventive tamoxifen therapy.

▶ Does it matter when in your life you start tamoxifen?

This is a very important question, and the answer depends heavily on your childbearing priorities. If a woman wants children, she should not start taking tamoxifen until after she has finished her family.

▶ Are there drugs other than tamoxifen that might help prevent breast cancer?

The ongoing STAR (Study of Tamoxifen and Raloxifene) trial is comparing tamoxifen with its close relative, raloxifene, in terms of breast cancer prevention. Raloxifene was designed to prevent osteoporosis and previously was studied only in postmenopausal women. Until the results of this trial become available, tamoxifen remains the drug of choice.

Breast Examinations and Mammograms

The three approaches to early detection of breast cancer are self-examination, examination by a physician, and mammography. It is vital to realize that no single method alone is sufficient; you should conscientiously pursue all three.

First is monthly self-examination. You know your breasts and their shape and feel better than anyone else. Although you may not know what a malignant lump feels like, you can detect subtle changes. The best time to do a monthly breast exam is right after your period, if you are still having periods, since a regular routine is easier to remember. If you are menopausal or are a perimenopausal woman on hormone therapy, just pick a convenient time.

In 2002, a study of female factory workers in Shanghai concluded that breast self-examination alone did not decrease the number of women who died of breast cancer, even though the researchers made significant efforts to teach the workers how to do the exams properly. The study lasted about eleven years and involved more than 260,000 women. The workers had no access to mammography, so self-exams were the only available screening tool. The study showed clearly that self-examination by itself was not an adequate tool.

However, the authors of the study pointed out that one of the striking changes over the past twenty-five years in the United States has been the reduction in the size of lumps women are discovering themselves. That is, over the past two and a half decades American women doing self-exams are finding smaller lumps, catching their cancers at earlier, more treatable stages.

Despite the results of the Chinese study, the American Cancer Society urges women to continue monthly breast self-exams. The method is inexpensive and noninvasive; used in conjunction with mammography, it can be a valuable tool.

The second aspect of the three-pronged approach is an annual breast exam by a physician, either your gynecologist or your internist. At the first exam, your physician will make a baseline study, perhaps jotting down notes or making diagrams, to establish a working knowledge of what your breasts are like. At future exams your doctor can note any changes. If such changes need to be followed more closely, your physician may recommend breast exams at six-month intervals instead of once a year.

Third is mammography, which is important in finding lesions or lumps that may be too small or too subtle to feel. Mammograms do not pick up all lumps, however, and sometimes you can feel a lump that does not show up on the X-ray; in fact, 7 to 10 percent of breast cancers that you can feel do not show up on mammograms. This fact does not mean that mammograms are useless. It means that you have to couple them with self-examination and examination by your doctor to get maximum protection. To minimize the discomfort of a mammogram, you can cut down on caffeine for a few days before the exam. Not only will this increase your comfort, but it will make the X-ray easier to read.

▶ *Do I need a mammogram if there is no history of breast cancer in my family?*

Absolutely. My patients ask me this frequently, and the answer is a resounding yes. Most women who develop breast cancer do not have a known family member who has had the disease.

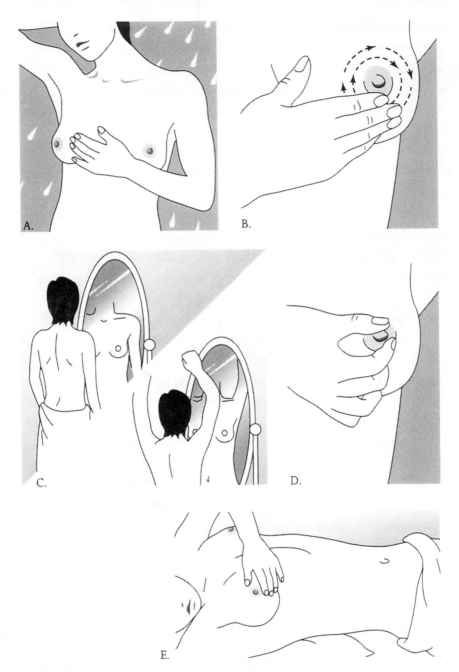

FIGURE 20. Breast self-examination. There are five simple steps to monthly self-examination:
A. Check the breasts while bathing; lumps may be easier to feel when your skin is wet.
B. Place your right hand behind your head and use the sensitive finger pads of your left hand to feel the right breast as you check for thickening, lumps, or other changes. Then use your right hand to examine your left breast in the same manner.

▶ *How often should I have a mammogram?*

The standard recommendations from the American Cancer Society are a yearly mammogram from age forty onward. The American College of Obstetricians and Gynecologists recommends a mammogram at least every other year between ages forty and fifty, and annually thereafter.

Mammography for women in their forties is currently controversial. The National Cancer Institute has stated that mammography during that decade does not increase life expectancy in women who are later diagnosed with cancer. Nevertheless, other major health organizations such as the American College of Obstetricians and Gynecologists and the American Cancer Society still believe that early detection is valuable and that it is worthwhile to have mammograms between the ages of forty and fifty. There is no argument that mammograms at least every other year for women in their fifties are of real value.

If a woman is at particular risk for breast cancer, her doctor will instruct her to get more frequent mammograms. Sometimes abnormalities are discovered on mammograms that are not significant enough for a biopsy but that should be followed on serial mammograms more frequently than once a year.

▶ *How reliable are mammograms?*

You have probably heard of someone whose mammograms gave a false negative (did not find existing breast cancer). Mammography is not a perfect diagnostic tool, having a sensitivity (the ability to detect existing cancer) of up to 94 percent, which means that about 6 percent of cancers will not be found. In particular, mammograms may not be able to detect a growth in dense breast tissue, the type of tissue often seen in young women's breasts.

On the other hand, mammograms have a specificity (the ability to find an absence of cancer when no cancer is present) of greater than 90 percent. Mammography can detect a cancerous growth as much as two years before it can be felt by a manual exam.

C. With your hands at your sides, examine your breasts in a mirror, looking for any change in size or contour, or any dimpling of the skin. Raise your hands over your head and again look for changes.
D. Gently squeeze each nipple, checking for discharge.
E. Lie flat and put a pillow under your right shoulder. Place your right hand under your head and use your left hand to feel the right breast and armpit for lumps. Then place your left hand under your head and use your right hand to examine your left breast and armpit.

▶ *Are mammograms safe?*

Since 1992, when the Food and Drug Administration required hospitals, breast clinics, and other facilities to meet specific standards in order to offer mammography, the quality and the safety of mammography have improved. The guidelines assure that the mammography equipment is safe and uses the lowest possible dose of radiation.

Many people are concerned about exposure to X-rays, but the level of radiation in up-to-date mammograms does not significantly increase the risk for breast cancer. A woman who receives radiation therapy for breast cancer will receive several thousand rads (a unit of energy absorbed from radiation). A woman getting yearly mammograms from age forty until age ninety will receive ten rads. The amount of radiation to which you are exposed during a single mammogram equals the radiation you get on a flight from New York to Los Angeles.

BOX 3.   When Your Mammogram Gives the Wrong Answer:
False Negatives and False Positives

False negatives (missed diagnoses) occur when mammograms appear normal even though breast cancer is present. False negatives are more common in younger women than in older women. The dense breasts of younger women contain many glands and ligaments, which make breast cancers more difficult to spot in mammograms. As women age, breast tissues become more fatty and breast cancers are more easily "seen" by screening mammograms. Screening mammograms miss up to 25 percent of breast cancers in women in their forties but only 10 percent of cancers for older women.

False positives (false alarms) occur when mammograms are read as abnormal but no cancer is present. For women at all ages, between 5 and 10 percent of mammograms are abnormal. Most abnormalities will turn out not to be cancer. False positives are more common in younger women than older women. About 97 percent of women ages forty to forty-nine who have abnormal mammograms turn out not to have cancer as compared with about 86 percent for women age fifty and older. But all women whose mammograms show abnormalities must undergo follow-up procedures such as repeat mammograms or biopsies.

▶ *Are there tests other than mammograms that can be used to detect breast cancer?*

Probably no one likes having a mammogram, and many women find them uncomfortable. Although no technique yet developed by modern science detects breast cancer as accurately as a mammogram, some techniques can be used as adjuncts to supplement what a mammogram shows.

If you have a lump that you can feel and want to know whether it is full of solid matter or filled with fluid, ultrasound can help. Sound waves outline the area that has a texture different from the surrounding tissue. Ultrasound does not detect the kind of small calcium deposits that often appear on a mammogram, sometimes triggering a diagnosis of breast cancer.

The reliability of an ultrasound study also depends on the skill of the person who reads the scan. This is far less true of mammograms, which are much easier to read and interpret. If you are in doubt, inquire about the training and experience of the ultrasonagrapher who will be reading your study. Here in New Haven, where I practice, we are fortunate in having some superb doctors who specialize in this field, but if you live in a small town or a remote area, check with your health care provider about the best place to have an ultrasound done.

Women occasionally ask about MRI, or magnetic resonance imaging, to evaluate the breast. Several articles have appeared in the media saying that MRI imaging is marvelous and that it is less painful than a mammogram; but in terms of evaluating the tissues, of pointing out areas in the breast that may be suspect, or of suggesting whether suspicious tissues are actually cancerous, MRI remains an experimental technique. It is also a very expensive test, costing more than a thousand dollars for a single study.

Thermograms measure heat production by tissues and were popular for a while, on the premise that cancer produces heat. However, the sensitivity of these tests did not prove helpful in the long run in screening for breast cancer.

A new technique called ductal lavage can be used to help diagnose or rule out cancer in high-risk people, such as women with the BRCA1 or BRCA2 genes, or to check on women who have an abnormal discharge from the nipple but no palpable mass. It can be considered a kind of Pap smear for the breast.

Ductal lavage is done by injecting a saltwater solution into the ducts of the breast and then sucking back the fluid to see there are if any abnormal cells. If there are abnormal cells, then further evaluation is in order. The test does not give a lot of false positives—

that is, it does not say you have breast cancer when you do not—but it does sometimes give false negatives—it fails to find existing disease. Currently ductal lavage is controversial and some breast surgeons doubt its usefulness as a screening tool. It is also moderately expensive, costing something in the hundreds of dollars.

For the present, mammograms remain the most important test for breast diagnosis, and no replacements are on the immediate horizon.

▶ What are fibrocystic breasts?

When you do your breast self-exam, you may find that your breasts feel lumpy or bumpy. You probably have also noticed that this condition changes throughout your menstrual cycle. About 60 to 70 percent of American women have lumpy breasts at one time or another. The lumps are caused by a high incidence of the fibrous tissue that is part of normal breast tissue; fibrous breasts are also prone to cysts, which are fluid-filled sacs.

This condition is sometimes called fibrocystic breast disease, but it is not a disease. Formerly it was known as cystic mastitis, which implied an inflammation of the breasts, but that is not the case.

▶ Are women with fibrocystic breasts at increased risk for cancer?

In general, you are not at increased risk for developing breast cancer if you have fibrocystic breasts. Some women, however, have fibrocystic breasts whose cells divide and reproduce faster than the cells of normal breast tissue. If these rapidly growing cells develop atypical changes, then these women are at a risk for cancer that is four times greater than the norm. The condition of overly rapid growth is called hyperplasia, and the odd-looking cells are called atypia. If you fall into this group of women who have hyperplasia with atypia, you should increase your attention to breast self-examinations and be sure you carry them out early in your menstrual cycle when your breasts are easiest to examine. If you find any subtle changes, call your doctor.

Fibrocystic breasts are harder to examine because they are lumpy to begin with. It is difficult in self-examination to tell a benign lump from something that might be potentially dangerous. It is also a little trickier for the radiologist to read a mammogram, because the breasts are a bit denser.

▶ *If I find a lump in my breast or have a mammogram that shows unusual areas of tissue, what should I do?*

You should first call your primary care physician, who can examine you and confirm that what you have found needs to be investigated. Your primary care physician will most likely refer you to a surgeon, who will set about determining what the lump is. Is it benign, perhaps a cyst? Or is it cancerous? Although gynecologists certainly examine a lot of breasts and order a lot of mammograms, few of them are trained to do breast surgery. In this country general surgeons perform almost all breast surgery.

The kinds of lumps that can be felt are called, in medical terminology, discrete or vague. Discrete lumps are very different from the surrounding tissue. Vague lumps are less distinguishable from their surroundings and usually not so hard.

If someone has a vague lump in her breast and is a heavy caffeine drinker, her physician may take her off the caffeine, give her vitamins E and B6, and see whether the lump goes away. If your doctor makes these suggestions, it is absolutely imperative that you take them to heart and that you follow the lumpy area closely yourself and call your doctor immediately should there be any change. You should also return for a breast exam in the next month or two, at some point early in the menstrual cycle.

Most lumpy areas or vague lumps can be followed safely through one or two menstrual cycles, but if after two menstrual cycles (with vitamin B6, vitamin E, and no caffeine) the lump has not gone away, it usually needs to be biopsied to be sure it is not a cancer. Although cancers can manifest themselves in very obvious ways, they can also be nebulous and indistinct. Therefore any lump, vague or discrete, has to be dealt with.

If the lump is discrete, it might be a cyst, which is a fluid-filled sac. One approach is to aspirate the lump with a needle. If the lump does not disappear, as a cyst does when it is aspirated, the specialist will recommend a mammogram (if one has not already been done) and perhaps an ultrasound study. An ultrasound will determine whether the lesion is solid or cystic but multiloculated; that is, whether it is a single cyst that has just one sac or has walls within it. Multiloculated cysts may not disappear when aspirated. If the lump is solid, the next step in the diagnosis is a biopsy.

Biopsies and Other Diagnostic Tools

▶ *What does a breast biopsy involve?*

If a lump persists and needs to be removed for diagnostic purposes, usually a surgeon will remove it surgically. This procedure, called an excisional biopsy, is followed when the lump can be located by palpation. It can be done in a surgicenter as an outpatient procedure, either with a sedative and local anesthetic or with a local anesthetic alone.

The anesthetics are injected into the breast; the surgeon makes an incision and removes the lump. It is taken out in its entirety, along with a rim of the normal tissue around it, to be sure that the whole lump is removed. The tissue then is sent to a pathologist for examination under a microscope.

Another kind of biopsy is a needle-localized biopsy. This technique is used on lesions that are too small to be felt (or cannot be felt for other reasons) but are seen on mammograms. When this happens, the surgeon uses the mammogram as a guide to find the lesion. This technique also is performed as an outpatient procedure, again with a local anesthetic with or without sedation.

Before the needle-localized biopsy takes place, the patient goes to the X-ray department of the surgicenter or hospital. Her breast is cleansed, a local anesthetic is injected, and with the aid of the X-ray machine a guide needle is inserted into the breast, to point toward the lesion. Once the guide needle is in place, the radiologist takes another mammogram to confirm that the needle has localized the lesion.

The needle is taped in place and patient goes to the operating room, where the surgeon uses the guide needle to locate the lesion. Sometimes after the incision has been made the surgeon can feel the lesion and can then be sure that all the suspect tissue has been removed. In other cases (for example, when the tissue in the suspect area looks different from the surrounding tissue) the surgeon will send the excised tissue back to the X-ray department to confirm that what was removed includes the entire suspect area. When the complete lesion has been removed, it is sent to the pathologist.

Another type of biopsy called a stereotactic needle biopsy is now being used in many institutions. It is similar to the needle-localization biopsy because it uses a mammogram as a guide, but in this case a needle is used to remove some of the tissue, which again is sent to a pathologist for examination. Although this technique is in the experimental stages and cannot be universally used, in some cases it eliminates the need to surgically excise the lesion.

▶ *Do women whose biopsies are diagnosed as benign need any special follow-up?*

The appropriate follow-up depends on what the biopsy showed. The woman whose biopsy was benign but displayed hyperplasia with atypia belongs to a group with somewhat increased risk and needs to be followed carefully. She should have a mammogram in six months; an annual mammogram is usually recommended thereafter.

If the lesion was a cyst and no other cysts appear, or if it was a solid lesion like a fibroadenoma or a fibrocystic tissue with no atypical hyperplasia, then the guidelines of the American Cancer Society suggest that routine mammograms are probably adequate, especially if there is no family history of cancer. Many physicians like to see such women six months after the biopsy, however, to check on the healing process and to note the appearance of the breast in the area where the biopsy was done. There can be significant scarring after a biopsy, and it is important to know whether that has occurred. The scarring will be a permanent feature of the breast and will figure in the physician's baseline assessment for future examinations.

Treatment

The purpose of surgery is to remove the original tumor so that it can't send cancerous cells to other parts of the body. Depending on the size of the tumor or the stage of the cancer, a woman and her doctor must make several decisions. First, how much tissue should be removed? Should it be just the tumor, the tumor and part of the surrounding breast, or the entire breast? If the cancer is found while the tumor is quite small, then treatment options include lumpectomy, mastectomy with immediate construction, mastectomy with later reconstruction, or mastectomy with no reconstruction.

In the past, the only treatment for ductal cancer considered safe in the United States was a mastectomy. The standard operation involved removing all the breast tissue of the affected breast and taking samples of the lymph nodes in the adjacent armpit. But in 1989 a large-scale scientific study, confirmed by subsequent studies, showed that a lumpectomy was as effective as a mastectomy. If a woman had one and only one cancerous area in the breast, if the area was smaller than 3 to 4 centimeters (about an inch and a quarter) and the tumor cells were not terribly aggressive (that is, they did not look particularly malignant under the microscope), then the lump could be removed safely without taking the entire breast. For many women this is a desirable choice, since cosmetically a lumpectomy is much less disfiguring.

▶ *What is the difference between a mastectomy and a lumpectomy?*

A mastectomy, which is the common term for a "modified radical mastectomy," is a surgical procedure that involves removing the breast tissue and sampling some of the lymph nodes in the armpit, or axilla. A lumpectomy, also known as a partial mastectomy, involves removing the cancerous lump along with a rim of normal tissue, plus axillary dissection. Axillary dissection refers to a separate operation in which the tissue in the armpit is removed along with anywhere from six to twenty-five lymph nodes. Radiation therapy after a lumpectomy usually lasts six weeks.

▶ Why are lymph nodes analyzed?

Lymph nodes are removed and biopsied to investigate whether the cancer has spread to other parts of the body. There are two methods for doing this. One, called lymph node dissection, involves removing a percentage of the lymph nodes and testing them to see whether cancer cells can be found there. The second technique, called sentinel lymph node biopsy, focuses on a single lymph node, the first one to receive drainage from the breast.

This single lymph node is identified through a special technology. A dye is injected into the breast, and special X-rays can be taken to see which lymph node picks up the dye first. This node is the most likely to be the first stopping site of any cancer cells. If the node is removed and found to be clear of cancer, then it is very unlikely that the cancer has spread to any other lymph node or any place outside the original tumor.

▶ Who is a candidate for a lumpectomy?

Despite what you read or hear in the media, not everyone is a suitable candidate for a lumpectomy, which will usually be accompanied by axillary dissection or sentinel node biopsy and radiation therapy. The two most important factors in determining who can have a lumpectomy are the number of cancerous areas and (if there is only one area) the size of the lump. If more than one spot of cancer exists in the breast, a condition that physicians call multifocality, radiation is not adequate therapy to prevent recurrence. If the lump is larger than 3 cm, or about an inch and a quarter, it is difficult to remove the lump cosmetically along with a rim of normal tissue. Even if a woman has a large breast, so that a lump bigger than 3 cm could be removed, a lump this size increases the possibility that there are other cancer cells within the breast.

▶ What kinds of breast reconstruction are available after a mastectomy?

Many women who have mastectomies want breast reconstruction. The time schedules for performing this procedure vary. One approach is immediate reconstruction, whereby the surgeon carries out the mastectomy and the plastic surgeon performs the reconstruction at the time of the initial surgery. Another approach is to wait six months to a year before doing the reconstruction.

Immediate reconstruction is a joint approach involving the cancer surgeon and the team of plastic surgeons who do the reconstruction. The decision is based on where the reconstructive tissue is going to come from. If someone with a tumor smaller than 3 cm has difficulty deciding whether she wants a mastectomy or a lumpectomy, she might speak to a plastic surgeon to learn the pros and cons of immediate reconstruction.

The pros are primarily emotional, doing away with the emotional stress that often accompanies the wait of six months or a year for reconstruction. Many women choose to wait, however, because with immediate reconstruction comes a 25 percent increase in complications, which can include infection and inadequate healing of the skin over the implant.

▶ *What materials are used for reconstruction now that silicone is no longer available?*

Depending on individual body type, tissue can be removed from other parts of the body, such as the abdominal wall. Saline (saltwater) implants are also used. And though silicone is banned officially for elective reconstructive surgery for cosmetic purposes, it is still technically available for cancer patients. Several of the companies that manufactured silicone in the past are no longer making implants, so availability is limited.

▶ *Where does chemotherapy fit into this scheme?*

Chemotherapy used to be reserved for patients whose cancer had spread to their lymph nodes. Today evidence from studies in this country and around the world shows that if a tumor looks even somewhat aggressive under the microscope, a woman is at increased risk of recurrence or of developing cancer somewhere else in her body, even though there may be no spread of cancer to the lymph nodes. Therefore the current recommendation is that chemotherapy is appropriate for many women with cancerous tumors, even if they have no lymph node involvement. So you need not worry that your doctor is hiding something from you if he or she recommends that you have chemotherapy.

▶ *What drugs are used for chemotherapy?*

In chemotherapy the needs of each woman must be considered individually. One kind of chemotherapy involves manipulating hormone levels. Some cancer cells have receptors called estrogen and progesterone receptors, meaning that estrogen and progesterone molecules attach themselves to the cancer cells and stimulate the growth of the cancer. Each cancer that is biopsied is examined for these receptors. If the estrogen receptors are positive, the patient may benefit from an antiestrogen drug such as tamoxifen.

Another approach to chemotherapy involves aromatase inhibitors including anastrozole, trade name Arimidex. These drugs also work by manipulating hormones to deprive estrogen-receptor-positive cancers of the estrogen that stimulates their growth. The main source of estrogen in postmenopausal women comes from the conversion into estrogen of androgens, male-type sex hormones produced by the adrenal glands and the ovaries. The process of conversion, called aromatization, takes place mainly in body fat and is carried out by an enzyme called aromatase. Anastrozole blocks this conversion, thus reducing the amount of estrogen in the body.

Other kinds of chemotherapy attack rapidly dividing cells regardless of their receptor status.

▶ *What are the possible complications of tamoxifen?*

There are two major risks from a gynecological point of view. One is the significant increase in cancer of the uterus; the other is the incidence of phlebitis, a potentially serious inflammation of the veins. There is also a possible benefit. In addition to its effectiveness in preventing recurrences of breast cancer, the drug reduces cholesterol levels, and it is hoped that it will reduce the risk of heart disease, the leading cause of death in older women.

Women should realize that taking tamoxifen is not a simple matter like taking a vitamin or an aspirin. Tamoxifen is a very complicated drug, both a form of estrogen and an antiestrogen at the same time. Its effects on veins and on the uterine lining come about because of its estrogenic qualities.

For women who have had breast cancer, the drug's proven benefit in preventing new cancers outweighs its risks. For women who have not had breast cancer, the preventive value of this drug is not yet known because the study is so new. Women who are taking tamoxifen should have regular checkups so as to treat any uterine cancer as early as possible.

Breast Cancer and Hormone Therapy

▶ *Can someone who has had breast cancer have HRT?*

The issue is highly controversial. Some oncologists believe that so little is known about the physiology of breast cancer and its relation to hormones that any woman who has had breast cancer should not be on hormonal therapy.

On the other hand, small-scale studies of breast cancer survivors comparing women who took ERT or HRT with those who took no hormones found no difference between the two groups in terms of risk of recurring cancer, a new breast cancer, or metastases. Some studies even found that women who were taking hormones at the time that their breast cancer was diagnosed had a better outcome than women who were not using hormones.

Many women with a severely compromised quality of life, because of significant hot flashes or vaginal dryness and discomfort, feel that their symptoms are so overwhelming that HRT might make sense for them. The risk-benefit relation must be carefully weighed by the woman and her health care provider.

▶ *Can someone who has had a biopsy that showed atypical hyperplasia have HRT?*

If a woman is at high risk for breast cancer, either because of her family history or because she had a biopsy that showed atypical hyperplasia, she should be aware of the risks of hormonal therapy. Again, the decision of whether or not to take HRT must be individualized; there is no one right answer for everybody.

UTERINE OR ENDOMETRIAL CANCER

Endometrial cancer is cancer of the lining of the uterus, the endometrium. It is a relatively rare disease, about five times less common than breast cancer, with an estimated 40,320 new cases in 2004 and 7,090 deaths. It is also a cancer that grows slowly and is likely to be diagnosed early. Unlike many forms of cancer (pancreatic, ovarian, or stomach cancer), endometrial cancer makes its presence known because most of the time it causes bleeding early in the process. With this early warning, uterine cancer is ordinarily quite easy to cure. When the disease is confined to the body of the uterus, cure rates are about 95 percent. A scientific study a few years back compared women with and without endometrial cancer who had similar risk factors for heart disease, diabetes, high blood pressure, and so on. Surprisingly, the group without endometrial cancer did worse statistically than the group with cancer. This finding certainly does not mean that endometrial cancer is good for you, merely that cancer did not prove to be the lethal issue for most of the women in the group.

Precursors and Stages of Endometrial Cancer

▶ *How does endometrial cancer develop?*

Before full-blown cancer of the endometrium develops, the tissues go through precursor stages just as they do with other cancers. Cancer is classified according to its location and its severity, that is, how far it has spread. These stages involve various kinds of hyperplasia.

Adenomatous hyperplasia refers to excessive growth of the glandular cells that make up the lining of the uterus. The term "adenomatous hyperplasia" indicates that a given sample of uterine tissue contains more than the normal number of glandular cells. Adenomatous hyperplasia with atypia means that there are more than the normal number of glandular cells and those cells look different, not ordinary. It is adenomatous hyperplasia with atypia that may lead to endometrial cancer. Many physicians believe that simple adenomatous hyperplasia is not a serious threat, that only when the pathologist starts seeing atypical cells is there reason to worry.

▶ *What are the stages once cancer does develop?*

As with most gynecological tumors, there are four stages of actual uterine cancer. Stage I disease is confined to the body of the uterus, also called the uterine corpus, and is easiest to treat. Stage II disease involves the cervix as well as the uterus. Although the cervix can be considered part of the uterus, there is an important difference. Lymph nodes are close to the cervix, and if these are involved it is possible for the cancer to spread from this location. In stage III disease the cancer is no longer confined to the uterus and cervix but has started spreading to other pelvic organs, to the ovaries, to the tissue around the uterus, to lymph nodes outside the uterus. Stage IV disease has distant metastases; fortunately we see very little of it. The vast majority of women who present with endometrial cancer are stage I, which means that they can be cured easily.

> Edith C. came to my office last year after a single episode of bleeding. She is seventy-three, postmenopausal of course, not using HRT, and healthy as can be. Edith is not fat; she is not diabetic; and she plays eighteen holes of golf several

times a week. In short, she is in great shape. We did a D&C and discovered that she had stage II uterine cancer; so I performed a hysterectomy. Fortunately, she came in with her first episode of bleeding; she did not delay; she did everything right, and there is a very good chance that she will be cured. She did have the bad luck to have her disease progress to stage II before she had any unusual bleeding. Now, a year later, her golf handicap is unchanged and she is as active as ever.

Life expectancies range from a 95 percent cure rate (which means that 95 percent of people with the disease will be alive in five years) with stage I cancer to a 10 percent rate with stage IV disease.

Risk Factors

Uterine cancer is a disease that has classic associated risks. Most women who get uterine cancer do so after menopause, with 95 percent of endometrial cancers occurring in women aged forty or older. The average age of diagnosis is sixty, but this rate does not increase with aging. While younger women can get the disease, they rarely do so.

Among the classic risk factors, obesity is far and away the most significant. Whenever I see a massively obese woman, I see a hysterectomy in the making. I must confess that I also feel a certain sympathy for the gynecologist who will have to penetrate all that fatty tissue to get to the uterus.

The reason fat women get cancer of the endometrium is that fat tissue makes estrogen, so their fat is making plenty of estrogen even when their ovaries are not. Women who are twenty-one to fifty pounds overweight triple their risk; women more than fifty pounds above normal weight increase their risk tenfold.

Two other risk factors, diabetes and high blood pressure, may be associated with obesity but may also be independent of body weight. That is, if you are obese you are at increased risk for high blood pressure and diabetes; but if you have one of these conditions even if you are not obese, you are still at increased risk for uterine cancer. If you are a slender diabetic, your risk of uterine cancer is higher than that of the average population. If you are an overweight diabetic, and many diabetics do have a problem with weight control, you are at significantly increased risk.

Not having children increases risk. A woman who has had four pregnancies is at much lower risk for cancer of the lining of the uterus than someone who has had one child. Delayed childbearing also seems to increase risk, but only minimally.

You might notice that this pattern of risk resembles the pattern for breast cancer. Factors common to both are increased risk with age, late age at first live birth or never having children, early age at onset of menstruation, and late age at menopause. The genetic factor is much lower in endometrial cancer, however. Because of the similarity in risk pattern, women who have had endometrial cancer are at high risk for breast cancer and should be sure to keep up their regular mammograms (but of course so should everyone).

The reason for the similarity in risk for the two diseases seems to have something to do with estrogen. Although pregnant women have high estrogen levels, the type of estrogen differs from that which nonpregnant women produce. Furthermore, progesterone is present in extremely high levels during pregnancy. It seems to be this profile of different hormones that offers a protective effect against breast cancer and endometrial cancer.

Women who take ERT but do not take progesterone are at some increased risk for uterine cancer. Depending on which scientific paper you read, that risk is estimated at anywhere from two times to as much as eight times that of the normal population. That may sound like a greatly increased risk, but if you are talking about a disease that affects one in a thousand people, as opposed to eight in a thousand people, you are still talking about a rare disease.

Taking progesterone and having periodic cleanout bleeds reduce risk to just about that of the normal population, although progesterone will not prevent uterine cancer in every case. Some women will get the disease regardless of their hormone status.

Taking tamoxifen as a prevention therapy for breast cancer increases the risk of endometrial cancer in that tamoxifen has estrogenic properties. However, raloxifene, which is similar to tamoxifen and presently is prescribed to protect against osteoporosis, does not increase the risk of endometrial cancer.

Prevention

The most important thing you can do to protect yourself from endometrial cancer is to maintain a normal body weight. Reliable studies suggest that birth control pills protect you against both uterine and ovarian cancer. Protection is greater if you take oral contraceptives for a long time, and the benefit lasts for at least ten years after you stop taking the pill.

▶ *What are the warning symptoms of uterine cancer?*

Irregular bleeding is the first warning. It is not the kind of bleeding you get when the length of time between your periods shortens from twenty-eight days to twenty-one days. Nor is it the heavy bleeding that women experience perimenopausally (though heavy bleeding does occasionally accompany uterine cancer). The bleeding that most women get with uterine cancer is sporadic spotting, the kind that comes for a few days or a week and then goes away and comes back again.

Treatment

▶ *If endometrial cancer is discovered in the precursor stages, is surgery necessary?*

Adenomatous hyperplasia, even with atypia, can be treated medically, without surgery. Many gynecologists treat it with progesterone. Since adenomatous hyperplasia seems to be a condition of excess estrogen, the addition of progesterone will bring the hormones into balance and actually reverse some of the hyperplasia changes.

> Ursula R. is forty-eight and perimenopausal. Fair and slim, she has a family history of osteoporosis. She has adenomatous hyperplasia with atypia. Ursula has tried progesterone in every known form, and whatever kind she takes, she feels awful. She gets headaches and she feels out of control emotionally, although when she is not taking progesterone she is a very stable, intelligent, responsible person.

Because she is fair and slender, Ursula is at high risk for osteoporosis and should probably consider taking HRT to protect her bones. If she could tolerate the progesterone, I would give her progestins and repeat biopsies and D&Cs to see whether the progesterone could get rid of her atypia. But because she cannot tolerate the progesterone, her only option is to have a hysterectomy.

The usual approach to adenomatous hyperplasia is to give progesterone and then do a biopsy in another three months or so, to see whether the extra growth is gone. Because this kind of cancer is not ordinarily fast growing, we have the luxury of time to try medical approaches before resorting to surgery.

▶ *What is the treatment for endometrial cancer that has developed beyond the precursor stages?*

The classic therapy for stage I disease is a hysterectomy. Unless there is some very good reason for not doing so, the ovaries are also taken out, since the estrogen they produce stimulates the cancerous cells. If cancerous cells remain anywhere in the body, the estrogen will cause them to grow. Sometimes the surgeon will take out a few lymph nodes. In any case, after removal the uterus is always sent to the pathologist, whose report will determine whether follow-up therapy is needed.

▶ *What does the pathologist look for?*

He or she will look at the tissue of the uterus under the microscope and grade the tumor according to several criteria. First will be an evaluation of how close to normal the cells within the uterus look. The least malignant tumors are called well differentiated; the cells in them look quite a bit like normal tissue, but there is more tissue present than under normal conditions. Poorly differentiated tumors, by contrast, contain cells that do not so closely resemble normal tissue.

The pathologist will also investigate the degree of penetration, how far the tumor has invaded the muscular area. Another term for penetration is myometrial invasion, which means penetration by the cancerous cells of the myometrium, or muscular wall of the uterus. Most of the time when the tumor is well differentiated, it has not penetrated very far through the wall of the uterus. Pathologists grade the penetration in percentages: taking the entire width of the uterus as 100 percent, the pathology report will state that the tumor has permeated or invaded 5 percent of the distance or 20 percent of the distance. A tumor that has penetrated only 5 percent of the distance through the uterine wall is very well confined.

Although a D&C will tell something about the differentiation of the cells and the rate of cell division, the only way that penetration can truly be evaluated is from the hysterectomy specimen itself. This grading or staging after surgery will often determine whether further therapy is needed.

If your doctor tells you that you have some abnormal cells in your endometrium, you needn't panic. You don't have to fear that because you have abnormal cells you will quickly die of cancer. Just as you have the luxury of time with abnormal Pap smears, you have a relaxed time frame to make decisions about adenomatous hyperplasia. You can treat it; you can try progesterone; you can have repeat biopsies. Unless your D&C has shown that you have invasive cancer, don't feel that you have to have a hysterectomy immediately.

> Liz H., a very chubby fifty-six-year-old, had a D&C in November that showed that she had stage I endometrial carcinoma. The treatment for it was a hysterectomy, but the proposed timing was unfortunate. She wanted to put off the operation for a month because the six-week postop recuperation period would take her into the middle of the Christmas season, and she wanted very much to be with her family during the holidays. I didn't see anything wrong with the slight delay, but I got some opposition from the oncologist. At any rate, we waited a month and performed her operation before Christmas. She had a very small focus of disease in her uterus. Now it is three years later and she is fine. Her cancer at the time of the surgery has not spread. The disease has not recurred, and her chances of remaining cancer-free are greater than 90 percent. However, I worry about her because her weight is 250 pounds and she is at high risk still for diabetes and high blood pressure.

▶ *What kinds of follow-up therapy might be recommended after a hysterectomy?*

One common follow-up, even for innocent-looking stage I disease, is radiation. Perhaps 8 to 10 percent of women with very mild-appearing disease get a recurrence at the top of the vagina after their hysterectomy. Gynecologists and radiotherapists have found that if you give some radiation to the top of the vagina, a very localized area, you can significantly reduce the chances of a recurrence.

Years ago physicians would put a bit of radium into the vagina and leave it there for a day. Now we use potent but very focused X-ray beams, given in three separate five-minute treatments. This gamma med, as the procedure is called, does not have side effects. There is no burning of the skin, and the patient does not lose her pubic hair. The top of the vagina is not scarred in a way that might make it difficult to have intercourse. The gamma med reduces the risk of recurrence from 8 or 10 percent down to 1 or 2 percent.

If the disease has progressed further, additional radiation therapy is usually recommended. Or different kinds of chemotherapy are given, some of which are very helpful. Hormonal therapies based on progesterone prevent hot flashes in situations where the gynecologist is not comfortable giving estrogen.

Among my patients are a number of nuns, all of whom because of their celibate lifestyle are at increased risk for endometrial carcinoma and breast cancer. (In contrast, their celibacy protects them from cervical cancer and sexually transmitted diseases.) One of the sisters is a little plump and has mild diabetes and hypertension, both of which are risk factors for endometrial carcinoma.

Ten years ago she did have endometrial carcinoma and I performed a hysterectomy. Since then she has been taking progesterone for prevention of hot flashes. Recently she developed breast cancer, which seemed independent of her progesterone therapy, and indeed it was progesterone-receptor negative. Nevertheless, her oncologist did not want her on any hormonal therapy. Without the progesterone she was having really unpleasant flushes.

We have been trying different medications to control the flashing and have settled on Bellergal. She feels better, but not as well as when she was taking the progesterone.

▶ *Are hysterectomies for uterine cancer ever done vaginally?*

Hysterectomies for cancer are almost always done abdominally, in part because an abdominal hysterectomy gives the best view of what is inside the pelvis. In rare conditions, for example if a woman is grossly overweight and her body fat is a real impediment to the abdominal procedure, or if she has had many children and her uterus is prolapsed, the surgeon may opt to do the procedure vaginally.

After a Hysterectomy
▶ *How do the treatments for endometrial cancer affect sexuality?*

Although women who have had gamma med basically experience no side effects, women who have had total pelvic irradiation can have some scarring in the vagina. For these women, it is important to continue to have intercourse to prevent further contraction of the vagina. If vaginal dryness is a problem, lubricants are available.

Many gynecologists would also feel comfortable recommending estrogen cream because of the small systemic absorption. Some would rule it out, because they believe that if even a small amount of estrogen is absorbed through the vaginal walls, it risks stimulating further cancer. Again, this is an area where each woman must discuss the issue with her gynecologist.

▶ *Can women who have had endometrial cancer take ERT?*

If the uterus and ovaries are surgically removed, menopause will come on immediately and often with significant symptoms. The question of estrogen replacement to relieve symptoms is controversial and centers on whether, after the hysterectomy, cancerous cells are left anywhere in the body. If there are none, then virtually every physician would feel comfortable giving ERT to relieve hot flashes and other symptoms.

In cases where it is impossible to be sure that every single cancerous cell has been removed, different doctors take different approaches. Some say that if the woman is free of cancer five years after the operation, hormone therapy is safe. Of course, by then many women no longer have hot flashes. Other doctors say that since most women with endometrial cancer are overweight and their fat produces estrogen anyhow, they will probably not have intense menopausal symptoms and will not need hormone therapy for relief. Certainly they won't have to worry about osteoporosis, because their fat protects their bones.

What about slim women? Although they are at lower risk, some of them do get endometrial cancer. Should they take ERT after their hysterectomies? Here the issue gets most controversial and there is no clear-cut right answer. The best procedure is for you to talk to your physician. If your symptoms are severe and your doctor does not want to give you estrogen, you might consider a second opinion.

▶ *Can women who have had a hysterectomy for endometrial cancer take*
testosterone to increase libido?

This issue is only mildly controversial. Many researchers feel that testosterone increases libido and find no reason why a woman who has had a hysterectomy for endometrial cancer cannot try testosterone therapy. If her doctor does not want to prescribe estrogen to oppose the testosterone, then the two of them will have to work through a period of adjustment to find just the right dosage: enough testosterone to increase sex drive, but not so much that it causes masculinizing symptoms.

There are physicians, however, who believe that since some of the testosterone will be metabolized into estrogen, women who have had endometrial cancer should not take testosterone or perhaps any other steroid.

CERVICAL CANCER

Cancer of the cervix, the neck of the uterus, most often afflicts women in their thirties and forties. If you are reading this book because you are a perimenopausal or menopausal woman, you most likely have passed your peak risk period for getting this disease, a rare form of cancer and generally a slow-growing one. An estimated 10,520 cases will be diagnosed in 2004 in the United States, and about 3,900 women will die of the disease. As Pap testing has become widespread, both the incidence rate and the death rate have fallen significantly, and between 1955 and 1992 the number of deaths from cervical cancer declined by 74 percent. Sadly, as many as 60 to 80 percent of the women diagnosed with invasive cervical cancer have not had a Pap smear in five years, and many have never had a Pap test at all.

▶ *What is cervical cancer and what causes it?*

Although the cervix, the opening of the uterus into the vagina, can be considered part of the uterus, cancer of the cervix is distinct from uterine cancer because the cells involved are very different.

The lining of the uterus (the endometrium) is composed of glandular tissue, made up of large, chunky, column-type cells. The outer part of the cervix is covered with squamous tissue, made up of flat cells like those that constitute skin. The tissue that covers the inner part of the cervix resembles the tissue that lines the uterus; it is glandular tissue.

There are two kinds of cervical cancer. The less common form is called adenocarcinoma of the cervix. This disease resembles cancer of the uterus and it affects the columnar, glandular cells that cover the inner part of the cervix. The other kind of cervical cancer is squamous cell carcinoma, which affects the flatter squamous cells, mainly on the outer part of the cervix.

Before puberty, however, the cells covering the outer part of the cervix are cube shaped. Right after puberty these cells transform themselves to flatter squamous cells. The technical term for the process is "squamous metaplasia."

During squamous metaplasia the cells already in the process of transformation may receive an insult of some kind that will cause them later to undergo further changes, though these further changes will not show up for decades, until a woman is in her twenties, thirties, or forties. It is easy to think of cervical cancer as a disease of younger women, because the further someone gets from the time when the cells are changing, the less likely she is to get cervical cancer.

Researchers are still trying to discover what agents produce the insult that initiates, however slowly, these cancerous changes. Are these agents chemicals or viruses or bacteria? Scientists do not know for sure, but they do know that the substances that trigger the changes are associated somehow with intercourse.

Right now the leading candidate is something called the human papilloma virus (HPV), the virus that gives you genital warts. Often women who have cervical cancer have had episodes of genital warts (researchers have actually been able to grow strains of the wart virus from tissue samples of women who have cervical cancer).

If you have had genital warts, don't assume that you will automatically get cervical cancer. More than fifty strains of condyloma or papilloma virus produce genital warts; only about three can give you cancer. In fact, the condyloma virus is very common. Many, many women carry HPV around with them, just as many people carry some other virus that doesn't always make them sick. Some experts believe that 100 percent of women who are sexually active in the United States have been exposed to HPV, but most women mount their immunological defenses against it and at worst have warts but often have no symptoms at all.

Other theories about the cause of cervical cancer exist, and the final answers are not yet in. As I explain to my teenage patients, we know that it has something to do with sex, but we don't know what.

▶ *How is cervical cancer diagnosed? Does it have symptoms?*

The vast majority of cervical disease in the United States is diagnosed through Pap smears even before it becomes cancerous. Since women routinely began to be given Pap tests, the incidence of cervical cancer has dropped drastically.

The classic symptom of established cervical cancer is abnormal vaginal bleeding. The bleeding patterns with cervical cancer are different from those of endometrial cancer. Women with cervical cancer often notice bleeding after intercourse; cervical cancer does not usually cause heavy periods (remember, cervical cancer is generally a disease of younger women), though endometrial cancer may do so. Sometimes there is a watery discharge, which may smell bad. Sometimes cervical cancer has no symptoms at all until it is fairly advanced.

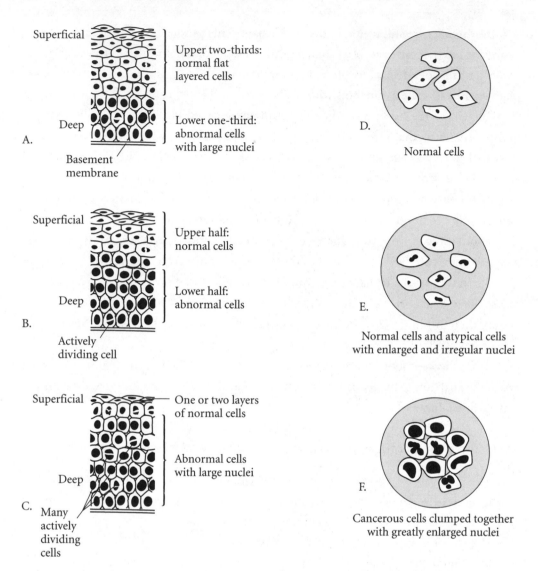

FIGURE 21. Development of cervical cancer. Like other cancers, cervical cancer develops by a series of gradual cellular changes. A, normal cells; B, normal cell and atypical cells with enlarged and irregular nuclei; C, cancerous cells clumped together with greatly enlarged nuclei.

Risk Factors

While we don't know the precise agent that initiates precancerous changes in the cervical cells, we know that women exposed to multiple sexual partners are at increased risk of cervical cancer. We also know that women who have early intercourse are at increased risk of cervical cancer, unless they protect themselves with condoms.

Because changes are taking place in your cervical cells when you are in your mid- to late teen years, you are more at risk if you have intercourse at that time. If you wait until you're twenty-two to have intercourse, most of these changes will have already taken place, so you are at lower risk than someone who has intercourse before she is twenty. To the question "Can sex give you cancer?" the answer is yes, absolutely. It matters how many different partners you have had and how early you began having intercourse.

Early childbearing also seems to have an effect. If you have children when you are young, obviously you have been having sex early also, but some factor in childbirth itself apparently increases risk. Women who have had many children are at higher risk than women who have had few children.

So if you began intercourse at age twenty-four, married, and then had only one partner for the rest of your life, you are a low-risk candidate—unless your husband has had multiple partners. In this case, the husband increases his wife's risk for cervical cancer.

Women who have had sexually transmitted diseases, including chlamydia and HIV infection, are at increased risk. Hispanic, Native American, and African American women have a higher incidence of cervical cancer than do white women, probably because these groups have less access to health care. Diets low in fruits and vegetables have been associated with an increased risk of cervical cancer and several other cancers.

Smoking increases risk, because it exposes the body to carcinogenic chemicals that are absorbed by the lungs and carried in the bloodstream throughout the body. Tobacco by-products have been found in the cervical mucus in women who smoke, and researchers believe that these substances damage the DNA of cells in the cervix and may contribute to the development of cervical cancer. Some researchers believe that a diet deficient in vitamins A and C may contribute to the development of cervical cancer, though this has not been proven. Poor nutrition may also contribute by depressing the immune system.

▶ *Does genital herpes increase the risk of cervical cancer?*

People used to think that getting herpes set you up for cervical cancer, but this is no longer considered to be the case. The data that led to the earlier conclusion were based on the fact that women who had had herpes seemed to have a higher incidence of cervical cancer. What is true is that women with herpes are more likely to have multiple sex partners, early intercourse, and more children. Thus the risks for cervical cancer are similar to the risks for genital herpes. Women who have genital herpes are likely, then, to fall into a high-risk category for cervical cancer.

Stages of Cervical Cancer

Like cancer of the uterus (endometrial cancer), cervical cancer is classified according to the amount of tissue involved. The first changes result in atypical cells (atypia)—not normal but not cancerous either—which can spontaneously revert to normal. The cell changes take place on the surface of the cervix at first, but as time goes on they can penetrate more deeply into the cell layers unless they revert to normal.

The atypical cells may progress to a state of precancerous change, referred to as dysplasia. As long as the changes are confined to cell layers above what is called the basement membrane, the condition is fully curable by local therapy. At the level of mild dysplasia some doctors will recommend observation only, because the cervix can heal itself spontaneously. Once moderate or severe dysplasia is diagnosed, most doctors will recommend intervention.

In the next stages, the precancerous abnormal cells can develop into a local condition called carcinoma in situ. The cells are not yet truly cancerous because they have not become invasive. Since all these changes are occurring slowly, you and your physician have plenty of time to deal with them. Indeed, it is highly unusual for somebody to proceed from mild to moderate to severe dysplasia to carcinoma in situ in a matter of months. Such changes usually take years. All the same, you should continue having Pap smears every year. If you do have an annual Pap test, your chances of getting invasive cancer are almost zero.

Microinvasion is a stage of minimal penetration of the basement membrane, which falls between carcinoma in situ and stage I cancer. Such cancers, although technically invasive, are still relatively easy to cure.

Stage I cervical cancer is confined to the cervix and the uterus. Stage II cancer has spread locally, to the top of the vagina. Stage III cervical cancer has spread a little farther, sometimes to the lower part of the vagina, toward the side walls of the pelvis, sometimes to the ureters, which enter the bladder right next to the cervix. Stage IV cervical cancer has spread still farther, perhaps extending backward or forward and involving the bladder or the rectum.

Pap Tests and What They Mean

Named for Dr. George Papanicolaou, the Pap test is a sampling of the superficial cells of the cervix. Your physician swabs your cervix, scrapes off some cells, and puts them onto a slide so that a pathologist can look at them and tell what kind of cells are being sloughed off. Are they normal-looking cells? Do they look like cancer cells? Or do they look like something in between, something on their way to becoming cancer?

I emphasize to my patients that a Pap smear is a guide. It is not a definitive test. It may suggest that everything is fine, that no cells are present that look at all cancerous or precancerous. But it may suggest that some cells should be further investigated. The test will not invariably show what is going on in terms of cell changes in the cervix, but it will show that there are changes and allow intervention before cancer develops. Most of the changes that we see on Pap smears are benign or precancerous; almost all can be cured with small interventions.

There are several systems for classifying the results of Pap tests, so the terminology can get confusing. Talk to your doctor about the precise meaning of your test results.

One system for grading Pap tests is called the Bethesda System (TBS). Its categories refer to the kinds of cell changes and the extent of the cervix affected by these changes. (The ratings in parenthesis refer to the former grading system, which rated Pap tests in Classes I to V.)

Normal: No evidence of malignant cells (Class I).

Atypical cells of undetermined significance: This category is sometimes called "reactive cellular changes." The cells look "funny," or abnormal, but probably aren't precancerous. The changes can be brought about by such infections as herpes, chlamydia, or yeast infection (Class II).

Low-grade squamous intraepithelial lesion (SIL): The squamous cells that cover the outer part of the cervix show abnormal changes that are not invasive but can become so over time. Sometimes these abnormal cells change back to normal cells on their own (Class III).

High-grade squamous intraepithelial lesion: High-grade SILs are less likely than low-grade SILs to go away without treatment and are more likely to eventually develop into cancer if untreated. Treatment, however, can cure all SILs and prevent true cancer from developing. A Pap smear cannot show for certain whether a woman has a high- or low-grade SIL (Class IV).

Invasive cancer (likely to be spreading into the cervix and potentially beyond): Since my residency days twenty-five years ago, I have never had a patient with a Pap smear that showed invasive cancer. The one patient with invasive cancer whom I did see during my residency was a woman who had four children and had not had a single Pap smear since delivering her last child ten years previously (Class V).

The most confusing of the Bethesda System categories for cells of the outer cervix is "atypical squamous cells of undetermined significance," which is often abbreviated as ASCUS and pronounced "ask-us." Pathologists use the category when the Pap test doesn't reveal whether the abnormal cells are due to inflammation or to a precancer.

The Bethesda System is not the only classification method for reporting Pap test results. An earlier system referred to "dysplasia," which literally means "abnormal growth." Changes in cervical cells were classified by degree, as showing mild dysplasia, moderate dysplasia, or severe dysplasia.

Another term you may hear is "cervical intraepithelial neoplasia" (CIN). The "intraepithelial" means that the changes are in the epithelium or outer layer of the cervix; these changes are not deep, and they are not invasive cancer. The word "neoplasia" connotes unusual cell changes but in this context does not imply invasive cancer. Although CIN is definitely not cancer, it is often classified in grades, as is cancer: CIN means mild dysplasia, CIN 2 is moderate dysplasia, and CIN 3 is severe dysplasia.

Some physicians refer to severe dysplasia as carcinoma in situ. I don't like to use that terminology, because the word "carcinoma" makes people nervous. Carcinoma in situ and severe dysplasia are essentially the same thing. What the "in situ" means is that the carcinoma is not invasive. If you take care of it, you should be cured, and unless you have HIV infection, you should never have to worry about the disease again.

▶ How often should I have a Pap test?

In 2002, the American College of Pathologists, the professional organization for physicians in that specialty, recommended that women at low risk who have had three consecutive normal Pap smears need be tested only once every three years; furthermore, women older than seventy can stop having Pap smears altogether. However, since most health care professionals recommend an annual pelvic exam beyond age seventy, my own feeling is that while I'm doing an exam anyhow, I might just as well do a Pap test.

> Monica D., fifty-three years old and two years past menopause, has come to me for her gynecological exams for more than twenty years. After twenty normal Pap tests, she had a very abnormal one, which really surprised me and I thought at first that the lab had mixed up the slides. She was also complaining of vaginal dryness. We tried treating that with estrogen cream, but it didn't help her. It turned out that she had a high-grade cervical lesion.

TABLE 4. Classification of Pap Test Results

PAPANICOLAOU CLASSIFICATION SYSTEM	OLD SYSTEM	BETHESDA SYSTEM
Class I	Normal	Within normal limits
Class II	Atypical	Benign cellular changes (or)
		Atypical squamous cells of undetermined significance (ASCUS)
Class III	Dysplasia	Squamous epithelial cell abnormality
	Mild	Low-grade squamous intraepithelial lesion (SIL)
	Moderate	High-grade SIL
	Severe	High-grade SIL
Class IV	Carcinoma in situ	High-grade SIL
Class V	Invasive squamous cell carcinoma	Squamous cell carcinoma
	Adenocarcinoma	Adenocarcinoma

To the best of everyone's knowledge Monica was in a mutually long-term monogamous relationship. Nevertheless, biopsies confirmed that she had carcinoma in situ of the cervix. We treated it with a cone biopsy, a minor surgical procedure, which confirmed the diagnosis. Since that time her Pap test has reverted to normal. Because Monica had her annual Pap test, she saved herself more invasive treatment: if she had waited a few years, she would have needed a hysterectomy instead of just a cone biopsy.

▶ *If I have an abnormal Pap smear, must I have treatment quickly?*

A few years back, Scandinavian researchers did a massive study on a group of more than ten thousand women. Several thousand had documented carcinoma in situ of the cervix, that is, carcinoma that did not penetrate the basement membrane. The researchers did nothing for these women; they simply watched them over a ten-year period to see what happened. One-third reverted to normal; they got well with no intervention. One-third stayed the same. The final third progressed toward cancer. But the time frame was ten years, not twenty minutes.

Although I am not advocating that we fail to treat carcinoma in situ just because the Scandinavian study said that some of these women get better spontaneously, I want to emphasize that if you have an abnormal Pap smear—and many women will at some time in their life—do not panic. Proceed slowly. Repeat the Pap test; have biopsies. But don't get involved with radical therapy because of one or two abnormal Pap smears unless a biopsy shows that you have invasive cancer. You have time to talk to your doctor and to get another opinion if you want.

▶ *What procedures may my doctor suggest if I have an abnormal Pap smear?*

Suppose your Pap smear shows a cervical abnormality. If the abnormality does not seem severe, your doctor may recommend repeating the Pap smear in another few weeks, because often the body can heal itself if left to its own immunological devices.

If you return in three months and the smear is still abnormal, what kind of evaluation is next? Most gynecologists will suggest something called colposcopy—looking at the cervix with a colposcope, which is a sort of giant microscope. The procedure can be done in the doctor's office without anesthesia. Through the colposcope the abnormal tissue really does look different from the tissue surrounding it. It has different blood-vessel patterns, and the cells vary in shape, size, and perhaps density. During the procedure the physician will snip off little bits of the most irregular-looking tissue and send them to a pathologist, who will look at them under a regular microscope and tell your gynecologist what is going on.

Often the pathologist will discover that the problem is merely an inflammation, not in any way linked to cancer. At other times the pathologist will say that the problem is caused by infection with the condyloma virus, hence the abnormal Pap smear, but there are no worrisome cellular changes.

Cervical biopsies are slightly uncomfortable, but from personal experience I can tell you that they aren't nearly as uncomfortable as endometrial biopsies; I was able to go right back to work in the clinic after I had my cervical biopsy, many years ago.

▶ *Is cervical dysplasia a forerunner of AIDS?*

It is true that cervical cancer is often associated with AIDS; that is, women who are HIV-positive are at increased risk for cervical cancer. But the opposite is not necessarily true. Just because a person has cervical dysplasia, she is not at higher risk for AIDS. Cervical dysplasia is much more common than AIDS; if you do have cervical dysplasia and you are worried about AIDS, have an HIV test. However, the vast majority of women with cervical dysplasia do not have AIDS.

Treatment for Cervical Abnormalities and Cervical Cancer

▶ *If I have cervical dysplasia, will I need to have a hysterectomy?*

The therapy for cervical disease depends on its severity. None of the several approaches to cervical dysplasia involve radical surgery. If a patient has severe dysplasia, desires sterilization, has painful menstrual periods, and really wants a hysterectomy, then she could have one. In general, few women end up with a hysterectomy for dysplasia.

▶ *What is cervical cryosurgery?*

Cryosurgery is a surgical therapy that involves freezing. The physician takes an instrument that looks like a magic wand and places it against the abnormal area on the cervix. Nitrous oxide gas is passed through the tip of the wand, which gets very cold and actually freezes the cells. Soon the abnormal area looks like a little iceball on the cervix. The frozen area is allowed to thaw and then is refrozen. This freezing and thawing kills the superficial cells, which are sloughed off, and the body generates new, healthy cells.

Another approach, which also kills the superficial cells so that the body sloughs them off, is laser surgery. This technique uses heat rather than cold and actually vaporizes the diseased cells.

Both laser surgery and cryosurgery can be done in an outpatient surgery center or in a physician's office.

▶ *What is a cone biopsy?*

Some physicians recommend taking out a chunk of the diseased tissue. This procedure, called a cone biopsy, is a little more complicated than cryosurgery or laser surgery, and it is a bit more aggressive in that more tissue is removed. A cone biopsy can be done in one of two ways, with a cutting tool—a scalpel or a laser—or with an electrical wire. The choice depends on your gynecologist's preference and on what your cervix looks like.

Either procedure can be done in an office setting, though most are performed in a surgicenter with a little sedation. Usually the sedation involves a local anesthetic such as Novocain for your cervix and something like intravenous Valium to calm your nerves, although some women elect to have general anesthesia.

With either a scalpel (a "cold-knife conization") or a laser, the surgeon removes a small, cone-shaped wedge of cervical tissue and inserts a few stitches around the area where the tissue was excised.

The newest technique is called a LEEP, which stands for "loop electrical excision procedure." A very hot tungsten wire with electric current passing through it is employed to remove a cone-shaped wedge of tissue. The advantage of the wire procedure is that it cuts through the tissue easily and cauterizes the blood vessels at the same time, thereby controlling the bleeding. There is very little of the charring of the edges of the incision that occurs when a laser is used for the cutting. For these reasons many physicians have switched to the LEEP procedure.

▶ What are the risks and possible complications of cone biopsy?

In terms of cure rates or complications after surgery, the procedures for cone biopsy are all comparable. As with any surgery, you should make sure that someone who has done it many times performs your operation, but the risks of cone biopsy are negligible. The risk of infection or bleeding is always present in surgery; but with cone biopsies, the risk is small and most people do well.

Many women do experience significant cervical or vaginal discharge for a few days or a few weeks after cone biopsy. The amount of discharge and the time it lasts differ from woman to woman, rather than from one type of procedure to another. The most significant discharge seems to occur after cryosurgery.

▶ Does a cone biopsy interfere with fertility or childbearing?

A cone biopsy does not affect your fertility. Nor does it give you an incompetent cervix, that is, a cervix that will not sustain a pregnancy. It is rare for women to experience problems with childbearing after a cone biopsy.

▶ *What kind of recovery period should I anticipate if I have a cone biopsy or LEEP procedure?*

Because the procedure is minor enough to be done in a surgicenter or a doctor's office, the recovery period is short. The vaginal discharge may last for a few weeks.

The only restriction on your activity is that you should abstain from intercourse while your cervix is healing, a period of two to three weeks. Usually your physician will check you at that point to be sure that you are healing well. A Pap smear is not useful as a diagnostic tool until the cervix is fully healed.

▶ *When should I have another Pap smear after a cone biopsy?*

Most physicians recommend waiting for about three months, but sometimes the cervix is not completely healed even then and the Pap smear is not readable by the pathologist.

The first accurate postoperative Pap smear usually shows that the abnormal cells are gone. After that, most physicians recommend a repeat Pap test more frequently than once a year, perhaps every six months for a year or two; thereafter, if nothing abnormal turns up, it is common to space the Pap smears further apart again.

▶ *Is a hysterectomy ever performed for cervical abnormalities?*

Some old-time physicians do not believe in cone biopsies and prescribe hysterectomy instead of the more recently developed procedure.

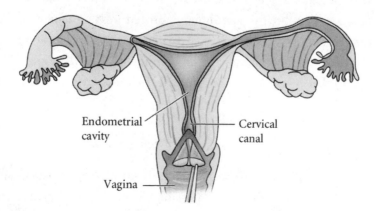

FIGURE 22. A cone biopsy involves removing a cone-shaped wedge of the inner cervix to eliminate and evaluate precancerous cervical changes.

If you have symptoms in addition to your cervical dysplasia, a hysterectomy, which removes the entire uterus along with the cervix, may be a better treatment for you than a cone biopsy.

Daisy M. is in her midforties and has six children. She is not particularly reliable about following instructions or taking her medication. She comes to the office complaining of periods that last ten days, with heavy flow and clotting. She doesn't want any more children and she is really incapacitated with her periods. It turns out that Daisy also has cervical dysplasia.

Daisy is a suitable candidate for a hysterectomy. Instead of removing part of her cervix and letting her cope with her heavy periods and with birth control, we can offer her a hysterectomy. It will give her the sterilization she would like and solve her bleeding problems as well.

Finally, a hysterectomy may be indicated if cervical changes have progressed beyond carcinoma in situ. Conservative therapy mandates a patient who will follow up and be reliable about coming in for examinations. If you don't wish to take on this responsibility, then conservative therapy is not for you.

▶ Is it appropriate to ask for a tubal ligation also, if I am having a cone biopsy?

Some women come into the office needing a cone biopsy and ask for a tubal ligation at the same time. They would prefer not to have their uterus removed, a personal preference that should be respected, but they would like sterilization. Fifteen years ago I seldom did a cone/tubal, because these are two very different procedures that achieve the same result as a hysterectomy, a single procedure. Today I do perform them. The two procedures are simple enough that doing both at the same time is not a problem. In general, recuperation from a cone/tubal is rapid. A hysterectomy is major surgery and requires a much longer recuperation period.

▶ What are the therapies for more advanced stages of cervical cancer?

Most women with cervical cancer are diagnosed early through Pap smears, usually in the precancerous stages. The early detection is possible because these women bleed.

With stage I cervical cancer there are two options for treatment. One is radiation therapy, which is quite effective. The other is radical pelvic surgery, which involves removing the uterus and taking out the lymph nodes next to it.

One advantage to surgery as a treatment for cervical cancer is that most women who get the disease are fairly young. They have functioning ovaries. Cervical cancer, unlike endometrial cancer, is not related to estrogen, so there is no reason to remove the ovaries. Radiation therapy, in contrast, will eliminate ovarian function, which is not desirable in younger women. Not only can the surgical approach preserve ovarian function, but it can usually preserve sexual function by keeping the top of the vagina intact without scarring.

Many physicians recommend some radiation therapy adjunctively because of the risk of involvement in lymph nodes that have not been taken out. And there are some new protocols that involve chemotherapy.

▶ What are survival rates for stage I cervical cancer?

They exceed 90 percent, which means that 90 percent of women treated for stage I cervical cancer will be alive five years later. In fact, if you have lived five years beyond your treatment, you are likely to live a great deal longer; cervical cancer, unlike some other forms of cancer, generally recurs quickly if it recurs at all. For women who are HIV-positive, survival rates are less reassuring.

▶ If I have a hysterectomy for cervical cancer, can I keep my ovaries?

One of the main reasons for performing a hysterectomy as opposed to radiation therapy for cervical cancer is that the ovaries can be preserved. Intensive radiation to the pelvis destroys ovarian function, which brings on premature menopause. Since cervical carcinoma is not estrogen sensitive, someone who has had a hysterectomy for cervical cancer can keep her ovaries and should be encouraged to continue having intercourse.

▶ What kind of physician should treat someone with cervical abnormalities?

Any board-certified gynecologist should be able to take care of cervical dysplasia and perform a cone biopsy or whatever therapy is appropriate. You do not need a cancer specialist for this kind of treatment.

If the cancer has spread beyond the cervix and become invasive, it is a good idea to consult a specialist—either a gynecological oncologist or someone who works in conjunction with one. Obviously radiation therapy should be directed by a specialist in this field. If you are going to have surgery for invasive cancer, you should choose someone who is a specialist in cancer surgery and has considerable experience. The kind of radical hysterectomy appropriate for invasive cervical cancer is different and technically more difficult than a simple hysterectomy for fibroids or for stage I endometrial cancer. Your surgeon need not be someone who has been board certified in gynecological oncology, but he or she should be skilled in radical pelvic surgery.

OVARIAN CANCER

Ever since Gilda Radner died of ovarian cancer in 1989, this disease has received serious publicity. Among gynecological cancers it is hardly the most common, far less so than breast cancer or uterine cancer. One woman in eight will have breast cancer over her lifetime (established for statistical purposes at 110 years), while only one woman in fifty-five will get ovarian cancer. Ovarian cancer accounts for only 4 percent of the cancers among women—with about 25,580 new cases of ovarian cancer estimated in 2004 and about 16,090 deaths from the disease.

It is not the incidence of ovarian cancer but its mortality rate that makes it such a threatening disease. Unlike uterine and cervical cancer, ovarian cancer is generally discovered late, often when it has reached stage III. Women with cancer of the uterus or cancer of the cervix tend to bleed at unusual times. Women with cancer of the breast may feel a lump or see some other worrisome change in their breast. Screening tests—Pap smears and mammograms—can pick up these diseases even before they have physical symptoms. Most of the time women with ovarian cancer don't have unusual vaginal bleeding or don't feel an abdominal mass. Nevertheless, if ovarian cancer is discovered while it is confined to the ovary, the cure rate is about 95 percent.

▶ *Does ovarian cancer have any warning signs?*

The symptoms that send women to their physician are usually the signs of extended disease; they are also signs that could indicate some condition other than ovarian cancer. The most common is a sense of abdominal fullness or bloating, caused not by the size of the cancerous mass itself but from fluid collecting in the abdomen, a condition called ascites. What makes diagnosis difficult is that most women regularly feel fullness or bloating at some time of the month. So if you are more than thirty years old and have vague digestive symptoms (stomach discomfort, gas, distension) that persist and can't be explained by another cause, talk to your gynecologist about evaluation for ovarian cancer.

Very occasionally established ovarian cancer will make itself known by pelvic pressure, back or leg pain, or, rarely, unusual abdominal bleeding.

Risk Factors and Prevention

The main risk for ovarian cancer is being a woman. Risk increases with age, and incidence of the disease peaks between the ages of seventy and seventy-five. This is a very important reason to see your gynecologist after menopause. Many women feel that when they reach menopause they don't have to keep on getting pelvic exams; after all, they aren't having difficulties with their periods. Nor are they at much risk for cervical cancer, which tends to be a disease of younger women. But if they haven't had their ovaries removed, those ovaries need to be checked, either by a gynecologist or by an internist who knows how to do a pelvic exam.

Women with a family history of the disease, as Gilda Radner's example suggests, have increased risk. If your mother or sister had ovarian cancer, your risk is multiplied almost three times and you should be closely followed; having additional relatives with ovarian or breast cancer increases your risk even more. The families in which ovarian cancer is a problem tend to have many members affected, not just one or two. The risk can be passed on by your father's side of the family as well as your mother's. Because the breast cancer genes are also implicated in ovarian cancer, women who have a family history of breast cancer are at increased risk for ovarian cancer.

> Amy L. is in her thirties. Her mother had ovarian cancer and her mother's sister died from it. Her mother's sister's daughter, Amy's cousin, was recently diagnosed with the disease. With this kind of strong family history it was clear how to proceed. Amy had her second child when she was about thirty-two. She waited until the infant was getting along well enough that Amy could go to the hospital and have her ovaries taken out. All the physicians treating Amy and Amy herself felt that this was unquestionably the right move.

Women who have had breast cancer are at increased risk for ovarian cancer, as are women who have never had children or who have had them late. Women who have used fertility drugs but not gotten pregnant have higher risk, and there is some speculation that infertility increases risk, even without the use of fertility drugs. Smokers are slightly more likely than nonsmokers to get ovarian cancer, although the increase in risk is not so great as it is with lung cancer or bladder cancer. Industrialized countries report higher rates of ovarian cancer than developing countries, and it is more common in Caucasian women than in African American women and in women of Jewish descent than in women of other ethnic backgrounds.

Some studies have suggested that using talcum powder on sanitary napkins or in the genital area increases risk slightly, but other studies have not confirmed this link. In the past talcum powder was sometimes contaminated with asbestos, a known carcinogen. For more than twenty years, however, body and face powders have been free of asbestos.

▶ *Are there ways to lower my risk for ovarian cancer?*

You can't lower your risk for ovarian cancer, as you can for cervical cancer, by postponing your first intercourse or limiting the number of your sexual partners, but there are factors that reduce risk.

Women who have never been pregnant are more likely to get ovarian cancer than women who have had several children. Some researchers theorize that the ovarian changes that eventually lead to cancer come about because of ovulation, and while a woman is pregnant she does not ovulate. Thus by reducing the number of her ovulations, she reduces the number of times when ovarian changes might take place. Breast feeding seems to reduce risk for similar reasons, and tubal ligation may also reduce risk.

Birth control pills also protect against ovarian cancer: women on the pill are about 50 percent less likely to get the disease than comparable women who are not. The protective effect seems to last for a considerable time after the woman has stopped taking the pill. Consequently, if someone tells me that she is terribly afraid of getting ovarian cancer, I suggest that she start taking birth control pills.

▶ *Are there ways to check on the history of ovarian cancer in my family?*

The Gilda Radner Familial Ovarian Cancer Registry at the Roswell Park Cancer Institute in Buffalo, New York, is a data bank of familial histories. The registry also maintains a help line (800.682.7426), education, and peer support. The head of the registry is Dr. Steven Piver, whose job it is to disseminate any information that you might need. When I called him about Amy, he concurred in the decision, believing strongly that Amy was at such high risk that she should have her ovaries removed even though she was only thirty-five years old.

▶ *Do people get ovarian cancer who do not have a strong family history of the disease?*

Familial cases make up only a small percentage of the women who have ovarian cancer. There is a good side and a bad side to this fact. The good side is that if you have just one relative who has ovarian cancer, perhaps your mother, it does not mean that you will get the disease. Your mother, or cousin, or sister—whoever—might be one of those nonfamilial, sporadic cases. If you have several relatives who have died of ovarian cancer, then you are at increased risk. The dark side is that you are not home free just because you do not have a relative who has had ovarian cancer.

▶ *Do fertility drugs increase my risk for ovarian cancer?*

A brouhaha erupted some years ago over whether fertility drugs such as Clomid and Pergonal increase the risk of ovarian cancer. Large-scale medical studies suggest that it is not the Clomid or the Pergonal that increases risk for ovarian cancer but the fact that women who have never been pregnant are at higher risk. Not surprisingly, many women who take these drugs are women who have never been pregnant; some do not succeed in becoming pregnant, unfortunately, and therefore fall into the higher-risk group.

A second connection between fertility drugs and ovarian cancer is that women who are taking fertility drugs to increase their chances of getting pregnant are not taking birth control pills, which would protect them from ovarian cancer.

Kinds of Ovarian Tumors

If your doctor says you have a mass on your ovary, chances are that it is not malignant. The overwhelming number of ovarian masses are benign, even in women who are as old as sixty.

To understand the different ovarian tumors, you need to know something about the structure of the ovary. It is made up of three kinds of tissue: the epithelium, the capsule surrounding the ovary; the tissue of which the eggs themselves are composed; and the inner stromal tissue that supports the eggs.

The most common tumors are epithelial tumors, on the outside rim of the ovaries. The most common epithelial tumors are called serous cyst adenocarcinomas, which means that they contain fluid or serum. Some cancerous tumors of the epithelium contain a jellylike substance; these are called mucinous cyst adenocarcinomas. Both mucinous cyst adenocarcinomas and serous cyst adenocarcinomas can also have solid material within them.

Tumors of the inner structure of the ovary are called stromal tumors. These tumors can make hormones and may cause hormone-related problems. Granulosa cell tumors, for example, produce estrogen. Women with such tumors may have symptoms such as bleeding, because they are producing very high levels of estrogen. Women who have tumors of the stromal tissue, which produce testosterone, may come into the office complaining of masculinization—excessive facial hair, acne, and aggressive behavior. These tumors, though rare, are occasionally seen in older women.

Tumors of the egg tissue itself are called germ cell tumors or egg tumors. The most common are cystic teratomas, also called dermoid cysts. They are rarely cancerous and are most common in younger women. They can have almost any body tissue inside them—hair, teeth, cartilage, neural tissue. After all, the egg is a totipotent cell, able to make any kind of cell found in the body; so it makes sense that disordered egg cells can also make body tissues. Because the diseased egg cells are not fertilized, they are not "turned on" in the normal way; indeed, scientists don't know what does turn them on and make them start dividing. One of the ways these tumors used to be diagnosed was by taking an X-ray and looking for teeth within the ovarian mass. Once I had a patient who had a whole palate in a cyst.

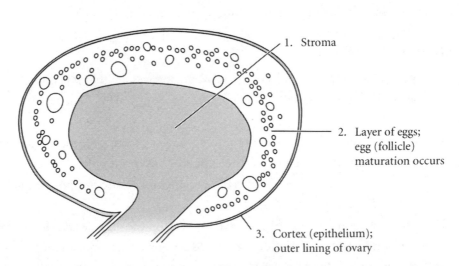

FIGURE 23. Structure of the ovary. The normal ovary contains three types of cells. The central supporting layer is made up of stromal cells; the cortical cells form the covering of the ovary. Between these two layers the egg cells (follicles) perform the actual business of the ovary.

Screening and Diagnosis

▶ *Are there ways to detect ovarian cancer early?*

Most ovarian cancer that is picked up early is found during routine pelvic exams. The American College of Obstetricians and Gynecologists recommends an annual exam to screen for ovarian cancer.

Some people believe that ultrasound technology can detect ovarian cancer, but its uses are limited. First of all, ultrasound is not cost-effective as a screening tool. A pelvic exam with ultrasound costs somewhere between two hundred and four hundred dollars. If the ovarian tumor is so small that a gynecologist cannot feel it, it may not be picked up by the ultrasound. This is very different from mammography, where X-ray technology is extremely helpful in detecting breast cancer.

Ultrasound is useful, however, in determining the nature of an ovarian growth. If your physician notes during an exam that you have an ovarian mass, ultrasound can help determine whether it is benign or malignant. Fluid-filled cysts are much less likely to be cancerous than those that have some solid components.

Certain blood tests have been given a lot of attention in the press, but these tests are not reliable enough to be used for routine screening. One is called a CA-125, and a newer one is known as a CA 19-9. These marker tests look for high levels of certain carbohydrates (CA-125 and CA 19-9) in the blood, since elevated blood levels of these carbohydrates are correlated with ovarian cancer.

The correlation is not like the association, for example, between spina bifida and alpha fetal protein. In the case of a fetus with an incompletely closed neural tube (the channel that holds the spinal column), the mother's blood shows an elevated blood level of alpha fetal protein because the fetus is making this protein. It leaks out through the opening in the defective neural tube and gets absorbed into the mother's blood, where it can be measured. It is logical, then, that a woman pregnant with a fetus that has spina bifida will have elevated levels of alpha fetal protein in her blood.

With CA-125, however, the association between the marker and ovarian cancer is not unique; the test gives many false positives and many false negatives. Women who have endometriosis often have elevated CA-125, as do some women who have fibroids. Occasionally women with chronic thyroid disease have elevated CA-125 readings. And many women who do have cancer of the ovary have perfectly normal CA-125 blood levels.

Because of the unreliability of CA-125 tests, they are not useful for screening the general population, but they can be helpful in particular situations. Suppose someone has had cancer of the ovary and her ovaries were removed. After the surgery her CA-125 level went down. Her doctor can use the test as a way to check for recurrence of the disease.

Or suppose someone has a familial history of ovarian cancer that is not clear-cut.

> Louise T. is in her early thirties. Her mother had ovarian cancer as a young woman. It is possible that Great-Aunt Natasha had it also, but since she lived in Russia and the stories about her are hearsay (no one in America ever met her), we can't be sure whether Natasha died of ovarian cancer or something else. Louise is anxious. She hasn't had her children yet and doesn't want to have her ovaries removed.

How can Louise's doctor monitor her closely? One way is to increase the number of pelvic exams to two per year. Another way is to alternate a pelvic exam with an ultra-sound every six months. A third way is to follow Louise's CA-125 level and observe possible changes. Finally, Louise could consider getting tested for mutations of the BRCA genes that are implicated in both familial breast and ovarian cancers.

A far more accurate test may be on the horizon. It uses proteomics (also called proteinomics), the study of proteins within cells, to detect the presence of disease in its early stages. Researchers "taught" a sophisticated artificial-intelligence computer program to distinguish between the profiles of proteins in blood of people who had ovarian cancer and those who did not. Rather than relying on a single marker—for example, CA-125—researchers looked at an entire pattern of proteins to make the diagnosis. Once the patterns had been identified, the researchers used them to test blood samples of women who did or did not have ovarian cancer; the researchers, of course, did not know which samples belonged to which group. The test correctly distinguished between all the cancerous and noncancerous samples, including all stage I ovarian cancers. Beyond identifying the presence or absence of ovarian cancer and other diseases, this diagnostic tool may help researchers evaluate how far disease has progressed by matching specific proteomic patterns to a particular stage.

▶ Is genetic testing available for ovarian cancer?

We know that there are relations between breast and ovarian cancer and that mutations in the BRCA genes are responsible for this link. (See the section, above, on genetic testing for breast cancer.) Testing is available for this gene, but the cautions that apply to genetic testing for breast cancer also apply to ovarian cancer screening. You should consider what you might do if you did have the mutated gene. Would you have your ovaries removed? And what about privacy? Do you want your insurance company to know that you have the mutated form of the gene?

Remember that most experts believe that only about 5 to 8 percent of breast and ovarian cancers are caused by BRCA gene abnormalities. Many women who have the mutated gene do not get either breast or ovarian cancer. Many women who do not have the mutated gene do get one of these diseases.

▶ *Are there tests that can determine without surgery whether an ovarian mass is cancerous?*

In recent years some fairly effective tests have been developed to differentiate between malignant and benign growths. One is the Doppler flow study, pioneered at Yale by the late Dr. Ken Taylor, which measures the blood supply to the ovarian mass. If the mass has normal flow characteristics and does not show signs of increased blood flow, it almost always proves to be benign.

However, the Doppler blood flow test sometimes shows false positives. That is, it will indicate that an ovarian mass has increased blood flow but the mass will turn out to be benign, not cancerous at all. Increased blood flow merely indicates the presence of rapidly dividing cells.

▶ *If a physician recommends ovarian surgery, is cancer the likely diagnosis?*

Although some physicians are beginning to rely more heavily on such tests as the Doppler, often it is difficult to tell with certainty whether a tumor is benign or malignant without resorting to surgery. The only absolutely sure diagnostic method is to remove the tumor or cyst, send it to a pathologist, and let him or her decide what is going on. So if your doctor recommends surgery, there is still a very good chance that what is happening is benign.

When one of my patients has to have ovarian surgery for diagnostic reasons, however, I do prepare her for the possibility of cancer. It is psychologically important to realize that the possibility exists, even though the chances are good that she does not have cancer. In a sense, I am overpreparing her.

▶ *What are the stages of ovarian cancer?*

The stages of ovarian cancer are similar to those of uterine or cervical cancer. Stage I disease is confined to the ovaries. Stage II disease extends through the pelvis to the uterus. Stage III disease involves spread through the pelvis to more remote pelvic organs such as the omentum, the fat that surrounds the intestines. Stage IV disease has spread beyond the pelvis to distant tissues, for example the lungs.

With endometrial or cervical cancer, the physician can often tell how far the cancer has advanced. Because the gynecologist has already done a D&C or taken a Pap smear, the extent of the disease may be fairly evident before any surgery. Unfortunately, with ovarian cancer this is not the case. Not until the surgery is performed can the physician know the extent of the disease.

Treatment

▶ *What is the usual surgical routine for ovarian cancer?*

For the majority of women who are perimenopausal to postmenopausal, most physicians recommend a total abdominal hysterectomy and a bilateral salpingo-oophorectomy—removal of not only the ovaries but also the fallopian tubes and the uterus.

Often women wonder why their uterus and both ovaries are removed because there is a mass on one ovary. There are several reasons. First, most women who are perimenopausal are not interested in reproductive function; if they are postmenopausal, it simply is not an issue.

Suppose the surgeon removes the ovary, sends it down during the operation for what is called a frozen section, and the pathology comes back benign. Later, during full examination of the entire tissue sample, the pathologist finds a spot of cancer somewhere else in the ovary. (In a small percentage of cases this does happen.) Then the patient will be subjected to a second surgery.

It is also possible that cancer is developing in the second ovary, even though that ovary looks normal. In a small percentage of cases the disease is bilateral. And someone who has had an ovarian cancer on one side has a higher chance of developing it on the other side, even if she does not have any active disease at present. So there is reason to remove both ovaries.

Why take out the uterus also? Occasionally there is microscopic spread of cancer to the uterus. But beyond that, many women who have their ovaries removed are candidates for HRT. If their uterus is removed, they will not have to take progesterone to protect them from uterine cancer.

At the beginning of the operation, the surgeon washes the interior of the pelvic cavity with water, which is then recollected and examined for evidence of cancerous cells floating anywhere in the pelvis. Such cells could attach themselves to a different organ and start cancer elsewhere. These floating cells are called washings; their presence suggests higher risk for the spread of disease.

Most surgeons also sample some lymph nodes in the pelvis during the operation. The nodes are sent to the pathologist, and their condition helps to decide the course of subsequent therapy—whether to have chemotherapy or radiation. Sometimes the surgeon also removes some of the fat inside the pelvic cavity—but not to make you more beautiful cosmetically. The omentum, a sheet of fatty tissue that lies around the intestines, is a common location for spreading ovarian cancer; so the pathologist checks fat cells from the omentum for evidence that the disease is metastasizing to other tissues.

▶ *If my doctor recommends a "bowel prep" before diagnostic surgery, am I likely to have a colostomy?*

Because ovarian tumors can attach themselves to the intestines or other internal organs, I often recommend a bowel prep to clear out the bowel before diagnostic surgery. If someone's tumor has adhered to her intestine, the surgeon may have to peel it off. For that reason it is advisable to have the bowel completely prepared. Few women end up with a colostomy, even if they have ovarian cancer.

Today, for a bowel prep, most physicians recommend a liquid laxative such as citrate of magnesia or a preparation called Go Lightly. Occasionally a bowel prep will also include oral antibiotics.

Many physicians recommend chemotherapy as a preventive step even though they are quite certain that they got all the cancer and even though there is no evidence that the cancer has spread.

In some cases the surgeon is unable to remove all the cancer. Then chemotherapy may well be recommended. It is worth knowing that often chemotherapy makes the remaining tumor dissolve and that there are recently developed chemotherapies to which ovarian cancer is highly responsive.

Still, chemotherapy can be difficult to endure and can have significant side effects. There is no way to prevent hair loss, although lost hair invariably grows back. However, chemotherapeutic agents are changing all the time, and major breakthroughs in nausea medications have occurred. A wonderful drug called ondansetron almost always prevents nausea in chemotherapy patients. It is extremely expensive, but it works.

▶ *What kind of follow-up is done after chemotherapy?*

After several rounds of chemotherapy, perhaps six months to a year after the original operation, the physician is likely to want a second look at the interior of the pelvis, to see whether the disease has completely cleared up.

There are two possibilities. Some physicians recommend a laparoscopy, which is basically a "Band-Aid operation," the kind of procedure that is used when someone's tubes are tied with the aid of a laparoscope. The physician makes a small incision, inserts a long tube with a light into the pelvic cavity, and looks around to see what is going on.

The older standard procedure has been a second-look laparotomy. The physician reopens the old incision and looks at the organs in the pelvis, taking biopsies, to see whether any evidence of cancer remains. Even if the second-look operation does not reveal any cancer, the physician occasionally recommends several more rounds of chemotherapy to make sure that there truly is no more cancer.

If the cancer is not gone at the time of the second-look operation, then the physician recommends more cycles of chemotherapy and perhaps a third-look operation. This may seem like heavy-duty therapy, but the reason for the second-look operation is that ovarian cancer is obscure and hard to track. The doctor wants to be certain that the disease is no longer present.

▶ *Is recovery from the second-look operation as difficult as recovery from the first?*

Generally not, for the surgery is much less intense. With a hysterectomy, I always recommend that women allow at least six weeks for recuperation; after a second-look procedure, women seem to be about their normal activities in three or four weeks.

▶ *Can women who have had ovarian cancer ever have children?*

Over the past two decades, attitudes toward surgery and ovarian cancer have changed. Twenty years ago, the standard recommendation was that if a woman had ovarian cancer, her ovaries, fallopian tubes, and uterus were removed—no exceptions. Physicians have become more open-minded and try now to adapt their recommendations to the specific circumstances. If a woman still wants to have children, often the surgery can be restricted to removing the diseased ovary and then following her progress very carefully. Many women who have had ovarian cancer can successfully reproduce, even women who have had chemotherapy. Often the physician will recommend that, after she has finished her childbearing, she have her other ovary removed inasmuch as her previous ovarian cancer places her in a higher risk category.

For this reason, younger women should be particularly careful about who operates on a pelvic mass. The surgery is probably best performed by a gynecologist, not by a general surgeon. At some locations in the United States general surgeons routinely do these operations, but they may not be as knowledgeable about the latest thinking on conserving ovarian function as gynecologists, who after all are specialists in this field.

Recently I called my esteemed colleague Dr. Peter Schwartz about a departmental matter and found him in a very good mood. Twenty-two years ago he had operated on a young woman who had a cancerous ovarian tumor when she was just sixteen. He had removed only the diseased ovary and had continued to monitor her carefully through the years. When she was thirty-eight, she delivered her first child; his only disappointment was that the baby was a girl and couldn't be named Peter.

VULVAR CANCER

This form of cancer is very rare, more so than breast, uterine, cervical, and ovarian cancer, accounting for 4 percent of cancer in the female reproductive organs and for only 0.6 percent of cancer in women. The most common symptom of vulvar cancer is itching. Occasionally the cancer will take the form of a lump or tumor, but most frequently it presents with a chronically irritated area that the patient scratches and scratches. It is not the scratching that causes the cancer; it is the cancer that causes the unremitting irritation that causes the scratching.

▶ *Who is at risk for vulvar cancer?*

Vulvar cancer is one of those diseases to which women become more susceptible as they grow older. Women in their seventies and eighties are more likely to have this kind of cancer than younger women.

▶ *Is vulvar cancer curable?*

Not only is vulvar cancer rare, but it is easily curable if caught early. It is treated by surgery, the extent of which depends on how deep the lesion is. Like other cancers, it has stages. If the disease is superficial, the doctor can just remove a small amount of the vulvar tissue around the lesion. If it goes deeper, the surgeon will do a vulvectomy, cutting into the fat under the vulva. Sometimes the disease spreads into the lymph nodes and a pelvic operation is necessary.

▶ *How do I recognize vulvar cancer?*

It typically presents with chronic itching that is resistant to the usual medications. Melanoma, a very malignant kind of skin cancer, can appear in the vulvar area. It does not produce itching but rather a dark spot or dark pigmentation on the skin and sometimes also on the mucous membranes.

If you see new dark pigmentation in your vulvar area, you should call your gynecologist to have it evaluated. Not every dark spot that appears on the vulvar tissues is cancerous. I must admit that I have had several patients about whom I was concerned because of dark pigmentation. After doing biopsies and sending off the tissue samples, I was able to come back with the diagnosis of a freckle. It is common knowledge that dark areas called liver spots appear on the hands of older people; they also can appear on the vulva.

▶ *What is a vulvar biopsy like?*

This procedure is not difficult and can be done in the physician's office. It involves putting a little Novocain in the area and taking a snip of the superficial tissue. Usually there is no scraping, just a little punch of tissue. Your physician may put in a stitch or two, though sometimes the sample is so small that stitches are not needed.

▶ *What is colposcopy like?*

Colposcopy is a common way of evaluating skin changes in the vulva, so if your doctor wants to use a colposcope to examine you, you should not be alarmed. The colposcope is a kind of giant microscope that the physician uses while you are in stirrups, to check around the vulva. Before examining with the scope, the physician may paint the vulvar area with vinegar. That sounds strange, but the acetic acid of the vinegar highlights certain cells to make changes in them more apparent. Instead of vinegar, the doctor may use a stain (for example, toluidine blue) to make cellular changes more evident.

► *What kind of doctor should treat gynecological cancers?*

If you have stage I disease, your regular gynecologist can probably handle the situation. Most gynecologists feel comfortable and competent performing an ordinary hysterectomy. If you have a satisfactory relationship with your gynecologist, you should be able to ask whether he or she feels comfortable doing the procedure. If the surgery is more complicated, it might be wise to seek out a specialist.

Within the field of gynecology are specialists whose expertise focuses on cancer. They have taken two years of training beyond the regular gynecological residency, training that involves pelvic surgery and radiation therapy, chemotherapy, and other treatments specifically related to cancer.

In my own town we have an active gynecological oncology service. Virtually all our patients who have positive biopsies are discussed by a gynecological tumor board, which then makes recommendations. Recently I biopsied one of my patients and the results showed atypical cells. The board members felt that it was likely that she had advanced pelvic disease. They recommended that they do the hysterectomy, so I consulted with my oncological colleagues on the board, who performed the actual surgery. In cases where the biopsy suggests that the disease is probably a stage I tumor, the board members recommend that I do the surgery but they remain available in case unusual problems arise.

14 Major and Minor Surgical Procedures

ABNORMAL vaginal bleeding may require surgical intervention for both diagnostic and therapeutic reasons. Surgical procedures range from minor operations, for example a D&C, which can be performed on an outpatient basis, to major surgery such as a hysterectomy, which involves a hospital stay and a significant recovery period.

DILATATION AND CURETTAGE

▶ *What is a D&C?*

The letters stand for dilatation and curettage. During the procedure, the cervix, the narrow opening to the main body of the uterus, is stretched or dilated, and then the lining of the uterus is scraped out with a curette. The old slang among physicians for a D&C was "dusting and cleaning," and although the term is not quite accurate, it describes the purpose of a D&C, which is to clean out the glandular lining and get back to the underlying muscular layer of the uterus.

▶ *What are the reasons for performing a D&C?*

In the context we are talking about, a D&C is performed for two principal reasons. The first and primary reason is diagnostic, to rule out or evaluate possible cancer of the uterus. The second is to help control bleeding.

A D&C is also the way most early term abortions are performed. The physician may use suction curettage, but usually after the suction is performed the gynecologist will use a sharp curette to make sure that no tissue remains in the uterus. If a woman has a miscarriage and the placental tissue needs to be removed, again a D&C is standard procedure.

▶ *Why perform a D&C for diagnostic reasons when there are so many modern and sophisticated techniques for looking inside the body?*

Modern technology has added refinements that are helpful in diagnosing possible uterine cancer, and there are many things a physician can discover by an examination that uses ultrasound or X-ray studies. Sometimes ultrasound can show the presence of polyps or other growths. Ultrasound technology can reveal the thickness of the uterine lining because the endometrium shows up on the ultrasound picture as a dark stripe. If the endometrial stripe is narrow, something less than 6 to 7 mm wide, then only rarely is there a chance of hyperplasia, a precancerous condition in which an abnormal number of cells is present. Ultrasound is especially useful in evaluating women who are on hormone therapy and have unusual bleeding, perhaps because of uterine atrophy. If the endometrial stripe is wider, say 1.5 cm, the physician may say, yes, this is a potential case of hyperplasia, let's do a biopsy and see what is going on inside the uterus.

CT scans and MRIs can also be helpful in looking at the inside of the body of the uterus and in diagnosing fibroids, for instance, but none of these fancy tests will show exactly what is happening to the individual cells that make up the uterine lining.

To rule out cancer, the physician must scrape out most of the lining, perhaps not every single cell but enough to get a generous sample of all areas of the endometrium. The sample is then sent to a pathologist, who looks at it under a microscope and decides whether the cells are totally normal or whether, though not actually cancerous, they show changes that could become cancerous. The variety of hyperplasia that concerns physicians most is a condition called adenomatous hyperplasia. Adenoma means "gland," so adenomatous hyperplasia means excessive growth of glandular tissue. Left unchecked, adenomatous hyperplasia can proceed to cancer.

▶ *Why isn't a biopsy always an adequate test for precancerous changes of the uterine lining?*

A biopsy is a mini-D&C. The physician dilates the cervix a bit and takes a pinch of tissue with a very small curette, an instrument about the width of a pipe cleaner with a sharp hook on one end. A D&C is a large-scale biopsy, and it takes tissue from all areas of the endometrium.

Most of the time a biopsy will suffice, because rarely is a cancer localized to one part or aspect of the uterus. Therefore in most cases a small sample will suggest what is happening throughout the uterine lining. If you are at high risk, however, a D&C may be preferable, to check out every part of the endometrium.

Over the years the tools have gotten more sophisticated. The pipelle, a relatively new gadget from France, is narrower than former tools and easier to insert through the cervix. It uses suction instead of scraping to sample tissue. My patients say it's much more comfortable than the older technology.

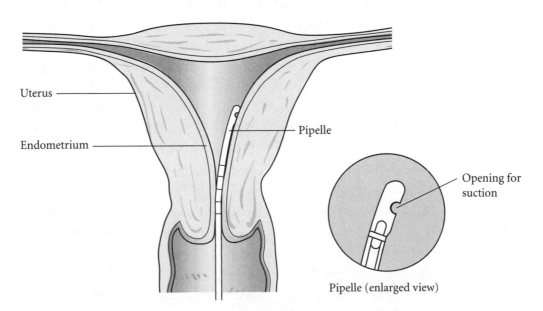

FIGURE 24. An endometrial biopsy involves removing a sample of tissue from the lining of the uterus. A new tool, the pipelle, makes the procedure more comfortable.

▶ *What is a hysteroscopy?*

Another refinement that modern technology has brought to the D&C is a tool called a hysteroscope. This is a long fiber-optic tube with a light at one end, and it is sometimes used in conjunction with video technology. What your doctor sees through the hysteroscope is projected onto a monitor, so that you can see the inside of your uterus on television.

With a hysteroscope the gynecologist can look into the uterus and see whether certain areas of the endometrium have abnormal-looking cells. If some areas look suspect, the gynecologist can scrape away that part of the lining. Hysteroscopes are especially useful to examine uterine polyps, growths on the endometrium. Hysteroscopes are also helpful for examining fibroids, since your gynecologist can see what the growth looks like. Although some gynecologists say that with the advent of hysteroscopy the D&C has become a thing of the past, most seem still to feel more comfortable scraping the lining to get a tissue sample and sending it to a pathologist to determine precisely what is going on.

▶ *What risks are associated with a D&C?*

The major possible complications of a D&C, as of any invasive procedure, are bleeding and infection. During a D&C it is possible for the physician accidentally to put a hole, or perforation, through the wall of the uterus. It is also possible to puncture the uterus with a hysteroscope, though this is less likely since that instrument is not particularly sharp. Perforations usually require no therapy unless they bleed, and even then a few sutures will usually do the job.

A few years ago a television documentary presented a special on hysteroscopy, with the message that hysteroscopies were good and D&Cs were not so good. For the next two weeks all my patients insisted on hysteroscopies and decided that they were definitely not going to have D&Cs. Television journalism aside, the prevailing opinion among American gynecologists seems to be that although hysteroscopy is a valuable adjunct, it should never replace the D&C as a bottom-line test for endometrial cancer.

▶ *How can a D&C be used to control bleeding?*

One of the tricks of old-time gynecologists (and by "old-time" I mean people like me, who were trained more than twenty years ago) was to use a D&C to help control heavy menstrual periods. Although there isn't any valid scientific basis for this, the technique often seems to help. If polyps cause the heavy bleeding, then the D&C will remove the polyps and help stop the bleeding; but even women who have totally benign pathology will sometimes improve after a D&C. I have worked with patients who had unpleasantly heavy menstrual periods; we have tried every trick known to modern science, and when all else has failed, a D&C has improved the situation. And of course recuperating from a D&C is a lot easier than recuperating from a hysterectomy.

> Yvonne P. is forty-seven. She is approaching menopause and having a few hot flashes now and again. Her menstrual periods are very heavy, and although we have tried to control her bleeding, nothing seems to help. She is a good candidate for a D&C, because classically the women who benefit from a D&C usually do well for a year, two years, or even three years before their periods start getting heavy again. Yvonne may be menopausal by the time her bleeding problem reasserts itself.

Some of my patients have had three D&Cs at about three-year intervals. Each time, they have improved for a long while, and in the nine-year period they have reached menopause. By having several D&Cs, they have avoided a hysterectomy, which was our goal. Sometimes, unfortunately, a D&C doesn't make much difference. Then we have to go on to the next step, which might be endometrial ablation (discussed below), which is more invasive than a D&C but less so than a hysterectomy. Or, it may be a hysterectomy.

Another advantage to a D&C is that for someone who is having unusual bleeding it will rule out endometrial pathology. Why is Yvonne, for example, having such heavy bleeding? Is it simply approaching menopause, or could she be harboring hyperplasia? The advantage of the D&C is that the pathologist gets tissue to look at. Whenever I do a D&C, I send tissue to a pathologist.

▶ What is the recovery time from a D&C?

If you have a D&C, you will not be out of commission for weeks and weeks. Most women will feel some cramping the day of the procedure, comparable to the cramping of a heavy-duty menstrual period. A mild painkiller such as Tylenol or Advil will probably take care of it. Most women feel pretty well the next day. I tell my patients that for up to two weeks after the procedure they may experience some spotting and staining; this is not uncommon or indicative of anything dangerous.

You can probably go back to work and resume normal activities in a day or two. A great deal of the recuperation depends on what type of anesthesia you were given.

► *Can a D&C be performed under local anesthesia?*

Yes, in most cases it can. The most commonly used anesthetic technique is a paracervical block, which means that something like Novocain is injected into the cervix. It is the same as dental anesthesia, only in a different location. If this kind of anesthesia is used, the procedure can be done in a doctor's office.

A D&C with a paracervical block does cause some discomfort. The block anesthetizes the cervix, but it doesn't do anything to the inside of your uterus. A biopsy usually involves taking samples from different parts of the uterus to ensure getting representative sections, and different people have varying sensitivities. How much discomfort a patient feels depends on the individual. I have had reactions ranging from "This is no big deal; why did you tell me it was going to be uncomfortable?" to "This is the worst thing that has ever happened to me in my life!" A middle-of-the-road group responds with "This is not fun, but who wants to go through general anesthesia?"

I tell any patient who is about to undergo a procedure under local anesthesia that if it gets too distressing she should say, "Stop, I don't like this; I'd rather be asleep." Sometimes I have had to abandon a procedure because the patient is too miserable. Especially with postmenopausal women who are being evaluated for unusual bleeding, the cervix may be so tight that to get inside the uterus I have to stretch it hard, which can be uncomfortable and unpleasant.

If for some reason or other you undergo general anesthesia, remember that anesthesia has changed dramatically. Twenty-five years ago, women would be admitted to the hospital the night before, have their D&C, and stay a day or two afterward. It was a big production. Nowadays, even with general anesthesia, the vast majority of D&Cs are done in surgicenters and other outpatient settings. You arrive at the center at about seven-thirty in the morning, your procedure is done an hour later, and you go home before lunch.

► *What kinds of anesthetics are used for a D&C?*

Several modern drugs can be used for sedation or anesthesia in this situation; deep anesthesia is not needed. The most commonly used sedative is Versed, generic name midazolam, a short-acting sedative something like Valium. Another agent is Fentanyl, a short-acting narcotic, which behaves somewhat like morphine but wears off more quickly. The usual anesthetic agent is propofol (Diprivan is the trade name); it has replaced sodium pentathol, which used to make some people feel drugged for days. Diprivan looks rather like a piña colada, a whitish milky liquid, and acts like one, too: it works quickly and wears off fast.

ENDOMETRIAL ABLATION

Endometrial ablation is a procedure that destroys the glandular lining of the uterus so that it won't bleed. The first techniques for doing ablation, more than fifteen years ago, used laser technology. The physician looked at the inside of the uterus through a hysteroscope and focused the laser beam to "fry" the glandular cells that line the uterus. Safer and simpler technologies have evolved.

Balloon ablation, the most popular technique nowadays, uses a device called the ThermaChoice balloon, a little sack at the end of a long, slender, insulated catheter (tube). The balloon is inserted into the uterus and filled with very hot water, which destroys the uterine lining. After eight minutes, the balloon is deflated and removed. The procedure gives good results for about 80 percent of women; it is about as easy for the patient as a traditional D&C and involves less bleeding. As in a D&C, the goal is to get back to the underlying muscular layer.

There are other means to achieve the same purpose. During cryoablation, a probe inserted into the uterus is gradually cooled to subzero temperatures to freeze the adjacent tissues. High-frequency radio waves can also be used.

Endometrial ablation is sometimes presented as a new high-tech panacea, an approach without risks or complications that can easily succeed where others fail. Although endometrial ablation has its place in the range of available procedures, it is not without risks or potential drawbacks.

▶ *Who might find endometrial ablation a suitable approach?*

Wanda C. is forty-seven and miserable with heavy periods. A D&C did not relieve her problem. A hysteroscopy showed no fibroids or polyps or anything pathological. She has tried progesterone and Ponstel, but they didn't help. Wanda is definitely not interested in a hysterectomy. She has heard that endometrial ablation can destroy the glandular cells of the uterine lining, which are causing the bleeding, and stop her heavy periods.

Virginia E. is forty-two. She is seriously overweight and has hypertension. Because of her obesity, she tends to bleed heavily. She, too, has tried progesterone and Ponstel; neither helped. Her obesity makes her a poor surgical risk for a hysterectomy.

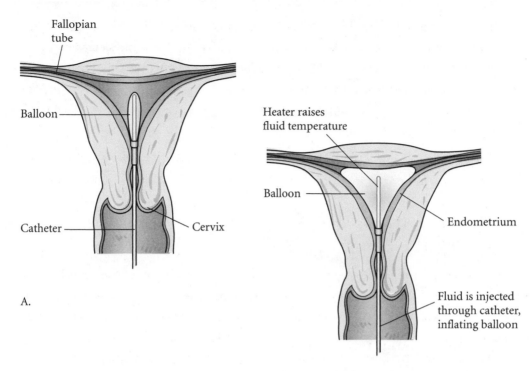

FIGURE 25. Endometrial ablation with a hot-water balloon. This is a new technique for destroying the glandular lining of the uterus to help control heavy bleeding. A, the balloon is inserted into the uterus with a catheter; B, it is inflated with fluid to the size and shape of the uterus. The fluid is then heated.

Endometrial ablation might be a reasonable option for either of these women. Women do not go into D&Cs lightly, nor should they approach endometrial ablation impetuously.

▶ Is endometrial ablation difficult to perform?

Like any surgical procedure, endometrial ablation should be performed by a skilled practitioner, someone who has done it many times before. The size or contour of the uterine cavity sometimes leads to a lowered success rate, because the procedure may not destroy the entire uterine lining.

Some physicians insist that a woman go on hormonal medication, say Lupron or danazol, for a month or two before the ablation. By suppressing FSH and estrogen production, which leads to stimulation of the lining of the uterus, the hormonal medication "flattens out" the lining and makes the procedure easier. The same physicians may also recommend continued hormone therapy for a month or two after the ablation, to let the endometrium scar and keep it from growing back.

▶ What are the potential complications?

As with a D&C or any procedure where instruments are used inside the uterus, there is a small risk of perforation or infection, though the risk is less than with a hysterectomy.

▶ What else should I consider in deciding whether to have an endometrial ablation?

If you are having an endometrial ablation because, like Wanda, you are perimenopausal and have heavy bleeding resulting from hormonal problems, you should realize that in a few years you will probably be menopausal. If you decide to go on hormone therapy after menopause, you will have to take progesterone, because no one can be certain that every gland in the uterus has been removed during the ablation. Suppose 5 percent of Wanda's endometrial tissue is left. That small amount will certainly not give her a substantial bleeding problem. But it can still become cancerous, so if she chooses to take estrogen, she will have to take progesterone and have a regular cleanout bleed to protect her endometrium.

HYSTERECTOMY

Hysterectomy, the surgical removal of the uterus, has become the center of a controversy almost as heated as the turmoil surrounding hormone therapy. Once the most commonly performed surgical procedure in the United States, hysterectomy was so routine that by 1975 one woman in three no longer had her uterus by age sixty. The attitude underlying this extreme willingness to perform hysterectomies was that once a woman finished with her last planned pregnancy, her uterus became a useless organ; it bled, produced unwanted symptoms, and was potentially cancerous. Therefore it should be removed.

More recently, hysterectomy has come under the scrutiny of women's health advocates, who believe that the operation is still performed much more frequently than is necessary. They note that the rate of hysterectomy (currently 5.6 per 1,000 women) is three times as high in the United States as it is in the United Kingdom and other nations of

Western Europe, where health care standards are presumably similar. Studies have shown that the incidence of hysterectomy varies widely from one region of the United States to another. In the Northeast, for example, the rate is lower than in either the Midwest or the South. Furthermore, the rate of hysterectomy can vary widely from community to community even within a small geographic region. Consequently, some observers believe that at least one-quarter of all hysterectomies done every year in the United States are unnecessary. These observers point out that the advice a woman receives about hysterectomy may depend on whether she has health insurance, on where she lives, and on the particular style of medical practice in her community. Finally, women's advocates have also attacked the medical profession for concealing from women the emotional and physical consequences of hysterectomy.

Perhaps because of the publicity generated by women's health advocates and perhaps because women in general are becoming more educated about their options, the annual number of hysterectomies declined from its high in the late 1970s (725,000 in 1978) to about 600,000 annually in the past few years. Women in their forties are at the prime age for hysterectomy.

All this controversy may complicate the decision on whether to have a hysterectomy, but it certainly brings the issues into sharp focus. Each woman should realize that it is her responsibility to understand the possible risks, benefits, and aftereffects of surgery; she should make her decision in conjunction with her caregiver on the basis of her own symptoms, her own habits, and her own preferences.

▶ *How do I know whether I need a hysterectomy?*

This question is one of the most common that women ask me. My standard answer is usually another question, "Do you think you need one?" In most cases hysterectomy is an elective procedure, not in the sense that a nose job or breast augmentation is elective, but in the sense that the reason for it is not life threatening. There is time to consider the options and make a thoughtful and informed decision.

Only on certain occasions must a woman absolutely have a hysterectomy. First and foremost is the presence of cancer. If a woman has cancer of the reproductive organs (uterus, cervix, ovaries, or fallopian tubes), she should in general anticipate having a hysterectomy. An exception might be a young woman in her twenties with certain kinds of ovarian cancer.

Another indication for hysterectomy is the presence of fibroids, benign tumors of the uterus, that have grown large enough to press on vital structures. Fibroids themselves do not inevitably necessitate a hysterectomy, for they can be small and cause little or no discomfort. However, large fibroids pressing against the ureters, the tubes that join the kidneys and the bladder, can cause compression of the kidneys or force the urine backward, which can lead to serious problems.

Another reason to have a hysterectomy is severe uterine prolapse. If the uterus has prolapsed to the point that it is actually out of the vagina, where it can become infected or ulcerated, a hysterectomy should be performed.

Finally, if a woman cannot keep up with her blood loss from severely heavy menstrual periods and is significantly anemic even though she is taking iron every day, she should think seriously about a hysterectomy if conservative therapies have not helped her.

The rest of the time the decision to have a hysterectomy is one that the woman herself should make in consultation with her caregiver. She has to feel that she is ready for a hysterectomy, that she wants it. The decision should not be made on the spur of the moment and it should not be made on a bad day. Suppose you have one or two days of very heavy bleeding every month; wait to decide about hysterectomy until a day when you are not bleeding.

Elective hysterectomy is determined by quality of life. The most common reason is the presence of fibroids that have not grown so large that they interfere with other important structures; the other principal reasons for elective hysterectomy are heavy bleeding and recurrent pelvic pain.

▶ Are there ways to avoid hysterectomy?

In many cases there are, but they may require patience and toleration of symptoms. In our culture, which admires getting things done and requires decisive solutions to problems, many women are reluctant to wait and unwilling to tolerate discomfort if they do wait. But if you are approaching menopause and your fibroids are causing heavy bleeding, backache, pelvic pain, or frequent urination, you might wish to consider watchful waiting. Most fibroids shrink after menopause because they are estrogen dependent. If you can live with your symptoms and if your physician has determined that your fibroids are not growing rapidly or becoming dangerous to you in any other way, you can wait until after menopause to make a decision about hysterectomy.

If uterine prolapse is the reason you are thinking about hysterectomy, you might

consider using a pessary. Although the pessary will not cure your prolapse, it may alleviate the symptoms by holding the uterus in place. Pessaries do not work for all women;
nor do all women like them.

If heavy bleeding not caused by fibroids is your reason for contemplating hysterectomy, hormonal and nonhormonal therapies are worth trying before deciding on
surgery. In many cases, the use of progesterone alone or of low-dose birth control pills
can bring heavy or frequent bleeding under control. Supplementing dietary iron with
iron pills can keep your hematocrit in a safe range. You can consider endometrial ablation by any of several techniques, a less invasive procedure than a hysterectomy.

▶ What are the risks of having a hysterectomy?

With any surgery there is always a risk of infection. There is always a risk of blood loss.
There is always a risk of problems with the anesthetic. And because the pelvic organs are
packed tightly in a relatively small space and sometimes adhere to other abdominal organs, there is a danger of an inadvertent puncture of the bowel, bladder, or ureters. The
risk increases for someone who has severe endometriosis or large fibroids. Obviously
such a puncture, if found, can be repaired at the time of surgery.

Sometimes holes, or fistulas, develop after surgery when things do not heal properly,
for example when a stitch gives way. The most common openings are between the vagina
and another structure: a vesicovaginal fistula is a hole between the vagina and the bladder, while a ureterovaginal fistula is between the vagina and a ureter.

Much as we would like to believe that everything always goes perfectly (in life as in
surgery), things do go wrong. Severe problems are very uncommon. And they can usually
be fixed. In general, however, additional surgery is required to repair the complications.

▶ Does hysterectomy have any effect on PMS?

Frances H. is forty and has PMS. She has finished having children and needs a
hysterectomy because of large fibroids. Because she is only forty, she can look
forward to ten more years of normal ovarian function. Should she have her
ovaries removed?

One advantage to many women is that when the ovaries are removed, PMS symptoms frequently disappear. If a woman with severe PMS needs a hysterectomy for bleeding or some other reason, she should seriously consider having her ovaries removed.

Some "PMS-ologists" have discovered that hysterectomy itself helps many but not all women with severe PMS, even though their ovaries remain in place. In light of our scientific knowledge today, this relief doesn't make sense, since PMS is a condition related to ovarian function and has little to do with the uterus. Perhaps the psychological dread of having a period is enough to trigger the PMS, or perhaps something subtle is happening hormonally that responds to the changed blood flow in the pelvis. No one knows, but physicians do report lowered PMS after hysterectomy.

▶ Do postmenopausal ovaries have any significant function?

Although the ovaries no longer produce estrogen after menopause, they do make small amounts of androgens, which some researchers believe may contribute to libido. Some feminist groups suggest that even postmenopausally the ovaries are functioning in ways that are not known or understood; but basically the understanding of the scientific community is that the postmenopausal ovary does not do a great deal beyond producing androgens.

▶ If I decide to have a hysterectomy, can I keep my ovaries?

This is another of the major questions pertaining to hysterectomy, one that I hear from patients at least once a week. If you are premenopausal and your ovaries are removed, you will undergo surgical menopause and can expect to experience hot flashes and other symptoms of menopause. Unless you are put on estrogen therapy postoperatively, the symptoms of menopause will be more severe than they would be if menopause were to occur naturally; for this reason women whose ovaries are removed usually elect to have ERT postoperatively. Occasionally women experience temporary hot flashes after surgery, even if the ovaries are left in place. This is not menopause, and the symptoms are usually alleviated with temporary ERT. Under certain conditions the ovaries absolutely should be removed. In other circumstances it would be better, but not essential, to remove the ovaries. And there are situations in which ovarian conservation is entirely a matter of personal preference.

> Alice D. is an eighteen-year-old who has not yet had her family. She came to one of my partners with a large ovarian cyst that had to be removed. In a patient so young, the goal is to conserve as much functional ovary as possible. Therefore my partner did not want to remove the second ovary and wanted to

save as much as she could of the ovary with the cyst. So she removed the cyst and sent a section of it to the lab for analysis while Alice remained in the operating room. When the pathologist examined the frozen section and found it benign, everyone was relieved. My partner finished the operation and closed the incision.

At the time of surgery the pathologist analyzing the frozen sections gives an instantaneous reading, which is not the final and decisive reading, since the frozen sections are only a few small bits of the diseased ovary. Later, in a more leisurely time frame, the pathologist looks methodically at every bit of tissue that has been removed. In most cases the instantaneous reading is the same as the final, decisive one.

Five days later, just as Alice was feeling better, the final pathology report came back. She had a borderline cancer, and the oncologists recommended that the rest of the ovary be removed. Unfortunately, Alice had to go back into surgery. The oncologists did not recommend removal of the other ovary.

Had Alice been forty-eight with the same grapefruit-sized mass on her ovary, the recommendation would have been to remove the uterus, tubes, cervix, and ovaries. Because Alice has had one ovarian cyst, she stands an increased chance, perhaps 5 to 10 percent, of developing a cyst on her other ovary and needing major surgery again. At forty-eight, Alice probably has only two or three more years of ovarian function. If she had been only forty, the recommendation might have been to remove the diseased ovary, not just the cyst, but to leave the second ovary intact.

The recuperation time of the second surgery, as in Alice's case, when the remaining ovary is removed is not significantly different from the recuperation time when ovary and uterus are removed together. The second surgery is also a major operation. The potential complications of removing just the ovary are similar to those of surgery that removes also the uterus, tubes, and cervix. If the uterus is removed, the woman will not have to take progesterone with her postoperative ERT. For this reason, many gynecologists prefer to remove the uterus, too, but the decision should depend on the patient's preference.

Sandy R. is thirty-two and has finished her childbearing. She has significant pelvic pain. She has bilateral endometriomas (ovarian tumors of endometrial tissue outside her uterus) and has decided to have surgery to remove her uterus. Even though she is only thirty-two, she is better off having her ovaries removed also.

Basically Sandy has come in for pain; if her diseased ovaries remain intact, she still has the possibility of pain from her ovarian tumors.

Cindy T. is forty-five. She is having a hysterectomy for heavy bleeding. Her ovaries are perfect; she has never had pelvic pain and has no reason to suspect she has endometriosis. Ten years ago she had a tubal ligation, and at the time her ovaries looked completely healthy. Now that she is forty-five, she has a small fibroid. Although she and her gynecologist have tried every approach to control her bleeding, nothing has worked, so she has decided to have her uterus removed. Should she have her ovaries removed also?

Statistically Cindy, like other women, has a 1 percent chance of developing ovarian cancer and a 5 percent chance of developing something on her ovary, for example a benign cyst, that will require surgical exploration. Therefore she is likely to be among the 99 percent of women who do not get ovarian cancer; she is also likely to be among the 95 percent of women who will go through their later years with perfectly normal atrophic ovaries.

How long can Cindy expect to continue to have ovarian function if she decides not to have her ovaries removed? If her mother started having menopausal symptoms when she was forty-three, or if Cindy herself has been having hot flashes, then her menopause might be imminent. She might want to hold off having a hysterectomy, hoping that with menopause the bleeding will abate. But if her mother went through menopause at age fifty-eight and Cindy seems nowhere near menopause, then she will be losing quite a few years of potential ovarian function. There are some data to suggest that women who have a hysterectomy with their ovaries left in place may undergo somewhat earlier menopause secondary to the blood flow changes consequent to hysterectomy. In essence, the decision is Cindy's.

A postmenopausal woman who is having an abdominal hysterectomy should consider having her ovaries taken out because they are no longer making estrogen. But personal choice enters into this decision also.

▶ *Do women who have their ovaries removed have problems adjusting to ERT?*

In general, women do well with postoperative estrogen therapy. In my many years of practice I have had only two patients who had tremendous difficulty finding an estrogen that agreed with them. One woman, a patient many years ago, finally decided on injectable estrogen, because it seemed to be the only thing that controlled her symptoms without giving her severe headaches. (Today, she would probably use the transdermal estrogen patch.) The other cannot tolerate any estrogen at all. She was in her late forties when I removed her ovaries and she has proved to be allergic to every form of estrogen available, including all brands and routes of delivery—patches, tablets, and shots. But of the hundreds of women on whom I have operated, only these two have had difficulties. I always tell patients who are premenopausal that it may take some time and experimentation to find the ideal estrogen regimen, but eventually we will succeed.

Types of Hysterectomies

Hysterectomies are performed either through an abdominal incision or transvaginally, through the vagina. A third type of surgery, a laparoscopically assisted vaginal hysterectomy (LAVH), has also become available. In this operation, a combination of the transvaginal and abdominal hysterectomies, the uterus and cervix are taken out and sometimes also the ovaries and tubes. The surgeon uses a laparoscope inserted through small abdominal incisions to visualize the upper part of the abdominal cavity. The uterus is detached from its support structures through the laparoscope but taken out through the vagina, as are the ovaries and fallopian tubes (if they are removed, too).

▶ *Are there conditions other than personal preference that determine which is the best procedure to use?*

Once you and your physician have decided that a hysterectomy is necessary, you must choose one of these three approaches. Some people are candidates for any of the three available operations: abdominal, vaginal, or laparoscopically assisted vaginal; for other women, one route is definitely preferable.

Part of the decision depends on your thoughts about ovarian conservation. You and your physician should also discuss the relative recovery times and the possibilities of complications such as bleeding and infection with each procedure.

Abdominal Hysterectomy

If you are going to have your ovaries removed, you should have either an abdominal hysterectomy or an LAVH. Although the ovaries can be removed vaginally, the process can be difficult, especially if their attachments are high in the pelvic cavity.

If there is a chance that endometriosis is involved (for example, if you are having significant pelvic pain), an abdominal hysterectomy or an LAVH is the best choice. If endometriosis is present, the physician will want to know about your ovaries. If the ovaries are involved and are attached by adhesions to other pelvic structures, they will be hard to remove vaginally.

If you have a cyst on your ovary, a growth that could possibly be cancer, you are a candidate for abdominal exploration. Some physicians would argue that an LAVH would be equally appropriate, but most oncologists prefer that the cyst or suspicious growth be removed intact. They believe that by removing in pieces something that is possibly cancerous, they risk spilling malignant cells into the abdominal cavity. People who favor LAVHs argue that it is all right to take out the questionable growth in pieces because the surgeon washes the interior of the pelvic cavity after removing the abnormal tissues.

Vaginal Hysterectomy

For other women, a straightforward vaginal hysterectomy is appropriate. Recuperation from this type is the easiest of all three procedures.

Diane T., a mother of three, has a problem with heavy bleeding. We believe the bleeding to be hormonally based, but after trying everything short of surgery, we have not solved her problem. Therefore we have decided to remove her uterus. She wants to retain her ovaries. Because she has had three pregnancies and deliveries, her uterus has descended somewhat into her vagina, so it should be easy to remove vaginally. Because she wants her ovaries to remain, there is no reason to use the laparoscope. This woman is a good candidate for a vaginal hysterectomy.

After the removal of her uterus by vaginal hysterectomy, examination of the uterine tissue by a pathologist revealed adenomyosis, that is, Diane's uterine muscle was penetrated throughout by endometrial tissue. This finding explained why our conservative attempts to stop the bleeding had not succeeded.

If you and your doctor decide on a vaginal hysterectomy, you should be aware that the procedure may turn into an abdominal hysterectomy once the operation has begun. I always tell patients that until they are in the recovery room I cannot guarantee that I will successfully complete a vaginal hysterectomy. The reasons for the change in procedure may be bleeding problems during the operation or difficulty with the uterus descending into the vagina, where it can be removed. When I am discussing with someone the possibility of having a vaginal hysterectomy, I sometimes give odds. I say that I am 90 percent sure that I can do this vaginally, but there is a 10 percent chance the operation will turn out to be abdominal. Or I may say that there is only a 20 percent chance that I can do this vaginally, but I am happy to give it a try.

Laparoscopically Assisted Vaginal Hysterectomy

The third group of women can have an LAVH; these women have no major abdominal problems, no large fibroids, no significant endometriosis, and no complicated pathology.

> I have already mentioned Grace Q., fifty-nine, who chose hysterectomy because she did not want to give up estrogen therapy. Grace has serious arthritis, which she keeps under control by daily exercise. She has taken estrogen since menopause, but progesterone in any form gives her severe headaches. We tried ERT without progesterone, but she developed endometrial hyperplasia and needed a hysterectomy if she wished to continue the estrogen. After considering her choices, she opted for the hysterectomy. A short recovery time was crucial because of her exercise regimen; since she had never had children, her uterus was quite small, which made her a good candidate for a laparoscopically assisted hysterectomy. She recuperated easily and was back working out at the gym in two weeks.

Grace is a woman who can't afford to be out of commission very long; she needs her daily stint in the gym to keep her joints flexible. Abdominal surgery would have kept her from her exercise routine for several weeks and thereby increased her suffering from arthritis. The LAVH allowed her to resume her daily exercises and whirlpool promptly. She was an ideal candidate for this procedure.

▶ *What are the advantages and disadvantages of an LAVH?*

The chief advantage is that the recovery time may well be shorter than with an abdominal hysterectomy. Many women do very well with an LAVH and are back in shape very quickly.

One of my partners has a patient whom I had seen at the local gym for quite a while; although I didn't know her name, we always nodded and smiled when we saw each other. One day she came up to me and said, "Tell your partner that Jennifer is doing fine." I was startled when I realized that she had had an LAVH two weeks earlier and was in the gym doing a full workout. Of course, she was in spectacular shape to begin with and she might have done just as well with an abdominal hysterectomy, but I think having the procedure done laparoscopically contributed to her quick recuperation.

By contrast, some patients are slow to recuperate after the operation; they have, after all, undergone major surgery. They may not have had an abdominal incision, but the interior surgery is the same as that of an abdominal hysterectomy. The surgeon is cutting the same veins, arteries, and ligaments. These things are painful, yet because the patient has no scar on her abdomen, she tends to get less sympathy.

Doctor Alan DeCherney, one of the foremost practitioners of laparoscopy in this country, has pointed out that this lack of sympathy is a real debit of laparoscopic surgery. One of his patients, from whom he had removed a benign ovarian cyst through the laparoscope, came back for her two-week postoperative checkup. He thought she would be happy about having had the procedure, but she told him that these had been the worst two weeks of her life. Even though she felt miserable, her friends and family had little sympathy for her; as far are they were concerned, she was feeling no pain whatsoever. If she had had a big scar on her abdomen to show for her trouble, she said, her friends and family would have been bringing her chicken soup and flowers instead of expecting to see her up and about.

Laparoscopic surgery certainly has its benefits, but it should not be considered painless surgery. For every Jennifer who is lifting weights at the gym two weeks post-op, someone else feels dreadful. You must take these variations into account in anticipating your recuperative course.

I have mentioned the slight possibility that an LAVH, like a standard vaginal hysterectomy, will change into an abdominal hysterectomy while you are on the operating table, that some problem or complication will necessitate an abdominal incision. Therefore no one can be absolutely sure in advance that she will be back at work in two weeks.

Since an LAVH is a relatively new operation and not all physicians perform it, you should be sure to determine whether your doctor is familiar with the procedure. As with any operation, especially one that has a steep learning curve, you want to be sure that the doctor who will be operating on you has performed the surgery many times successfully, that is, without a significant rate of complications. You should find out whether your physician is credentialed to perform an LAVH. You should also determine whether you are a suitable candidate for the procedure, and if not, why not.

In group practice, often one doctor is better at a particular procedure and another specializes in something else. My own senior partner is one of the best abdominal surgeons I know, but he is not a vaginal surgeon. I do most of the vaginal surgery; he does our complicated infertility cases, which require special abdominal procedures. A third partner in our group is skillful at LAVH.

You may find it difficult or embarrassing to ask your doctor these questions, but it is worthwhile to do so. If you are an appropriate LAVH candidate but your own gynecologist does not routinely perform this surgery, ask for a referral to someone who has significant experience in the procedure. If you have a reputable physician and your relationship is solid, you should be able to get a satisfactory answer to your questions. If your physician is not experienced in performing LAVHs, he or she should be willing to tell you, "Yes, you are a reasonable candidate for an LAVH; no, I am not an experienced LAVH doctor." Fortunately, as time goes by more and more doctors are becoming skilled in laparoscopy.

▶ Are laparoscopic hysterectomies less expensive?

Unless you have adequate health insurance, cost can be a major factor in health care decisions. Although it would seem that shorter hospital stays would make an LAVH cheaper than an abdominal hysterectomy, this is not the case. LAVHs are done with disposable surgical instruments (except for the laparoscope itself), and these instruments—the probes and stapling guns and suture devices used to tie off the blood vessels—cost about two thousand dollars Because these instruments are hard to sterilize and must be extremely sharp, they cannot be reused. Therefore the economic gain of a shorter hospital stay is more than offset by the cost of surgical instruments.

BOX 4. Questions to Ask Your Physician Before Hysterectomy
or Other Surgery

How long is the surgical procedure?

Is it advisable to store my own blood?

How long will I be in the hospital? What complications can arise?

How will you deal with these complications if they do arise?

What type of pain will I have after surgery?

What will you use to alleviate the pain?

What type of anesthesia will be used?

How long will I be under anesthesia?

Will I have stitches?

Will I have a catheter or an IV in me? For how long?

When will I be able to return to my normal routine, which includes work,
exercise, sex, and driving a car?

When will I visit you postoperatively? How often will I see you after my first
postoperative visit?

Source: Adapted from Karen Giblin, founder PRIME PLUS/Red Hot
Mamas.

▶ *Is there such a thing as a laser hysterectomy?*

Sometimes patients ask me about a laser hysterectomy. There really isn't such a thing.
What most people are talking about is the LAVH, which uses a laparoscope, clips, and sutures, but not a laser. Lasers are used for other surgery, of course, but in many cases they
do not have significant advantages over more traditional techniques.

General Surgical Questions

▶ *How can I prepare for a hysterectomy?*

The better shape you are in, the better you will withstand the surgery and the more
quickly you will recover. Being in good shape means getting aerobic exercise rather than

doing sit-ups or push-ups to strengthen particular muscles. If you smoke, stop; or at the very least, cut down on the number of daily cigarettes. Smoking increases problems with anesthesia and causes additional discomfort after the surgery. If you have a smoker's cough, you will really feel it postoperatively.

Get in good nutritional shape. Try to stay close to your ideal weight. If you are forty, fifty, or one hundred pounds overweight, lose as much as you can; significant overweight is a major risk for anesthesia and other surgical complications. Take iron to build up your hematocrit. The average American woman is well nourished and probably doesn't need too much in the way of supplemental vitamins, although taking extra vitamins in moderation can't hurt. Get enough rest before the operation so that your immune system is not stressed by fatigue.

▶ *What should I discuss with my physician before surgery?*

If you are taking medications, you should find out which are safe to take before surgery. Medicines that could be hazardous include common anti-inflammatories: aspirin, Motrin, Naprosyn, and similar drugs that many people use for arthritis, headaches, and other conditions. These drugs interfere with clotting, and your doctor may ask you to stop taking them a few days in advance. You can ask for alternatives. Tylenol, for example, is perfectly safe.

Other drugs that you absolutely should not take if you are undergoing surgery are MAO (monoamine oxidase) inhibitors. People taking these uncommon drugs are restricted in their intake of cheese, wine, and nuts. If these foods are off-limits to you and you are taking medication, be very sure that your physician knows about it. There are other drugs whose dosage your physician may wish to lower.

Be sure to tell your doctor about any herbal products you are taking. Many can be associated with clotting abnormalities.

If you have allergies to any medications that your physician does not know about, you should mention them. Some people are allergic to iodine, which is sometimes used as a surgical scrub. If your physician knows, another antiseptic solution can be substituted.

If you have serious heart or lung disease, it is probably prudent to schedule a meeting with the anesthesiologist well before surgery so that everything can be understood and planned before the day of your operation.

▶ *What are autologous blood donations?*

In this AIDS-conscious era, many women donate blood for themselves preoperatively. Since a hysterectomy is generally an elective procedure, you will have time to make what is called an autologous blood donation. As soon as you decide to have a hysterectomy, start taking iron. A few weeks before the operation, you may wish to donate a unit of blood at your hospital's blood bank, then build yourself up with more iron, and a few weeks later donate another unit, continuing this routine until you have given an adequate supply of your own blood (usually one or two units are enough). You can safely give blood about every two weeks; since the hospital and operating room will be booked for you three or four weeks in advance, you will have plenty of time.

Not every hospital has the facilities for autologous donations, but most do. If your physician doesn't discuss this issue with you, you should raise it yourself if you are concerned.

If you are unfamiliar with the blood supply laws in your state, ask your physician. In Connecticut, where I practice, the state's blood supply is extremely safe because all of the blood in the state blood bank is donated at Red Cross centers. Drug addicts who might sell their blood to make money have to go elsewhere. Furthermore, the word is out in the gay community not to donate. By law all blood in Connecticut since 1985 has been screened for syphilis, for HIV, and for hepatitis.

In other states not all blood is donor blood. If you live in one of those states and cannot donate an autologous supply for some reason, you may want to contact the Red Cross about directed donation, that is, having your friends and relatives donate blood. Even this tactic is not without risk. Some blood bank directors believe that directed donations can be riskier than the donations from the general blood supply. Suppose you ask cousin George to donate blood for you. If, unbeknown to you, he has participated in risky activities, such as unprotected homosexual sex or intravenous drug use, he may feel pressured to donate anyhow. It is naive to think that you can be sure about anyone else's sexual habits and experiences; I have seen many women who discovered after years of marriage that their husbands were bisexual.

▶ *What tests and evaluations are done before surgery?*

Before you undergo anesthesia, your doctor will want you to have a cardiogram to be sure your heart is sound and a chest X-ray to be sure your lungs are clear. Usual pre-op blood evaluations include a blood count to see that you are not too anemic to withstand surgery. A clot of blood is sent off to the blood bank so that in case you need blood in an emergency (and you have not made an autologous donation), the blood bank will be able to give you blood that matches yours. Some doctors ask for a clotting study (called a PT and PTT) to see how long it takes your blood to coagulate.

Although the blood that is drawn for these tests may look like a lot to you, it really isn't. Three of the standard tubes contain just one ounce (30 ml) of blood.

▶ What preparations are required the day before surgery?

People undergoing surgery should not eat after midnight the night before. If you're making your children's lunches the morning of the operation, don't even lick the peanut butter knife! If an anesthetized patient vomits, what is thrown up may be aspirated into the lungs and cause serious problems. Under elective circumstances no anesthesiologist will give anesthesia to anyone whose stomach contains food or liquid. Occasionally, however, the anesthesiologist will tell you that it is all right to take your normal medications with a sip of water.

Another thing you should do before surgery is take an enema. One of the major complaints after abdominal surgery is gas pain, and you can save yourself a lot of discomfort if you have an empty bowel. Usually I tell people to use a Fleet enema, which is all that is needed for most hysterectomies.

If your physician thinks you may have cancer of the pelvic organs, you will probably be asked to have a bowel prep, just in case the surgeon needs to do bowel surgery. Occasionally ovarian tumors can spread to the bowel, and in some instances the surgeon may have to take out part of the bowel. This does not mean that you are going to have a colostomy, but if your doctor is working near the bowel, it is advisable that the bowel be cleaned out.

Years ago it was standard procedure to come to the hospital the night before surgery. This practice allowed for the necessary tests and ensured that you didn't eat or drink anything after midnight. Today, because of hospital costs, most patients come in on what is called express admission. They have their blood tests, cardiograms, chest X-rays, and other preoperative evaluations as an outpatient in the week to ten days before surgery.

▶ What kinds of anesthesia are available and what are the risks?

Most gynecological procedures can be done either under a general anesthetic or with an epidural or spinal anesthetic. General anesthesia puts the patient completely to sleep; she is hooked up to respirators that do her breathing for her, monitored by the anesthesiologist. When a spinal anesthetic is used, a small amount of Novocain or a similar drug is put into the space around the spinal cord. With an epidural anesthetic, a larger amount of the same type of medication is injected into the area outside the spinal space. A small, soft tube, or catheter, remains in the back, so that the anesthesiologist can administer more medication as needed. Both a spinal and an epidural cause numbness from the chest down. In addition to the anesthetic itself, the anesthesiologist usually gives intravenous medications to make the patient oblivious to her surroundings. Although she continues to breathe on her own, she is not alert and not counting the minutes as they pass.

In most hysterectomies, the choice of anesthesia is up to the patient and what she feels most comfortable with. If you are deeply anxious about surgery and don't even want to see the inside of an operating room, you are probably better off having a general anesthetic. Occasional patients who have epidurals are aware of tugging and pulling; they are not in pain, but they do feel something happening. If this would distress you, general anesthesia is a better choice.

One advantage of a spinal anesthetic is that it wears off gradually. With a general anesthetic, you wake up and immediately feel the full brunt of the surgery. With a spinal, you are brought to the recovery room and the effects of the surgery assert themselves little by little.

There is little difference in risk between a general and an epidural anesthesia. With recently developed anesthetic agents, anesthesia is extraordinarily safe. Although death from anesthesia does still occur, it is extremely rare. People who had surgery twenty-five years ago should know that the agents used today for general anesthesia are very different from the old-fashioned ones. So much surgery is done in outpatient clinics that it has been important to develop anesthetic agents that act quickly and wear off quickly. Formerly, when a patient stayed in the hospital for three days after a D&C, it did not matter that she was groggy. Nowadays, when she goes home right away, she needs an anesthetic that will wear off rapidly so that she can take care of herself at home. These quicker-acting agents have fewer side effects than the old ones did.

Furthermore, scare stories used to circulate about people who were paralyzed by spinal anesthetics. With current methods and techniques, there is no such danger. In the past, people often had severe headaches following spinal anesthesia, caused by a leak of cerebrospinal fluid from the puncture where the needle introduced the anesthetic. Today's needles are so small that postoperative headaches are a rare complication, and anesthesiologists have medications that can alleviate the few spinal headaches that do occur.

What Happens During a Hysterectomy

Technically the word "hysterectomy" means removal of the hystera, the Greek word for "uterus," but today the operation almost always includes the cervix; the fallopian tubes and the ovaries may also be removed.

The technical names for these operations describe the organs that are involved. If the entire uterus (that is, the fundus, or body, of the uterus) and the cervix are removed, the operation is called a total abdominal hysterectomy, abbreviated in the gynecology literature as TAH.

About fifty years ago one of the commonly performed procedures was something called a supracervical hysterectomy, which meant that the uterus was taken out but the cervix was left in place. Another name for this operation was subtotal or partial hysterectomy. Common sense lay behind this approach, since most of the maladies that necessitate a hysterectomy are remedied by taking out only the fundus of the uterus. Without the uterine corpus, symptoms such as bleeding, fibroids, and pain usually can be cured. Still, the cervix in and of itself has no function, and now physicians tend to take it out routinely as part of a hysterectomy, because it can become cancerous. An occasional physician will perform a supracervical hysterectomy if a patient specifically asks for it; I have only done three in all my years of practice. The issue has become somewhat controversial for two reasons: some women believe that the presence of the cervix contributes to sexual satisfaction; and a few investigators believe that it helps support the vagina when the uterus has been removed.

A supracervical hysterectomy may be appropriate in an emergency, perhaps when someone is bleeding postpartum. Sometimes the patient is critically ill, and a hysterectomy is easier if the cervix remains in place. Removing it may increase the risk of infection or further blood loss.

When women speak of a "total" hysterectomy, they usually mean the uterus, the cervix, both ovaries, and the fallopian tubes. In strict medical terminology, however, a total abdominal hysterectomy means removal of the entire uterus including the cervix. The abbreviation for removing everything—uterus, cervix, ovaries, and tubes—is TAH and BSO, total abdominal hysterectomy and bilateral salpingo-oophorectomy. The term "salpingo" comes from the Greek word for "tube," while "oophorectomy," sometimes called ovariectomy, refers to removal of the ovaries. In terms of the risk of complications and recovery time, the procedures are basically the same whether or not the ovaries and tubes are removed.

Often when a gynecologist is performing a hysterectomy, he or she will talk about taking out the appendix at the same time, which adds perhaps five or ten minutes to the operation. Sometimes patients request it, and although appendicitis is more common in young people, it can strike at any age. Although the appendix does not serve any biological function, some people have an emotional attachment to it; others as a matter of policy want nothing removed that absolutely doesn't have to be removed. It is very important that your physician respect your wishes and do what is emotionally comfortable for you.

▶ *What exactly does the surgery involve?*

The most common form of hysterectomy is abdominal. After the patient has been anesthetized, the surgical team washes the vagina with an antiseptic solution. The reason for this prepping is that later in the operation an incision will be made in the vagina, and decreasing the germ count lowers the risk of infection. The physician then inserts a catheter into the bladder to keep it empty and minimize the space the bladder occupies in the pelvis.

The abdomen is then cleaned and the top part of the pubic hair shaved off. Whereas formerly the whole pubic area was shaved, now only enough shaving is done to keep hair from getting into the incision. The rest of the abdomen is draped with towels to create a clean field around the incision.

The surgeon then makes the incision. Two kinds of incisions can be made for an abdominal hysterectomy. One is up and down, going from just beneath the belly button down toward the pubic bone. An up-and-down incision is useful if the surgeon needs a large area within the pelvis to work, for example to remove a large fibroid or if there is strong suspicion of cancer. Otherwise many surgeons favor a Pfannenstiel incision, a low transverse incision popularly known as a bikini cut. A Pfannenstiel is more attractive cosmetically than an up-and-down incision and tends to heal a bit faster.

Beneath the skin is a layer of fat. Some people have a little; others have a lot. The surgeon cuts through the fat and encounters the fascia, the layer that holds other structures together. Fascia is like tendon tissue, shiny and white and tough. Usually the surgeon incises the fascia sideways and removes it from the muscles beneath it.

The rectus muscles beneath the fascia are two straplike muscles that run up and down parallel to each other, from the ribs to the pubic bone. In the midline there is a little space between the two rectus muscles; sometimes in a late pregnancy, the uterus bulges out in the separation between the rectus muscles. In a nonpregnant woman, the rectus muscles are quite tight and lie close together.

The surgeon separates the rectus muscles and pushes them to the two sides. Occasionally, to get more room, the surgeon will have to cut the rectus muscles a little, but at the end of the operation the muscles will be sewn together and will heal. Patients do not have to worry about having their strength diminished or their abdominal wall permanently weakened.

The next layer is the peritoneum, which lines the body cavity. Since the intestines and other structures lie right beneath it, the surgeon carefully makes a little nick in it, then extends the incision with direct visualization. Usually this incision is vertical. The surgical team moves the bowel and the muscles out of the way with sterile packs, all of which are numbered and labeled, so that they will not get stuck or lost in the belly. The team puts in retractors to hold the abdominal wall and the bladder out of the way for better visualization.

After the physician manually palpates the organs in the pelvis—the liver, the intestines, the lymph nodes, the kidneys, and so on—checking for abnormalities, the hysterectomy proper begins.

If there is a lot of scar tissue or adhesion, the surgeon removes it to restore normal anatomy. Working from the top down, he or she locates and cuts the round ligaments that support the uterus at the top. If the ovaries are being removed, they are isolated from their blood supply (the ovarian artery and vein) and from their attachments in the pelvis and removed. If the ovaries and fallopian tubes are to remain, they are isolated from the uterus. Since the bladder sits right on top of the uterus and cervix and is attached to them, the surgeon must separate these organs, a procedure known as taking down the bladder flap.

Next, the uterus and the cervix are divided from the broad ligament, the uterine blood supply, and the cardinal ligaments that attach them to the side wall of the pelvis. The surgeon has now reached the level of the top of the vagina. Unless the patient has cancer, no vaginal tissue will be removed, so the surgeon makes an incision at the cervicovaginal junction and divides the cervix from the vagina.

Since the uterus is now separated from the vagina, from the side walls of the pelvis, and from the ovaries, it can be removed through the abdominal cavity. The surgeon puts several stitches at the top of the vagina to stop bleeding and to reattach the vagina to the ligaments that formerly supported the uterus. The vagina is now attached to the cardinal ligaments and the round ligaments.

Once that is done, the bladder flap is tacked back over the top of the vagina. This procedure creates a significant change in the anatomy of the bladder, which is now sitting more or less where the uterus was located. Accordingly, women who have had a hysterectomy will be aware for a week or so after surgery that urinating feels different.

When the vagina has been resuspended, the surgeon may do an appendectomy, detaching the appendix from the fat surrounding it and from the bowel and snipping it off. The surgeon then removes the packs and the retractors and closes the various layers, starting with the peritoneum and working outward, closing and stitching the muscle layers, the fascia, the fat, and finally the skin. There are several ways of closing the skin. If you prefer one way to another, talk to your surgeon beforehand. If you don't like clips or you want a specific kind of suture, let your surgeon know.

A vaginal hysterectomy is an abdominal hysterectomy in reverse. The patient is in stirrups and usually two assistants are holding retractors to keep the side walls of the vagina out of the way while the operation proceeds. The operation begins at the cervix, with an incision all the way around its circumference. After pushing the vaginal tissue away from the uterus, the surgeon makes a small incision in the posterior cul de sac, which opens into the abdominal cavity. The patient's position, with her head a bit downward, keeps the intestines out of the way. Much of a vaginal hysterectomy is done by feel. After pushing the bladder off the uterus from below, the surgeon makes an incision anterior to the uterus. Through these incisions the surgeon feels along the uterus, working upward to its top, clamping and cutting and stitching, until the uterus is detached from its pelvic ligaments. Because all of this is done as much by feel as by direct visualization, the pelvic structures have to come down easily. If the patient proves to have endometriosis or adhesions, it is at this point that a vaginal hysterectomy may become abdominal.

Interestingly enough, one of my patients who has fared the best after a hysterectomy was a woman on whom we intended to do a vaginal hysterectomy. Her uterus did not descend, so we had to make a change partway through. Logically her swift recovery makes sense. We did vaginally what is easy to do through the vagina. Then we did abdominally what is easy to do via that route. She was home from the hospital in three days, eating, and feeling comfortable. At her post-op check three weeks later, she said that she had never felt ill for even one day.

The procedure for an LAVH is a combination of the two previously described. The surgeon begins at the top, making two small abdominal incisions through which the laparoscope is inserted. The cutting of the ligaments near the top of the uterus and division of the uterine artery and vein are done via the laparoscope, through which the surgeon can visualize the interior of the pelvis to see whether there are adhesions. The bladder flap and uterine vessels are taken from above. From below, the surgeon takes the cardinal ligaments and withdraws the uterus through the vagina.

Once the uterus has been removed in a vaginal hysterectomy, the surgeon sews up the peritoneum and reattaches the ligaments to the top of the vagina. When all the reattachments have been made, the surgery is complete. There is no skin, no fascia, nothing else to close. For this reason the healing process often takes less time with a vaginal hysterectomy.

▶ How long does a hysterectomy take?

The length of surgery depends on whether other procedures, for example a bladder repair, are being done at the same time. The average hysterectomy takes anywhere from an hour and a half to three hours, depending on how much surgery is undertaken. Ask your physician for an estimate. But remember to tell the relatives or friends who are waiting for you to add an hour or two to that time. You may spend a little while waiting outside the operating room; once inside, it takes a half-hour or longer for the IV to start and the monitoring devices to be hooked up.

Anesthesiologists as a group are chatty people, and they may spend time talking with you to help you relax. Some hospitals have more rigid schedules than others; your physician can give you an estimate of how long relatives may have to wait beyond the scheduled operating time.

▶ What can be done for postoperative pain?

Thirty years ago the standard treatment for post-op pain was Demerol or morphine, given by injection every three or four hours—sometimes with an antihistamine such as Vistaril added to give better pain relief, sometimes just straight Demerol. When the pain decreased, oral pain medications were substituted.

Nowadays there are better ways to administer these drugs. Among the most significant improvements is something called patient-controlled analgesia (PCA), which means that you are hooked up to a little pump and given a controller. You can push this "joy buzzer" every six to ten minutes and a dose of painkiller drips right into the IV. If you push the button more frequently, say every minute, the pump will dispense the drug only every six to ten minutes. Interestingly enough, it turns out that people require less analgesia if they can control its frequency.

Before the pump came into use, the posthysterectomy patient would get her shot of morphine or Demerol, go to sleep for about two hours, wake up in pain and get another shot, go back to sleep, wake up in pain again, and so on. But with the PCA, she can keep dosing herself and control the pain. Because the doses are small, she remains more alert. Most women need to keep the PCA going for a day or two after surgery, though some use it for longer or shorter periods.

Another modern technique for pain control involves giving a spinal containing narcotic medication before the surgery. This kind of medication is called intrathecal narcotics and gives pain relief for up to twenty-four hours after surgery. You can have intrathecal narcotics even if you are going to have a general anesthetic. Some physicians even keep the epidural in place after surgery so that more medication can be introduced. The advantage of putting the narcotic into the spinal or epidural space instead of the brain is that it doesn't cause grogginess. The patient is alert but the pain is deadened.

Recovery and Recuperation

▶ *What pain medications are available to take at home?*

The two major categories are narcotics and anti-inflammatories. Narcotics include codeine, Demerol, Percodan, and Vicodin. A narcotic nasal spray called Stadol is absorbed through the nasal mucosa and gives satisfactory post-op pain relief. Anti-inflammatories include Motrin, Naprosyn, Toradol, and a host of other widely available drugs. For postoperative pain the drug of choice depends on what kind of hysterectomy you have had and how much pain you are experiencing. If you have had an abdominal hysterectomy, you will probably need a narcotic for a few days beyond surgery. Some physicians send patients home with both narcotics and anti-inflammatories.

▶ *Is there a danger of becoming addicted to pain medications?*

Although people worry about addiction, it is not a real danger. Studies have shown that you have to use painkilling narcotics every four hours for a month to become addicted. After the first week or two, most people don't need much in the way of pain medication.

Narcotics do cause constipation by decreasing the activity of the bowel. Since many people have difficulty getting their bowel function back to normal after surgery, overuse of narcotics can increase the problem. There is a delicate balance between being comfortable and not drugging the bowel. The major advantage of anti-inflammatories is that they don't usually cause constipation.

You can mix and match your pain medications. If you are reasonably comfortable during the day with a couple of Tylenol or a couple of Motrin, stick with those medications. At night, when pain tends to increase and you are trying to sleep, take a Demerol or Vicodin or use your Stadol.

▶ *What is the recovery period after hysterectomy?*

If you have had an abdominal hysterectomy, you should anticipate a six-week recovery period. That time frame is based on the healing of the stitches that hold the fascia. Recuperation time is an individual matter dependent in part on your age, in part on your physical shape, and in part on factors that perhaps cannot be anticipated. If you are a debilitated fifty-year-old, you will probably take considerably longer to recover than a sixty-five-year-old who is in great shape.

Even if you are having a vaginal hysterectomy, you should anticipate six weeks' recovery time. Part of the reason is that a vaginal hysterectomy can easily turn into an abdominal hysterectomy, and your post-op schedule should reflect this possibility. A second reason is that I don't think women should make unreasonable demands on themselves. I want them to be kind to themselves and enjoy the luxury of an available six weeks. If you feel terrific and want to go back to work earlier, all right. But if you don't, you won't have to be angry with yourself or disappointed with the pace of your recovery; such moods are far from therapeutic.

Most of my patients are eager to know in advance when they can go back to work. A hysterectomy is major abdominal surgery, and though you may not be in actual pain two weeks after surgery, you are sure to be tired and need a rest period in the afternoon, no matter how tough-minded you may be. If your job is fairly sedentary and does not involve lifting, it is probably all right to go back to work two weeks after surgery as long as you limit yourself to half-days. If your job involves sitting in front of a computer managing your accounts or writing your novel, work from nine to noon but plan to take a nap in the afternoon. If you work in a nursing home and have to lift patients, you should wait six weeks before resuming your regular job activities. Whether you have had an LAVH, an abdominal hysterectomy, or a vaginal hysterectomy, the six weeks' prohibition before lifting still applies.

After six weeks you may think you are back to normal in terms of energy and comfort, but about three months after surgery, you may wake up one day and really feel completely recovered. About twenty years ago, before gallbladders were removed by laparoscopy, I had mine taken out. I was back at work in three weeks and was running in four. If you had told me that I didn't feel 100 percent recovered, I would have disagreed. But, retrospectively, about three months after surgery, I was out running one day and it hit me that I felt better. I hadn't felt bad in the interim, but suddenly I felt truly recovered. This seems to happen to most people after a hysterectomy.

In general, during this interim period you can do whatever you normally do, but you might want to do it less intensely than you did before surgery. Yes, you can go skiing, but you might not want to do the giant slalom. Yes, you can go bowling, but you might not want to bowl the three games you normally do.

Therefore you should organize your life around this projected recovery time. If you are a schoolteacher and don't want to miss school, have your hysterectomy at the end of June. I have one patient who skis avidly all winter and goes boating all summer. I performed her hysterectomy between the two seasons. Some women prefer to have their children in school during the recovery period; other mothers find the school year busier than summer as far as child care is concerned, because heavily scheduled activities involve more driving.

▶ What symptoms should I watch for after a hysterectomy?

Be alert for bleeding. Most people have some staining or discharge from the vagina as the stitches at the top of the vagina dissolve, but the discharge is usually less than the bleeding of a normal menstrual period. Occasionally a stitch gives way and the vaginal area can bleed; this kind of bleeding may happen weeks after surgery and may be as heavy or heavier than the flow of a menstrual period. Report it to your physician.

You should not be having fevers higher than 100 degrees. If you do, call your doctor. As far as pain is concerned, you should be feeling better, not worse, as each day goes by. You will probably go home from the hospital with pain medications; if you find that you need them more rather than less, call your doctor. Pain and fever could be signs of infection.

You may also feel some hot flashes related to changes in your estrogen levels, whether or not your ovaries have been removed. If you did have an oophorectomy and your ovaries were working full tilt before they were removed, you may need a fairly large dose of estrogen. If you were going through menopause at the time of your hysterectomy and oophorectomy, you may need less estrogen. But if you notice menopausal symptoms—

hot flashes, sleep problems, and so on—call your physician about these also, as they probably indicate that your estrogen dosage needs adjustment.

If your physician has put you on ERT after your hysterectomy and you notice unpleasant side effects of the estrogen (for example, queasiness or headaches), let him or her know. You can have your dosage changed or switch to another route of administration. For these reasons you should keep an open dialogue going with your physician during the early weeks of recovery.

▶ *What restrictions are there on diet or physical activities?*

You can eat and drink whatever you wish, but until your bowels are working well you should avoid onions or broccoli or whatever makes you feel bloated. Gassiness isn't dangerous, but it is uncomfortable after surgery. If you are no longer taking narcotics for pain control, alcohol in moderation is all right, but if you are taking narcotics, you should be very careful about drinking. Pain medications and alcohol can interact strangely and can even be dangerous, so do not take your two Demerol tablets with a glass of wine.

Avoid strenuous activities or anything that will put your abdominal muscles in jeopardy. Don't do your sit-ups; don't do your laundry; don't pick up your vacuum cleaner or your thirty-two-pound grandchild. I had a patient who saw her granddaughter every day. The child, who was as attached to her grandmother as to her mother (an operating room nurse), even came into the waiting room outside the operating room and sat on the stretcher, unable to let her grandmother out of her sight. My principal post-op instruction to the patient was that she could not pick up the child, though she could hold her on her lap.

Although doctors used to tell women not to go up and down stairs, the current feeling is that stairs are all right if you do them slowly and infrequently. Take one step at a time. Don't go up and down twenty-seven times a day; two or three times a day is enough for the first week or two. Don't carry anything. Plan your day so that you don't find yourself wanting to run upstairs for your book and then your glasses and then something else. You can sleep upstairs, but you may want to take your afternoon nap downstairs in the living room.

I don't want my patients to drive for the first week or two after surgery. The rationale for this restriction is that it is fine to drive under normal conditions, but if a child darts in front of your car and you have to slam on the brakes, I can guarantee that it will hurt.

In addition, I tell my patients not to have intercourse until I have had a chance to see that everything is healing well. Some doctors say their patients should wait a month; others say six weeks. This is not to say that you can't have sexual stimulation or orgasmic responses, it just means that you should not have anything in your vagina until you are well healed.

I tell my patients that it is all right to shower and even to get the incision wet, though some surgeons would disagree. Taking a tub bath is different, because it is difficult to get into and out of the bathtub. Sitting in the water is not a problem and won't lead to infection; the difficulty is the climbing over the edge of the tub.

▶ What are the emotional aftereffects of hysterectomy?

This issue is a delicate one and of course differs from woman to woman. In my own experience as a physician, few patients have regretted the decision to have a hysterectomy as long as the decision was theirs to begin with. Most women are very accepting of the idea of the operation once they have decided to have it.

When my patients who have had a hysterectomy come back for a routine annual checkup, I ask each how she is doing and (as a joke) whether she wants a uterine transplant. The answer is usually along the lines of "Are you crazy?" Another answer I hear frequently is, "I should have had this done a long time ago." My standard comeback is, yes, but a long time ago you weren't ready for it. Although the quality of your life is much better now without the heavy bleeding or the backache or whatever, emotionally you were not ready for the hysterectomy until you decided to have it.

The emotional issues can be particularly strong when the ovaries as well as the uterus are removed. Questions of femaleness, of sexuality, and of sexual response should be addressed before the operation. They are so complex that for some women who have finished their childbearing, even having a tubal ligation brings a lot of concern. (Many men do not want to have vasectomies for similar reasons.)

For other women a hysterectomy is nothing more than an operation, a physical procedure akin to having an appendix removed. They must decide whether they want to go through the operation and whether they have time for the recovery period, but the decision doesn't carry a lot of emotional weight.

Because the operation is usually an elective procedure, the decision is harder than some to make. If gallstones in your common duct are causing you significant pain, it is easy to say to the surgeon, yes, take them out. If they are just sitting there in your gallbladder and not bothering you, the decision is more difficult. Do you want to go through all that pain and discomfort when you don't feel bad in the first place?

If you have decided to have a hysterectomy and you mention it to friends, you will soon discover vast numbers of women eager to discuss their experiences with you. Many will tell you that their operation was no problem and assure you that you will feel great afterward. But others will tell you horror stories. They will pull out the tale of Great-Aunt Julie's hysterectomy, how awful it was, and how it ruined her life. Much the same kind of thing happens when you are pregnant, and in both cases it is wise to listen with a grain of salt and keep in mind the source.

If something really gets under your skin, call your doctor. If you feel foolish calling your physician with your worries, call your doctor's nurse, who will probably know the answer to your question. Most nurses have been through a lot of patients' hysterectomies and can tell you what goes on.

▶ *Is there such a thing as posthysterectomy depression, caused by the physical effects of the procedure itself?*

Some experts believe the depression some women feel after hysterectomy may have a biochemical cause. They reason that pelvic surgery causes a drop in beta-endorphins, those natural "feel good" chemicals released by the brain, and that this decrease could cause the depression.

▶ *Will having a hysterectomy interfere with my sex life?*

Many women experience some pain during intercourse the first few times after a major operation. This response is temporary.

Other women find permanent changes. If as part of your usual orgasmic response you have uterine contractions, obviously you will not have them after a hysterectomy. After a hysterectomy you will have no cervix, but unless you are among the women whose pleasure involves pressure against the cervix, the hysterectomy should not affect your sexual response. Most of my patients tell me that their husband or partner is not markedly aware of the cervix being gone. If you retain your ovaries, you probably will notice little change as far as libido is concerned. If you had your hysterectomy because you were troubled by endometriosis or fibroids, you may be much more comfortable during intercourse because this painful tissue is not being jabbed.

The other issue is the ovaries, which affect vaginal moisture and, possibly, libido. Estrogen keeps the vagina moist, and if your ovaries are taken out, you will have to deal with the problem of vaginal lubrication. If you do not go on ERT postoperatively, your choices are standard lubricants such as K-Y Jelly or vaginal estrogen. The ovaries are also implicated in libido or sexual desire. In addition to estrogen, they produce small amounts of testosterone, even postmenopausally. Some researchers believe that androgen production by the ovaries is responsible for libido, although others believe that testosterone only heightens aggression.

If you find that you suffer from loss of libido, estrogen preparations that also contain small amounts of testosterone may be helpful. One of the most commonly used is Estratest, which contains testosterone—not enough to give you a beard, facial hair, or acne, but enough, supposedly, to increase libido if lack of androgens is responsible for your disinterest in sex. Some postmenopausal women who still have their ovaries find it helpful. A small percentage of women who take testosterone notice an increase in aggressive feelings.

In addition to these physical issues surrounding hysterectomy and sexual response are the psychological issues, which can be complex. Consider the analogous situation of a man who has a vasectomy and thereafter finds himself impotent. Is his impotence related to his vasectomy? Not anatomically, but if his self-image requires that he be able to impregnate women to be truly masculine, his vasectomy may well interfere with his sexual functioning. If, before vasectomy, he fears he will have a problem functioning sexually, then he probably will.

The same thing can be said of a hysterectomy. If a woman thinks she will have a problem with sexuality after she has a hysterectomy, then she probably will. If her self-image as a sexual being is tied into having a uterus, even though she may be past her childbearing years, hysterectomy may well be a problem for her. Therefore a woman for whom hysterectomy is an elective procedure should make her decision very carefully; she might want to consider going to a counselor before her operation.

15 You and Your Doctor

IN recent years the American health care system has come under scrutiny and criticism by patients, consumer groups, feminists, the government, the media—in short, by practically everyone. As the old-time family doctor who knew you and your children, and possibly even your parents and your siblings, has evolved into a "primary health care provider," the whole health care system has become more complex and more bureaucratic. You can expect this pattern to continue at a more rapid and bewildering pace as health maintenance organizations (HMOs) increase in power.

As a practicing gynecologist, I've watched these changes, many of them distressing for my patients and difficult for me as well. Most HMOs are run for cost effectiveness and many to make a profit. So cost considerations come into decisions where ideally they should not.

Even the choice of whether to take hormone therapy can be affected by these economic factors. Suppose you have decided that your symptoms make HRT a reasonable choice for you. You and your doctor should sit down and discuss the pros and cons, what you can and what you shouldn't expect from estrogen. Finding just the dosage and just the approach that are right for you is a delicate process. You should know what potential side effects you may experience and what you can do if they occur. Perhaps you get some bleeding while on HRT. Maybe this happens because you are not taking enough proges- terone, or because you are not taking enough estrogen. Maybe you should try a different regimen. Or does the bleeding signify some serious condition? (Usually it does not.) Your doctor will have to decide whether you need a biopsy. If efficiency is the main considera- tion, your doctor may chose a biopsy because he or she doesn't have the luxury of time to explore all the options.

You may have questions and want to talk to your physician about your hormone therapy. If you belong to an HMO, you may be talking, not to your own doctor all the time, but to someone who has not followed your health year after year. It would be more efficient for your doctor simply to say, "Okay, you're menopausal; come back next year for your annual checkup."

But is that approach penny-wise and pound-foolish? In the long run, estrogen re- placement may indeed be cost effective. Estrogen prevents osteoporosis and just possibly may delay the onset of coronary artery disease. If women end up with fewer fractures and perhaps fewer heart attacks, they save the health care system a lot of money. Treating a heart attack in a major medical center costs more than twenty thousand dollars. Treating a hip fracture is about the same just for the acute event itself, without factoring in that many of these older women must remain hospitalized for a long time. If HRT costs about a dollar a day, or $365 a year, then at today's prices you could have HRT for about fifty-five years for the cost of one heart attack or one hip fracture.

There is also the matter of quality of life. One of my mentors was John McLean Mor- ris, by then an elderly and well-respected figure in his field. One of Dr. Morris's favorite statistics was that if every American woman took HRT, it would increase the average life span of American women by four months. Four months, of course, is not statistically sig- nificant: what was important, he said, was the quality, not the duration, of that average American life. If that life, whether four months longer or shorter, is lived in a nursing home, then its quality may be doubtful. But if that life can be lived with the energy and zest that good health provides, there is little doubt about its quality.

Another reality in the practice of medicine today is malpractice insurance, which weighs heavily on obstetricians (and on the many gynecologists who are also obstetri- cians). This, too, affects the time your doctor can spend with you. In 2001, my insurance was $32,000 yearly. In 2002, it rose to $50,000, and by 2003, it was $58,000. This year it rose to $100,000. Surprisingly, these are "bargain" rates because the practice with which I'm associated is connected with the Yale University School of Medicine. Some gynecologists in my state paid $100,000 yearly and their insurance can be expected to rise accordingly.

Given the increasing reduction in HMO and Medicare reimbursements to doctors, physicians must see more and more patients to cover the malpractice insurance. When we reach the limits of how many hours we can work, we are faced with the choice of seeing fewer patients, spending less time with each one, or leaving our specialty, which some doctors in my state are already doing. (This is a good reason for everyone—patients as well as doctors—to push for malpractice reform.)

THE DOCTOR-PATIENT RELATIONSHIP

At the core of the system remains the doctor-patient relationship. Your personal dealings with your doctor are certainly among the most important elements of the system. You want competent, intelligent care; you want a physician whose personality you find pleasant and who inspires your trust and confidence. As health care plans limit your choice of personal physician, it may become harder to find one who suits your needs and your personality. Nonetheless, the relationship between you and your doctor should remain at the center of your health care plan.

That relationship is quite complex, both personal and impersonal at the same time. On one hand, it is professional, similar to the interaction you might have with a lawyer whom you pay for services and of whom you demand technical knowledge and expertise. On the other hand, the doctor-patient relationship is more than a simple liaison between a buyer and a seller. It contains elements of caretaking, like the relationship between a parent and a child or between a teacher and a student.

In fact, these days it is common to speak of someone's doctor either as a health care provider (a term that emphasizes the marketplace aspect of the relationship) or as a caregiver. The old-fashioned word "doctor" comes from a Latin verb meaning "to teach." The word "patient," another Latinism, comes from a root that means to "suffer" or "endure." So when you spoke of your doctor, the word implied that he or she knew something that you did not and was therefore an authority who taught or told you something you needed to know. You, as a patient, were someone who suffered or endured something; you were basically a passive receptacle for your doctor's wisdom. (The word "client" seems to be coming into use today as a substitute for "patient"—a word that again stresses the impersonal, economic aspect of the relationship.)

Today, however, the relationship between doctor and patient, caregiver and client, is changing, pushed into new shapes by the rise of consumerism and of feminism. Doctors have been toppled from their pedestals, and patients have demanded a voice in their medical care. The previous attitude whereby the physician dogmatically said, "I will tell you what is right and you will listen to me and do what I say," has changed.

Even something as apparently simple as the form of address between doctor and patient has changed. It used to be that the patient called the doctor Dr. So-and-So, while Dr. So-and-So called the patient whatever he (or occasionally she) decided was appropriate.

Today our culture has changed. We are far more informal than we were a decade or so ago: people use first names in relationships where their parents would have used surnames. When rules or customs change, situations can be tricky. Some women, particularly older women who are accustomed to a different tradition, object to being called by their first names; some women prefer the informality. Some physicians do not mind being called by their first names; others do. Many of my patients call me by my first name and I respond in kind. It is usually worthwhile to state your preference; if you wish to call your physician something other than Dr. So-and-So, simply ask.

▶ *What qualities should I seek in a physician?*

As the bottom line, you want medical competence. How can you find out whether your doctor is competent? First, every state has a licensing board, and you can call the department of health to determine whether a particular individual is licensed by the state. Most counties in this country also have medical societies, and the county societies, too, can tell you whether someone is licensed.

Because physicians must do something outstandingly bad to lose their licenses, some less-than-ideal doctors do have state licenses and are in practice. If you do not have the opportunity to get a referral from another doctor whom you trust (if, for example, you have just moved to a new community), you might try calling the county medical society. Talk to the secretaries. Because they are the people registering the complaints, they know who does not have a reputation for competence. Ask them whom they would go to if they had your problem.

Another aspect of technical competence is credentials. If you are having a laparoscopically assisted vaginal hysterectomy (LAVH), a relatively new surgical procedure, you want someone who has done that operation successfully many times. As far as new procedures are concerned, reputable hospitals and surgicenters have strict credentialing procedures. Jane Doe or John Doe, gynecologist, cannot just walk in and say, "I am an LAVH surgeon." To be credentialed, doctors must go through a course, usually two to four days long, that teaches them how to perform an LAVH. Most of these courses are sponsored by the various surgical companies. Afterward the physician has to do a preceptorship, performing the procedure in two, four, or six operations overseen by or working with someone who does the operation regularly. The number of cases that the physician in training must perform under the guidance of an experienced doctor depends on the credentialing program. Today, of course, some doctors just coming out of their residencies are routinely trained in such procedures as part of their education. These people are automatically credentialed because they have learned and practiced the technique during their residencies.

Any competent and conscientious physician will improve with practice. So when you are contemplating a new or relatively new procedure, ask your doctor whether he or she is credentialed. Ask how many times he or she has done a specific procedure. Most physicians will not take offense.

▶ *What qualities are important beyond technical skill?*

One of the first things people seek is a doctor who will listen to them. Some studies have shown that physicians typically interrupt patients after the first eighteen seconds of an interview; even though he or she may be interrupting to get further details or to confirm a hypothesis, you do want your physician to listen as you explain your symptoms or the reason for your visit.

You also want a physician whose personality complements yours, with whom you will feel comfortable discussing what might be significant and even intimate problems. Frequently my own patients come to me with questions about referrals, and I am happy to help. I am also willing to suggest which physicians might appeal to a particular patient in terms of personality. Patients will say, "Well, you know what I'm like; would I do well with Dr. So-and-So?" When it is possible, I will try to match them with someone whose personality will mesh with theirs. This is especially important with regard to an internist, who most often will become someone's "primary health care provider," now that the old-fashioned family doctor no longer exists.

You also will hope to find a physician who respects your tolerances. For example, people have very different thresholds for surgery. Some have tremendous fear of it, and although no one eagerly seeks major surgery, some would rather have a procedure that causes temporary pain and discomfort in order to gain a long-term benefit. There are women, for example, who absolutely do not want a hysterectomy, so for them I would not encourage surgery except in a life-or-death situation.

Sometimes it is not possible to find the caring practitioner you are looking for in the specialty you need. It is a well-known cliché in the medical profession that few neurosurgeons could be nicknamed "Mr. Personality." For various reasons, this specialty seems to attract people who are brusque (which could be considered the down side of being decisive) and aggressive (the down side of being assertive and self-confident—which seem to be requisite qualities in someone who is going to take a knife to a person's brain).

I will tell a patient looking for a referral to go see Dr. So-and-So; he will not coddle you, and he may not be the friendliest person in the world, but he will give you advice you can trust. If he says you don't need surgery, you can trust that judgment. If he says you do need surgery, you probably do, and he will perform it capably.

The stereotype holds that cardiothoracic surgeons are even more lacking in personal friendliness than neurosurgeons. You will seldom if ever find one who will sit and talk to you about the emotional aspects of your coronary bypass graft. A competent cardiothoracic surgeon will tell you whether you need surgery and give you a good idea of your statistical odds with the procedure proposed; a good CT surgeon will competently perform the operation and may well prolong your life or drastically improve its quality. But you should consider yourself extremely fortunate if your CT surgeon is emotionally supportive as well.

Another vital factor in choosing a physician is your preference for male or female caregivers. Many women today want female physicians. Many men prefer male doctors and feel uncomfortable with a woman physician. These preferences are relevant and should be honored.

Individuals may have preferences about the age of the physician. Some people feel that a younger doctor is up on current developments and aware of the latest advances. Other people prefer a doctor with more years in practice, someone who has seen more and can rely more on previous experience to make judgments. Doctors vary in their attraction to technology, which might affect your preferences. Some are drawn to the newest techniques; others are more conservative and traditional in what they recommend. The same doctors who prefer to do LAVHs often control heavy bleeding with endometrial ablation, a technique that uses a hot-water balloon to burn the lining of the uterus, instead of an old-fashioned D&C.

At a medical meeting some years ago, my female colleagues and I were talking about our practices, asking one another about standard procedures in different parts of the country. From our conversations (and of course these observations are merely anecdotal) it seemed that male gynecologists are more attracted to new high-tech techniques than we women are. Maybe this bias comes from the sex stereotyping in our society: women are encouraged to develop relationships and men are encouraged to take action.

All physicians should keep up on current developments, but it is not always easy to know whether your physician does so. If you have an ongoing relationship with your doctor, sometimes conversations can be revealing. He or she may say, "I heard about this at a meeting; let's try it and see whether it works." Or, "In England the latest therapy is this, and it sounds promising." When you are looking for a referral, ask whether the doctor in question stays abreast of new advances; physicians know which of their colleagues do their homework, they know who attends meetings of their professional society and who does not.

The way a doctor runs his or her practice is also important to many patients. Some physicians are precise and orderly; barring emergencies, they keep everything running smoothly. In other doctors' offices you can count on waiting two hours every time you have an appointment. If you are the kind of person who feels the pressure of time and is annoyed by waiting, find another physician or try making an appointment the first thing in the morning, the first thing after lunch, or the first evening slot if there is one. You can also call the office a while before your appointment to see whether the doctor is on schedule.

Remember, though, that no one can schedule perfectly. Emergencies happen, even in specialties where they are not frequent. If your gynecologist is also an obstetrician and is in solo practice, you should realize that he or she may be performing a delivery when your appointment is scheduled. If you choose a doctor in group practice, you are more likely to be accommodated at the time you have arranged, but your physician still may be away taking care of someone with a ruptured ectopic pregnancy.

I confess that I often run fifteen minutes or half an hour late. But I think that I get behind because I listen to my patients, and statistically, a doctor who listens will run late more frequently than one who does not. My patients come in and tell me things that really need to be listened to; sometimes in the course of an appointment I will hear that someone's husband is beating her or that she is an incest survivor and having flashbacks. These are not trivial problems, and clearly we have to talk about how to get her to appropriate counseling and other issues. Some physicians will say, "Yes, this is obviously bothering you and we need to talk more about it; make another appointment and come back."

I can't do that. If somebody is pouring her heart out about having just realized that she is an incest survivor, I can't tell her to come back next week.

Even if a woman comes in for her regular appointment and tells me that she is feeling seriously depressed because her child flunked math or her dog died or her father-in-law is impossible to deal with, I listen. These may not seem like the world's greatest problems, but different things distress people, and sometimes they need to talk about them.

I always apologize to the next patient, the one I kept waiting. But I expect understanding from that patient, too. If I spend a half-hour talking to someone else when I have scheduled fifteen minutes, I will also spend that time with you if you need it. If you are a person who expects her doctor to be absolutely on time, you should not expect that doctor to listen to you if your cat dies or your daughter does not get into Harvard or your mother-in-law is causing you grief.

In general (and I base this generalization only on my experience), women physicians seem more willing than men to hear about their patients' emotional problems. If punctuality is important to you, you might think twice about going to a female health care provider. At the meetings of our local women's medical society, we commiserate about the fact that we all tend to run late.

▶ *Once I know what I want, how do I find the right physician?*

This is one of the most difficult questions. If you have a warm relationship with one doctor, for example your gynecologist, you can ask him or her for referrals to other physicians. Suppose you are developing chronically painful knees; call your gynecologist or your children's pediatrician and ask for a lead or two.

Physicians know other physicians. The gynecologists in your area or town know who are the good orthopedic surgeons or the good ophthalmologists practicing nearby. But remember that it is hard for one practitioner to criticize others who practice in their town. So you might want to present an alternative: "Do you think I would prefer Dr. Jones or Dr. Smith?"

If your physician suggests a specialist whom you like, or dislike, you can do your part to keep the network going by providing feedback. When I recommend someone to my patients, I later ask them how they got along with that person. If they did not hit it off, I try to channel them to someone else. My patients' feedback is important to me because people change, doctors included. Someone who might have had an amiable personality five years ago may have burned out, or turned into a money-grubber, or worse.

Choosing a physician becomes truly difficult when you move to a new area where you have not established a relationship with any physician and have no friends or relatives with whom to network. I have several tricks that I recommend to patients who are moving and will have to find new doctors for themselves. None of these subterfuges, I must admit, originated with me.

If you are going to a location with a medical school nearby, call the school. Find out, if you can, what department in that school is especially good. A number of my patients have moved to Florida, a common relocation area, and although I don't happen to know any physicians in practice on the west coast of Florida, I do know that the University of Southern Florida has a well-respected ob-gyn department. So I tell my patients to call the Department of Obstetrics and Gynecology at the university and ask for recommendations. Frequently the department will know doctors who were residents in their training program and have settled in the vicinity. Physicians tend to stay in the area where they trained, and it is a statistical likelihood that the school will be able to recommend an admirable former resident. When I first started in practice, I got a number of referrals from the ob-gyn department at Yale, where I had trained. At the time I was one of the few women in practice in the New Haven area, and I had a reasonable reputation; I was flattered that the department thought well of me.

Another trick, helpful for women who are looking for a gynecologist, is one I learned from a nurse-midwife colleague who used to be a labor-floor nurse. Whenever she moved to a new place, which she did frequently as a young woman, she called the labor floor at the local hospital and asked to talk to the charge nurse. She asked, "Whom do the nurses prefer as their ob-gyn?" For the most part, her referrals were quite successful. The nurses in labor and delivery are in the know; they see the doctors delivering babies and they see them operating. Since they are trained caregivers themselves, they know what to look for and fully understand who is a reputable doctor and who is not so great.

▶ *How long can I expect my appointment to be?*

At our office we schedule patients at fifteen-minute intervals for regular yearly checkups, though some doctors schedule ten minutes. There may be instances when your regular checkup requires more time. When you are attempting to choose a physician, it is worth asking about the routine office schedule. With the changes currently taking place in health care, physicians are under pressure from HMOs and insurance companies to schedule more patients in less time. The standard office visit may be cut to five minutes in the future, which would certainly interfere with the quality of care.

▶ *What rights do I have as a patient?*

You, and all patients, have a right to the best medical care available. You have a right to understand your own medical situation and the treatment recommended by your doctor.

My job as a physician is to perform an examination and then explain to you, in terms you can clearly understand, what is going on with your body. If I find endometriosis or fibroids or vaginitis, I explain what is happening and tell you whether I think you need treatment or not. If I think you do, I'll suggest what that treatment should be and explain its risks and benefits.

Obviously you are entitled to have your worries taken seriously. If someone comes to me with concern about a symptom or a physical change that is not harmful or pathological, I need to reassure her and let her know that something either ordinary or nonthreatening is happening. In the late 1980s the television drama "thirtysomething" had two episodes in which a character developed ovarian cancer. The show must have aired on Tuesday evening, because on both of the following Wednesdays many of the patients who came in suspected that they had ovarian cancer. Although it may have been exasperating to me after the sixth or seventh "case" of this rare Wednesday cancer, the show raised real concerns and fears in the women who watched it. And those anxieties deserve to be taken seriously.

The next step is to decide whether the situation needs intervention. I'll often ask someone, "Does this symptom drive you crazy? Is it something you can live with, or something you should make a decision about?" If your period is lasting seven days and you are going through six boxes of tampons every cycle, this blood loss may well bother you. If you can live with the inconvenience and are keeping up with your blood loss by taking three iron tablets a day, then the situation is under control.

One of my standard lines goes, "Is the cure worse than the disease?" A lot of people, for example, don't like to take medicine.

> Theresa D. has a terrible fear of cancer, actually a phobia about it. She also has a strong family history of osteoporosis. Taking estrogen, which would protect her bones, would make her extraordinarily anxious and might well provoke true disease. At her annual checkup I told her that since she didn't want to take estrogen, she should start exercising—taking a two-mile walk every day instead. I assured her that the walk could help her bone strength and give her cardiovascular protection as well, at no risk.

▶ *What responsibilities do I have as a patient?*

I in turn expect certain things from my patients. Occasionally people adopt the attitude that they have fulfilled all responsibility for their own health care when they (or their insurers) pay for it. In actuality the process demands work on both sides.

I believe that you have a responsibility to know what is going on with your own body. By this I do not mean that you are expected to examine yourself, diagnose what is wrong, and simply go to your doctor demanding a prescription. I see the procedure as one of give and take.

A couple of decades ago, in a particularly intense period of feminism, some of the women's health cooperatives used to teach women to do vaginal self-examination with a speculum and a mirror. The fact is that women really can't examine themselves very well. Nor can most women be expected to know much about menopausal physiology, although fortunately more information is available to the public nowadays. Examining the patient, I think, is my role.

But I do expect my patients to keep track of what is happening to them. If you are concerned about heavy periods, you should know how long the periods are continuing and how many tampons you are using. Write things down. Keeping calendars is helpful both for yourself and for the doctors who take care of you.

I expect patients to follow the advice I give them. If your physician tells you to do something, or stop doing something because it is important for your health, then you should comply. Of course, I am realistic about the difficulty of some changes. Suppose someone comes to the office who is, say, one hundred pounds overweight. If I say to her, "Please lose a hundred pounds; it would be good for you," it would be unrealistic for me to expect that she will lose that hundred pounds. It has taken her a long time to gain so much weight and she has entrenched habits that have brought on her obesity. Still, if she comes in the next year and has lost ten pounds, I congratulate her. She has been trying and is certainly headed in the right direction.

As a physician (and I am sure many other physicians feel this way), I find it distressing when a patient rejects the therapies I suggest but continues to complain about the symptoms. Someone will come in and say, "My breasts are killing me." I advise that she stop drinking coffee and start taking 400 units of vitamin E a day. Neither is difficult to do: there are some flavorful decaffeinated coffees on the market today, and taking vitamin E is certainly painless. (You brush your teeth twice a day; keep the vitamin bottle next to the toothbrush to remind you.) Yet the same woman will call me back the next month with the same complaints. If she hasn't followed my advice, it is distinctly frustrating to me and there is nothing I can do for her.

In contrast, someone else may call and say, "Well, I cut out caffeine. I am down to one cup of coffee a day, which I dilute with decaf, and I am taking 400 units of vitamin E. And my breasts still hurt." This is a call I want to receive. We can go on and try the next step. Or someone can say, when I recommend cutting out coffee, "I love my coffee, I love my tea. I've decided that I can live with the tender breasts since they aren't going to cause anything life threatening."

The same is true of PMS. You cannot expect your physician to make something improve if your lifestyle contributes to the problem. If you have PMS and you sit around eating bonbons before your period and don't go out and get a bit of exercise, you don't have a legitimate complaint. One patient became a marathoner to get rid of her PMS. This is drastic, and most women aren't going to become marathoners, but exercise is a key to controlling PMS. This woman tried running a little and she felt better, so then she tried running farther and felt still better. She is in her seventies now and has run the New York marathon five or six times and the Boston marathon, too. But even someone who regularly walks a couple of miles or joins an exercise class will feel better.

Physicians are also distressed when patients ask the same questions over and over again. I have people who call me on the phone every few weeks with the same queries. Some of these women have Alzheimer's disease, and for them the repetition allows me to keep track of the progress of their disease. I understand their problem and am sympathetic with it. But if you have normal mental capacities and are told something that you do not understand, you should ask questions until you do understand. It is far better to do that than to call repeatedly with what seems to your physician to be the same inquiry.

Doctors also are likely to be upset if patients fail to do the appropriate follow-up. If you are to be responsible for your health care, then you are responsible for getting yourself to the doctor. If your doctor says to call in six weeks, you should call in six weeks. If you are the kind of person who gets mixed up or if you are in the midst of a menopausal period of forgetfulness, write down the need for an appointment on your calendar six weeks or six months ahead. Most physicians send out notices of annual checkups and many physicians have tickler files for appointments at shorter intervals, but patients should realize that the physician's need for such files adds to the cost of health care. Every time I have my nurse or secretary call a patient to remind her of what should have been her own responsibility, it costs money. Too many times I am forced to consider myself a high-class baby-sitter.

You must also realize that your doctor cannot make you feel 100 percent wonderful 100 percent of the time. There are trade-offs, as in everything in life. But you have to know what is important to you, where your tolerances lie. Suppose you love potato chips. If the salt makes you feel bloated, you can try drinking lots of fluids, and maybe this will relieve the discomfort. If not, you have a choice: give up the chips and live without the bloating, or enjoy your chips and put up with discomfort.

The same can be said for medications. Just as you have to be willing to invest in some lifestyle changes that will help you, you have to be willing to take the medications your doctor recommends, or at least to understand that without them your symptoms may not change. I recognize that some women have social or cultural or biological reasons for not wanting to take estrogen. That is their prerogative, and it is my responsibility as a physician to try to help them with their hot flashes and other symptoms in different, non-hormonal ways. It is my responsibility to explain the pros and cons of a medication. But if I suggest a medication that has no social stigma or significant risk, I find it difficult to be sympathetic with a patient who will not at least give it a try.

Nor can a doctor make everything work perfectly for everyone all of the time. This applies both to medical situations, for example where you are taking a medication for some distress, and to surgical situations. If you have an operation and there are complications, it does not necessarily mean that the physician is careless, wrong, or incompetent. Different procedures have known and accepted complications. In the jargon of lawyers, these events are "maloccurrences": bad things that happen, but they are not malpractice. Patients of the best gynecologists in the world will sometimes get an infection after a hysterectomy, for example; this doesn't necessarily mean that the physician did something wrong.

▶ *Are there special considerations to think about if my doctor is a woman?*

Many female patients want female caregivers. It is definitely a trend in this country, and understandably so. If you choose a female doctor, you should remember that she is a woman as well as a physician: if she is in the appropriate age bracket, she may well get pregnant; if she has young children, she will occasionally be involved in the same situations faced by other mothers of small children.

I have had patients who were very irritated when I took maternity leave, strange though that may seem. Most patients are considerate, but occasionally someone has called repeatedly and told the office staff that her problem was "special" and needed my personal care. Some went so far that their behavior could be considered harassment. Such conduct does not happen frequently.

If you trust your doctor, you can trust that she will arrange for a competent replacement to handle your problem while she is off having her baby. The substitute may not know your entire sociobiological and ethnic background, but if you are having a problem with bleeding because of your estrogen prescription or you have had a heavy period that is worrisome, he or she can help you out. If you suddenly discover that you are an incest survivor and are having flashbacks, the interim physician probably cannot deal with it as well as the doctor who has known you for the past ten years; but in truth your problem might well wait six weeks until your doctor is back from maternity leave. Your physician's partners can probably steer you to appropriate counseling, but if you feel that you really want to talk to your own doctor about it, you will have to wait until she returns from her leave. Just as your physician will understand if you have to cancel your appointment because your six-year-old has chickenpox or your teenager has an emotional crisis, you should extend the same understanding to her.

In recent years I have cut down on my hours. I have not stopped taking care of women who were already my patients, but I have not taken on new patients. Before I was married and before I had my family, I was willing and eager to work sixty hours a week in the office plus many hours on call. Now I want to have some time with my children and my husband; we need one another. Most of my patients understand these feelings, but a few are angry because I will not see their daughter. If I were to take on everyone's daughters and mothers and mothers-in-law, my time would have to be infinitely expandable. Again, if you trust your physician, you can trust her to recommend someone who will be competent to treat your daughter.

Since our biology and our society are structured as they are, female physicians have some problems that male physicians do not have. Some time ago, I organized a medical group for women doctors practicing in New Haven. We were all dealing with the demands our patients, our children, and our spouses were making on us. We were all feeling that we were alone in coping with these problems, but we discovered through the group that the problems are common to us all.

▶ *What should I look for in a gynecologist as I approach menopause?*

Basically, you should find a doctor or health care provider whom you can trust and who can guide you through the morass of popular knowledge (or rumor) and scientific literature. You need someone who is interested in menopause, who keeps up with the profusion of scientific papers that are published every year, someone who can interpret all these data for you in terms of your own life and help you make good decisions for yourself.

Although I am not yet menopausal, I do feel qualified to talk about menopause. First of all, I have spent almost twenty-five years listening to women discuss their experiences. So I have considerable secondhand knowledge. I use the analogy of my car to suggest what the doctor-patient relationship is like in many cases. I don't have to know everything about an automobile engine in order to drive a car. I don't have the interest, I don't have the time, I don't even know if I have the ability. But I have a capable mechanic who has never led me astray; who, when something is wrong with my car, will tell me what to do in order to fix it; who gives me the available options and lets me decide: should I scrap the thing, or should I spend money having it repaired? Should I get rust treatment for the underbody, or should I go on as I have been, without it?

The car analogy isn't perfect, because more is at stake with your health than with your car. I have two children. Though I know something about pediatrics, I don't consider myself an expert, and I wouldn't want to be my children's pediatrician. So I take them to a doctor who keeps up in that area and tells me what she would do in certain situations.

Likewise, with menopause I can only tell my patients what I would do in a certain circumstance. Would I take estrogen? If I were menopausal today and had annoying symptoms, yes I would take estrogen. I have big bones, I drink a quart of milk a day, and I run about twenty miles a week, but aside from being a bit fair-skinned, I have absolutely no risks for osteoporosis. Cardiovascularly speaking, my family is healthy. Still, based on what I know about estrogen, I would take it. If in eight or ten years we find out things that are different, that estrogen does not provide the benefits we think it does, or that it poses risks we have not yet understood, then I will take the new evidence into consideration.

MAINTAINING YOUR GENERAL WELL-BEING

Since menopause is an appropriate time to reevaluate your general well-being, it is also an appropriate time to set up a schedule of regular physical exams with your internist, if you have not done so already. The risks of many diseases increase with aging, and the best way to prevent sudden and unexpected problems is to keep up a regular plan of maintenance, just as you do with your car. As a gynecologist, I serve as the first-line health care provider for many women, because a great many young women in their childbearing years simply do not see other physicians. But there are things that a competent internist can do for you that your gynecologist cannot do as well, and as you get older you perhaps need more attention than you did as a younger person.

▶ When should I establish a relationship with an internist or a family care practitioner?

Although you probably see a gynecologist regularly during your childbearing years, you should establish a relationship with an internist when you are about thirty-five years old. Many internists feel that certain women's problems, for example, of sexual dysfunction, surface in the thirties when many women are spending a lot of time taking care of their children and less time taking care of themselves and their relationship with their spouse or significant other. Furthermore, it is important to get baseline readings on several factors related to your general health.

Your internist serves as the coordinator of your care, an important consideration in these days of managed care. If you suddenly have a problem that needs the attention of a specialist, your internist can help you find an appropriate person and, if your problem needs prompt attention, get you an appointment in a reasonable time frame. He or she can also see the "big picture" as far as your health is concerned—putting together all the pieces from different doctors you see for different problems, which might (or might not) be related.

▶ How often should I have a physical exam?

A very healthy woman in her thirties should have an exam every three to five years. If you are in your forties, you should be examined every two to three years. After age fifty an annual examination is a good idea. If you are obese at any age (more than twenty to thirty pounds overweight), you should have an annual exam. Some doctors make an exception to the yearly examination rule for women in their thirties and forties who are obese but whose weight is stable and who exercise regularly.

▶ What procedures are recommended for a baseline physical?

First, you should have your weight checked. Many women keep the extra weight they gained during pregnancy. Once the pattern of overweight is established and supported

TABLE 5. Medical Tests for Women over Fifty

TEST	HOW OFTEN
Breast exam by caregiver	Every year
Mammogram	Every year
Breast self-exam	Every month
Pap test	Every three years, after three consecutive normal tests
STD (including HIV)	Whenever a woman has had multiple sexual partners, especially without condom use
Pelvic exam	Every year
Bone density test	Every two years, if a baseline test at menopause shows bone loss
Colonoscopy or sigmoidoscopy	Every five to ten years
Fecal occult blood test	Every year
Cholesterol (total and HDL)	Every five years
Blood pressure	Every visit to doctor
Immunizations	Every ten years for tetanus and diphtheria
Eye exam	Every year
Dental exam	Twice a year
Urine test	Every year
Skin exam	Every year
Diabetes screening	Every three years
Thyroid stimulating hormone test	Every three to five years

by ingrained eating habits, it is hard to lose the excess poundage. By the time you are fifty, losing extra weight that you have been carrying around for fifteen or twenty years is extraordinarily difficult. Therefore many internists feel that early intervention, when you are in your thirties, for example, is helpful.

Interestingly, during these baseline exams physicians also identify women who are anorectic. They tend to be borderline anorectics, not in such difficulty that they need hospitalization. Often they are women who have been so involved with their families that they have neglected themselves.

A baseline physical should include a cardiogram. If you don't have any cardiovascular symptoms, it is not necessary to repeat the cardiogram, but obviously if you do, a cardiogram will be part of your routine physical. Internists also recommend a chest X-ray as a screening device for lung disease. If you are not a smoker, you probably won't need another X-ray for five years, but if you do smoke, you probably should have an annual chest X-ray. If you have just quit smoking, for a few years you remain statistically a smoker in terms of your risk for carcinoma of the lung, so an annual chest X-ray for the first three to five years after quitting is in order. After that you can go back to an X-ray every five years.

Also as part of your general screening, a baseline cholesterol check is a good idea. If you are not obese, have no family history of coronary artery disease, and so on, you can probably go three to five years without another screening. But if you are at risk, either because of your family history or because you have high blood pressure, then an annual cholesterol test is quite appropriate.

Nowadays a PPD (purified protein derivative) test for tuberculosis exposure is sensible. It should be repeated annually for people who are at high risk for the disease, for example health care workers, people who ride buses or subways every day, and those who work in soup kitchens and other charitable endeavors. Some of my patients out of a sense of civic duty volunteer in hospitals and literacy programs, thereby exposing themselves to the possibility of tuberculosis.

Physical examinations can be important for checking up on immunizations. Many women, though conscientious about their children's schedule of shots, are remiss in keeping their own tetanus immunizations, for example, up to date. A tetanus booster every ten years is a valuable precaution. Flu shots, while not recommended for the general population, are worthwhile for many women in their sixties and for younger women, say single mothers, who cannot afford to be laid up for a couple of weeks. Women whose activities or work expose them to large numbers of people (health care workers, teachers, and the same people who are at risk for tuberculosis) should consult their internists about the desirability of flu shots.

Another test that is performed at routine physicals is a CBC (complete blood count). This test turns up a significant amount of anemia. Because people are eating less red meat than formerly, many women are becoming anemic and have to get iron in their diet by other means.

Diabetes screening probably is not necessary as a general measure. If you have a family history of diabetes, a fasting glucose test, which simply tests the amount of sugar in your blood at least eight hours after eating, is probably adequate to determine the presence of diabetes. If your doctor has any misgivings, then a blood glucose measurement two hours after eating or even right after eating (a postprandial glucose) is likely to clear up any doubt. A full formal glucose tolerance test is probably not necessary, even for people with a family history of diabetes.

▶ *Should I have a bone density test?*

Many internists recommend bone density studies perimenopausally in women who are not planning to take hormone therapy. If you do plan to take estrogen, you don't have to worry about a bone density study; but if you do not, especially if you are at high risk for osteoporosis, then you should consider having one.

COLONOSCOPY AND SIGMOIDOSCOPY

▶ *At what age should people start having tests for bowel cancer?*

Colon cancer is the second largest cancer killer in the United States. It usually develops slowly and, when caught early, is 95 percent curable. Because it often doesn't have symptoms until it has been present for quite a while, it is important to get tested.

Most internists feel that checking the stools for blood, the so-called guaiac testing, is an important part of routine screening for everyone in their forties. Sigmoidoscopy or colonoscopy are more invasive, and internists recommend one or the other for people between ages forty-five and fifty if they have a family history of bowel or colon cancer, especially if more than one relative had the disease. Doctors start recommending testing for everyone at the age of fifty and start twisting arms after the age of sixty.

There are two major tests for bowel cancer, one more extensive than the other. Both tests check the inside of the colon for polyps or other abnormalities. Polyps are growths that arise in the lining of the intestine and protrude into the intestinal canal. Some are flat and others have a stalk. Most are harmless, but some can develop slowly, over ten or fifteen years, into cancer. Since there is no way of telling which polyps will become cancerous and which will not, the usual procedure is to remove all polyps. Most of the time this is a fairly simple procedure and can be performed during a colonoscopy or a sigmoidoscopy.

The less invasive of the tests, sigmoidoscopy, uses a flexible tube to look at the left side of the colon, about 30 percent of its entire length, where most of women's colon cancers occur. A flexible tube is inserted into the sigmoid colon, and a tiny camera projects an image of the interior of the intestine onto a screen. The test takes about twenty minutes and can be done in your doctor's office. You do not need anesthesia.

The full-scale test, the gold standard of diagnosis, is colonoscopy, which involves looking at the entire length of the colon from the rectum all the way up to the lower end of the small intestine. The procedure is basically the same as for a sigmoidoscopy, except that a colonoscopy usually involves intravenous sedation.

Neither colonoscopy or sigmoidoscopy is particularly uncomfortable or risky, but people understandably are not eager to have them. The only hard part, as we can tell you from experience, is the preparation, which involves cleaning out the bowel with laxatives so that the scope can get a true picture of its interior.

In recent years virtual colonoscopy has become a possibility, a technique that combines a CAT (computerized axial tomography) scan with sophisticated image processing computers. The CAT scanner provides the X-ray images, which the image-processing computers manipulate to create a three-dimensional display of the colon. A skilled radiologist then interprets the processed image. Virtual colonoscopy is less invasive than the standard procedure, but is probably not as accurate and is not yet widely available. Although the virtual colonoscopy is done from outside the body, you must still have an empty bowel. If polyps are found, they cannot be removed during the virtual colonoscopy, so you will then have to have the standard procedure.

Television host Katie Couric "popularized" colonoscopy by having one on the "Today" show. Since her husband died of colon cancer at age forty-two in 1998, Couric has devoted considerable energy to educating the public about this disease; after her colonoscopy was televised, colonoscopy rates jumped about 20 percent.

▶ Which is better, a colonoscopy or a sigmoidoscopy?

Your gastroenterologist is probably the best judge. A colonoscopy has slightly greater risks, the main one being perforation of the intestine, and it is more expensive, but many gastroenterologists recommend colonoscopy for older people or for those who have a strong family history of colon cancer.

OTHER TESTS

▶ *Are there blood tests for cancer that I should have?*

There are blood tests that will reveal the presence of various kinds of cancer markers, but many of these tests are not very accurate. Blood screening markers for ovarian cancer, for example, have gotten a lot of attention in the media even though they are not too reliable. The CA-125 test looks for high blood levels of CA-125, because women with ovarian cancer often have high blood levels of this carbohydrate. Unfortunately, the test gives many false positives (false alarms) and false negatives (false reassurances). Women with endometriosis, or even fibroids or chronic thyroid disease, sometimes have elevated CA-125. And many women who do have ovarian cancer have perfectly normal CA-125 levels. A more recent test, for the carbohydrate CA19-9, has proven to be too inaccurate to be useful.

In the near future we may see the use of proteomics (also called proteinomics) to detect cancer in its early stages. Rather than relying on a single marker—for example, CA-125—these tests look at an entire pattern of proteins to make the diagnosis.

There are also blood tests for bowel cancer, the CEA (carcinoembryotic antibody) test for cancer of the bowel, which may be useful in checking for recurrences in people who have had bowel cancer, but is not accurate enough to be used for routine screening.

One of my internist colleagues believes that if she can get her patients to wear seat belts, she is probably saving more lives than by any blood testing she may recommend. And I continue to think that one of the most crucial tests for women is the mammogram.

For men older than fifty (and this is something you should mention to your partner and other significant males in your life), a PSA (prostate-specific antigen) blood test for prostatic cancer is worth having.

▶ *What are the costs of a full physical exam?*

The average comprehensive physical exam, including a chest X-ray, an electrocardiogram, basic blood work, and the time of the physician, runs somewhere between $300 and $500. The price varies widely depending on where you live and which doctor you visit, so you can expect a routine physical to cost more on Park Avenue in New York than on Main Street in rural Maine. Most HMOs will cover a full physical exam; others do not, even at a time when health care professionals are highlighting the importance of preventive health maintenance.

Remember that for many people a routine physical exam can be considered treatment for a symptom, in which case the care is reimbursable even if your plan doesn't cover preventive care. And almost everybody has some kind of problem. Women with heavy periods often have iron-deficiency anemia, and testing has to be done to evaluate the anemia. Former smokers need to have a follow-up, because even though they have quit smoking, they still should evaluate their increased risk of lung cancer from smoking. People with strong family histories of coronary artery disease need to be followed. For some women, a baseline bone density test can rule out osteoporosis.

There are many things you can do to take good care of yourself in midlife, but one of the most important is to set yourself on a course of overseeing your own well-being. Establish a relationship with an internist whom you like, have the tests you need, and enjoy the well-being and peace of mind you have earned.

16 Lifestyle

IN 1900, when the average woman could expect to live only about fifty years, menopause came toward the end of life. Women who died in their fifties or early sixties survived a few years or perhaps a decade beyond menopause. With increased life expectancy, however, everything has changed. Today the American woman can expect to live until about age eighty and will spend fully one-third of her life as a postmenopausal woman.

Menopause used to be called the change of life. Although the term was a euphemism, it did express a certain basic truth, for menopause is truly a marker of change. And because it does signal a boundary, as does pregnancy (or even New Year's Day, for that matter), it is a suitable time to take stock, to evaluate your daily habits and try to prepare yourself for many healthy years to come. It is a time to evaluate your diet, your exercise routine, and your other life habits to maximize the possibility that the ensuing years will be healthy and productive.

Speaking physiologically, the "change" that happens to women at menopause is fairly clear-cut: women who have passed through menopause are no longer producing significant amounts of estrogen on their own. During their reproductive years, estrogen has protected them from certain diseases to which they become vulnerable as they age. Heart attacks and cardiovascular disease are relatively rare in premenopausal women, though they are a threat to men throughout their adult lives. Osteoporosis is not a threat to younger women (or men), but it is a concern for older women and to a lesser extent for older men. So although women do not have to worry much about coronary artery disease or osteoporosis before they are fifty, they become more vulnerable to these diseases as they age. Prevention, ideally, should have started years before, with a healthy diet and an exercise regimen, but the years surrounding menopause are critical in paving the way for the future.

In recent years Americans have become more conscious of what they need to do, especially in terms of diet and exercise, to provide the foundation for physical well-being. With the barrage of information in the media, we would have to be willfully ignorant not to know what is good for us. The concepts are simple, at least on paper. Implementing them in your own life may be a lot harder.

▶ What can I do to prepare myself for menopause?

Suppose you are a woman in your forties, and you come to my office wondering what you can do to prepare yourself for menopause. My answer is that you should begin the healthy regimens that will stand you in good stead for the rest of your life. My single most important recommendation is that you make sure you are getting adequate calcium, either in your diet or with dietary supplements. The recommended amount for women who are still menstruating is 1,000 mg a day; for postmenopausal women not taking estrogen, the recommendation is 1,500 mg.

To my way of thinking, you should follow two basic principles for a healthy life, either before or after menopause. First of all, keep yourself in shape by staying close to your ideal body weight and getting enough exercise. The two are related, for numerous studies have shown that you can only maintain desirable body weight by a combination of a moderate caloric intake and exercise. Second, stay away from destructive habits: don't smoke, don't abuse alcohol, and don't use illicit drugs.

HEALTHY BODY WEIGHT

As far as female body weight is concerned, our society has in recent decades been torn between an unreachable (and ultimately undesirable) ideal and a less-than-healthy reality. In terms of the ideal, society as reflected in the media proposes a slenderness that borders on emaciation. In the fashion magazines the only models we see are barely postpubescent women with prominent cheekbones, protruding collarbones, and thin, coltish legs. In reality, however, many Americans are overweight and becoming more so as time goes on.

In 2000, 38.8 million American adults were obese, that is, they had a body mass index, or BMI, score of 30 or more. (By that standard a woman who is five feet, five inches tall would have to weigh at least 180 pounds to be obese.) In the year that followed the prevalence of obesity climbed from 19.8 percent of American adults to 20.9 percent. And currently more than 44 million Americans have reached that undesirable status. This is a 61 percent increase in the past decade, since in 1991 only 12 percent of American adults were obese.

Years ago, back in 1988, the Surgeon General's report pointed out that as a statistical pattern the more overweight you are, the greater is your risk of premature death. Obese people are at increased risk for diabetes, heart disease, high blood pressure, some kinds of cancer, back pain, gallbladder disease, and even chronic degenerative arthritis.

In addition to the increased health risks of obesity, enormous social consequences begin in adolescence and continue throughout life. According to a study published in 1993 in the *New England Journal of Medicine,* young women who are overweight are less likely to marry and will have lower household incomes and higher rates of poverty than women of normal weight. These consequences, which hold true regardless of socioeconomic origin and ability as measured by aptitude tests, are only magnified over a lifetime. Because there is a strong cultural bias against overweight people, heavy women are discriminated against in the job market.

That is the bad news. The good news is that our notion of what is defined as overweight has been revised.

▶ *How do I know if I'm overweight?*

Because overweight increases health risks and lowers life expectancies, some life insurance companies publish charts suggesting appropriate body weights. In the years since the 1960s, the Metropolitan Life Insurance Company, whose statistics were standard throughout the industry, revised its tables to reflect a wider interpretation of what an appropriate weight might be for a given height. Back in 1968 a woman five feet, four inches tall with a small frame weighing between 108 and 116 pounds would fall within the guidelines established by the actuarial tables. Today that same woman can weigh between 114 and 127 pounds and still be within the suggested range. If you are five feet, eight inches and have a large frame, nowadays the life insurance companies consider you a good risk, other factors aside, if you weigh between 146 and 167 pounds; in 1968 you would have had to shed 8 or 9 pounds and get down to somewhere between 137 and 154 pounds to meet the requirements.

Individual differences in bone diameter and in the relative proportions of muscle

TABLE 6. MetLife Height and Weight Tables [portion for women reproduced here] Weights at ages 25–59 based on lowest mortality. Weight in pounds according to frame (in indoor clothing weighing 3 lbs; shoes with 1″ heels).

HEIGHT FEET	INCHES	SMALL FRAME	MEDIUM FRAME	LARGE FRAME
4	10	101–111	109–121	118–131
4	11	103–113	111–123	120–134
5	0	104–115	113–126	122–137
5	1	106–118	115–129	125–140
5	2	108–121	118–132	128–143
5	3	111–124	121–135	131–147
5	4	114–127	124–138	134–151
5	5	117–130	127–141	137–155
5	6	120–133	130–144	140–159
5	7	123–136	133–147	143–163
5	8	126–139	136–150	146–167
5	9	129–142	139–153	149–170
5	10	132–145	142–156	152–173
5	11	135–148	145–159	155–176
6	0	138–151	148–162	158–179

Source: Reprinted courtesy of Metropolitan Life Insurance Company. Source of basic data: 1979 Build Study, Society of Actuaries and Association of Life Insurance Medical Directors of America, 1980.

and fat account for the wide ranges of acceptability on the chart. If you are a strapping, heavy-boned woman of five feet, six inches, you can weigh more than a delicately boned woman the same height and still be close to your desirable body weight. Since muscle weighs more than fat, you will weigh more inch for inch if you are muscular and athletically trained than if you are sedentary.

In addition to the general guidelines established by the chart, there are other tests for overweight. Physicians specializing in weight control sometimes use calipers to measure the thickness of skinfolds on various parts of your body. Another method is to immerse you in a tank of water to find the volume of your body and, relating it to your weight, calculate your percentage of body fat.

Nowadays the standard for assessing weight status is the body mass index. This number is calculated by plugging your weight and height into an arithmetic formula.

$$\text{BMI} = (\text{weight in pounds}) \times 703 \,/\, (\text{height in inches}) \times (\text{height in inches})$$

So if you are five feet, six inches tall (66 inches) and weigh 140 pounds, your BMI = 140 pounds × 703 / (66 inches) × (66 inches) = 22.6.

A BMI of 22.6 falls within the normal range, which is from 18.5 to 24.9. In fact, if you weight anything between 111 and 150 pounds you will be within your normal weight. A BMI above 30 indicates obesity.

If you don't feel like doing the math, you can check a BMI table.

The Gerontology Research Center of the National Institute on Aging suggests that as we grow older a certain amount of weight gain is normal. It says that men and women who are just slightly overweight based on the standard height and weight charts have lower mortality rates than those who are precisely on target. So their system also includes the factor of age and often gives a slightly higher desirable weight than the standard BMI. By their formula the same woman at age fifty would have a desirable weight somewhere between 136 and 154 pounds.

If, in fact, you are overweight, you probably already know it and feel guilty about it; a National Institutes of Health study on obesity suggests that of all its effects, none is more adverse than the psychological suffering it entails. The most intuitively obvious test is a quick look in your full-length mirror or, even more revealing, in the three-way mirror in your local department store—the one you stand in front of when you try on a bathing suit. If you look fat and flabby to yourself (unless you are anorectic and would look fat to yourself no matter how thin you were), you are probably overweight.

TABLE 7. Body Mass Index

Body Weight (pounds)

BMI Height (inches)	NORMAL						OVERWEIGHT					OBESE										EXTREME OBESITY														
	19	20	21	22	23	24	25	26	27	28	29	30	31	32	33	34	35	36	37	38	39	40	41	42	43	44	45	46	47	48	49	50	51	52	53	54
58	91	96	100	105	110	115	119	124	129	134	138	143	148	153	158	162	167	172	177	181	186	191	196	201	205	210	215	220	224	229	234	239	244	248	253	258
59	94	99	104	109	114	119	124	128	133	138	143	148	153	158	163	168	173	178	183	188	193	198	203	208	212	217	222	227	232	237	242	247	252	257	262	267
60	97	102	107	112	118	123	128	133	138	143	148	153	158	163	168	174	179	184	189	194	199	204	209	215	220	225	230	235	240	245	250	255	261	266	271	276
61	100	106	111	116	122	127	132	137	143	148	153	158	164	169	174	180	185	190	195	201	206	211	217	222	227	232	238	243	248	254	259	264	269	275	280	285
62	104	109	115	120	126	131	136	142	147	153	158	164	169	175	180	186	191	196	202	207	213	218	224	229	235	240	246	251	256	262	267	273	278	284	289	295
63	107	113	118	124	130	135	141	146	152	158	163	169	175	180	186	191	197	203	208	214	220	225	231	237	242	248	254	259	265	270	278	282	287	293	299	304
64	110	116	122	128	134	140	145	151	157	163	169	174	180	186	192	197	204	209	215	221	227	232	238	244	250	256	262	267	273	279	285	291	296	302	308	314
65	114	120	126	132	138	144	150	156	162	168	174	180	186	192	198	204	210	216	222	228	234	240	246	252	258	264	270	276	282	288	294	300	306	312	318	324
66	118	124	130	136	142	148	155	161	167	173	179	186	192	198	204	210	216	223	229	235	241	247	253	260	266	272	278	284	291	297	303	309	315	322	328	334
67	121	127	134	140	146	153	159	166	172	178	185	191	198	204	211	217	223	230	236	242	249	255	261	268	274	280	287	293	299	306	312	319	325	331	338	344
68	125	131	138	144	151	158	164	171	177	184	190	197	203	210	216	223	230	236	243	249	256	262	269	276	282	289	295	302	308	315	322	328	335	341	348	354
69	128	135	142	149	155	162	169	176	182	189	196	203	209	216	223	230	236	243	250	257	263	270	277	284	291	297	304	311	318	324	331	338	345	351	358	365
70	132	139	146	153	160	167	174	181	188	195	202	209	216	222	229	236	243	250	257	264	271	278	285	292	299	306	313	320	327	334	341	348	355	362	369	376
71	136	143	150	157	165	172	179	186	193	200	208	215	222	229	236	243	250	257	265	272	279	286	293	301	308	315	322	329	338	343	351	358	365	372	379	386
72	140	147	154	162	169	177	184	191	199	206	213	221	228	235	242	250	258	265	272	279	287	294	302	309	316	324	331	338	346	353	361	368	375	383	390	397
73	144	151	159	166	174	182	189	197	204	212	219	227	235	242	250	257	265	272	280	288	295	302	310	318	325	333	340	348	355	363	371	378	386	393	401	408
74	148	155	163	171	179	186	194	202	210	218	225	233	241	249	256	264	272	280	287	295	303	311	319	326	334	342	350	358	365	373	381	389	396	404	412	420
75	152	160	168	176	184	192	200	208	216	224	232	240	248	256	264	272	279	287	295	303	311	319	327	335	343	351	359	367	375	383	391	399	407	415	423	431
76	156	164	172	180	189	197	205	213	221	230	238	246	254	263	271	279	287	295	304	312	320	328	336	344	353	361	369	377	385	394	402	410	418	426	435	443

Source: Adapted from Clinical Guidelines on the Identification, Evaluation, and Treatment of Overweight and Obesity in Adults: The Evidence Report.

A second test you can perform is the pinch test. Extend one arm and pinch the flesh on its underside halfway between your shoulder and your elbow. If you pinch more than an inch of fat, then you should think seriously about weight reduction.

▶ *Which is more important, the total amount of fat on your body or its distribution?*

Scientists have suggested that fat distribution as well as its total amount affects the risk of disease, particularly coronary artery disease.

Researchers have described two general silhouettes in overweight people: the pear and the apple. Pear-shaped people carry their extra weight low, around the hips, buttocks, and thighs; apple-shaped people carry their weight around their waists. Typically, overweight premenopausal women are pear shaped, while overweight men (the sagging belly syndrome) and postmenopausal women (the potbelly syndrome) are apple shaped.

How do you know whether you are an apple or a pear? Measure your waist at the navel. Then measure your hips at their fullest point. If you divide your waist measurement by your hip measurement and the result is less than 1.0, you're a pear. If it is greater than 1.0, you're an apple. For women, if your waist-to-hip ratio is greater than 0.8, you are at increased risk of heart disease.

Having a large waist, not even counting its relationship to your hips, can put you at risk for metabolic syndrome, also called Syndrome X, a collection of health factors that increase the likelihood that you will get heart disease or diabetes, or have a stroke. More than one in five Americans has metabolic syndrome, which increases with age, affecting more than 40 percent of people in their sixties and seventies.

You have metabolic syndrome if you have more than three of the following:

- A waistline of forty inches or more for men and thirty-five inches or more for women
- A blood pressure of 130/85 or higher
- A triglyceride level above 150 mg/dl
- A fasting blood glucose (sugar) level greater than 100 mg/dl
- A high density lipoprotein level (HDL) less than 40 mg/dl (men) or under 50 mg/dl (women).

Researchers don't know the exact cause of metabolic syndrome, but it seems to be caused by a combination of your genetic makeup and your lifestyle choices—the types of food you eat and your level of physical activity. If you have metabolic syndrome, your body experiences a series of biochemical changes that are ultimately destructive. If you find that you do have this problem, work with your internist to get out of the category; diet and exercise alone may succeed for you.

▶ What is the best way to lose weight?

Although genetic inheritance has a great deal to do with body shape and you can do nothing to change the tendency to heavy thighs that you inherited from Great-Aunt Tilly, with effort you can maintain something close to your ideal body weight.

There are two basic ways to lose weight, and to succeed you have to do both: follow a moderate diet with not too many calories, and increase the amount you exercise. Although it may be possible to lose weight by doing one without the other, it certainly is difficult. Restricting calories without exercise usually results in frustration and failure, because the body in its wisdom turns down its metabolic regulator when it senses lowered caloric intake, trying to save you from what it interprets as incipient starvation. If you exist on, let's say, a thousand calories a day for a week or so, your body begins to believe that a thousand calories is all it's ever going to get, so it readjusts its metabolic set point to maintain itself on a thousand calories.

Nor does exercise alone seem to do the trick. It is generally believed that just as the body shuts down its metabolic regulator if it becomes accustomed to a low caloric intake, the body will boost its metabolic thermostat if it gets accustomed to a high-energy output, for example needing to supply extra calories for regular exercise. However, there are some data to the contrary. In a study published in the *International Journal of Sports Medicine* in 1989, researchers followed a group of male and female novices who were training for their first marathon. The athletes trained for a period of eighty weeks, with no control over diet. During the training regime, the men lost weight and fat, but the women, alas, did not. A study in 1992 reported in the *Journal of Applied Physiology* showed similar results among female runners whose weight was tracked for a year. In a study from 1984 in the *Journal of Obesity and Weight Regulation,* both men and women were monitored in a continuous exercise program for twenty weeks, again with no control over diet. The men showed significant decreases in body weight and percentage of fat mass, but the women experienced no change. Apparently exercise alone may result in decreased body weight for men, but not for women.

So the only answer has to be the two-pronged attack, controlling caloric intake while increasing exercise. More exercise helps counter the diet doldrums and, we hope, resets the metabolic regulator, helping you to burn more calories for the same amount of physical activity.

You should aim for only a pound or two of loss per week. After all, your objective is a new set of habits that will keep you where you want to be for the rest of your life. If you are losing weight, even though you are doing it slowly and steadily, you will eventually reach your goal and maintain it if you continue your improved habits.

HEALTHY DIET

Just as the notion of ideal body weight has been revised, so has the notion of what we should eat. Most women now approaching menopause were born in the 1950s, when a healthy diet consisted of a lot of meat and potatoes, plenty of milk, cheese, and dairy products, as well as fruit and vegetables. Protein was "in." Starches, as complex carbohydrates were called, were "out" because they were thought to be fattening. Potatoes and pasta were definitely regarded with suspicion. There were seven basic food groups and you were told to eat a certain number of servings of each one.

Then, in 1992, the Department of Agriculture came out with new guidelines based on a food pyramid. Basically, the guidelines said that fat was bad and carbohydrates were good. People were encouraged to eat six to eleven servings of complex carbohydrates (bread, cereal, rice, pasta, and so on), less fat, and less protein than formerly. Potatoes and pasta had moved from bad to good; dietary fat had acquired a sinister reputation as a leading cause of heart disease. Research in the past decade has shown that the 1992 USDA food pyramid was seriously flawed.

We now know that that all fats are not bad for you, and most are not as bad as previously thought, especially if consumed in moderation. By contrast, complex carbohydrates are not as good for you as we used to think. The general feeling nowadays is that your diet should emphasize weight control, first of all through exercising daily and keeping your calorie intake down. The bulk of your diet should consist of healthy fats (liquid vegetable oils including olive, soy, corn, canola, sunflower, and peanut) and healthy carbohydrates (from whole grain foods, including whole wheat bread and brown rice). You should include moderate amounts of healthy protein (from nuts, legumes, fish, poultry, and eggs), perhaps one or two servings daily. And you cannot eat too many servings of fruits and vegetables (potatoes count as starch rather than vegetables). If you get your fats and carbohydrates from healthy sources, you probably don't have to worry about the exact percentages of each in your diet.

Minimize your intake of red meat, butter, potatoes, and sugar; stay away from refined grains (white bread, white rice, and white pasta), and avoid altogether foods that have trans fat—the kind produced by partially hydrogenating liquid vegetable oil—to solidify it. Trans fat is used in many margarines, commercial baked goods, and fried foods. These fats are especially bad for you because they raise your LDL (bad cholesterol) and triglycerides while reducing HDL (good cholesterol).

▶ *What is an appropriate caloric intake for a fifty-year-old woman?*

Unfortunately, our caloric needs decline by about 100 calories per day for each ten years of age over twenty-five. So if the average woman at age twenty-five needs about 2,000 calories to maintain her body weight and keep up her energy, she needs only 1,800 calories for the same activities at age forty-five. When she is in her midfifties, she needs only about 1,700 calories daily, unless she increases her exercise level.

If you are trying to lose weight, remember that you are working toward slow loss, maybe one or two pounds weekly, which is brought about by a change in your eating habits.

▶ *How much calcium should I be getting?*

Although the subject of calcium metabolism is complex and the evidence is somewhat ambiguous, it seems that estrogen makes it easier for the body to absorb calcium from the diet. Therefore the current recommendation is 1,000 mg daily for premenopausal women and for postmenopausal women who are taking estrogen, and 1,500 mg for postmenopausal women who are not taking estrogen.

▶ *How can I work 1,500 mg of calcium into my diet?*

Dairy foods are the main sources of calcium, but many other foods are rich in this mineral. Certain green and leafy vegetables, such as broccoli, collard greens, and kale (which may not be a part of your regular diet), are good sources of calcium. Canned fish, such as sardines and salmon (which are canned with the bones), is another source. Any vegetable with high oxalic acid is less desirable as a source of calcium, because the oxalic acid interferes with calcium absorption; among these are spinach, beet greens, rhubarb, parsley, and chard. In case you had hoped to get your calcium from chocolate, you should know that it, too, is high in oxalic acid. If you don't like milk or dairy products, remember that some orange juice now comes with added calcium.

To ensure effective calcium absorption, you must get adequate vitamin D. Good dietary sources include fortified milk, "oily" fish such as sardines and salmon, and cod liver oil, once the bane of millions of American children (a single teaspoon of it contains as much vitamin D as a quart of fortified milk). Another source is sunlight, whose ultraviolet radiation converts a complex fatty component of skin into vitamin D, hence the name sunshine vitamin.

You can see from the accompanying table that you have to be very conscientious if you are to get adequate calcium from your diet: two cups of milk, a cup of yogurt, and a cup of fortified orange juice will give you a baseline 1,320 mg of calcium.

▶ What about calcium supplements?

Since the average calcium intake in the United States is something like 400 to 500 mg daily, only about a third of what a postmenopausal woman needs if she is not taking estrogen, many women who do not like milk and other dairy products find it difficult to get adequate calcium in their diet.

Fortunately, calcium supplements are available. A single chewable tablet of calcium carbonate or calcium citrate will supply an additional 200 to 300 mg of calcium beyond what you have in your diet. Some physicians recommend extra-strength Tums, the over-the-counter antacid used by many people to counteract heartburn and indigestion. Since

TABLE 8. Foods High in Calcium

FOOD	QUANTITY	CALCIUM (MG)
Milk, 1% fat	1 cup	350
Yogurt	1 cup	300
Cottage cheese, low fat	1 cup	120
Collard greens, cooked	1 cup	360
Broccoli, cooked	1 stalk	160
Kale, cooked	1 cup	200
Sardines, canned	8 medium	350
Salmon, canned with bones	3 ounces	170
Tofu (soybean curd)	4 ounces	150
Orange juice, natural	1 cup	30
Orange juice, calcium fortified	1 cup	320

your body best absorbs calcium in an acidic environment, you should take Tums after meals, when your stomach is producing copious amounts of acid to digest your food. Instead of an after-dinner mint patty, try an after-dinner Tums tablet. A single "Tums 500" tablet contains 500 mg of calcium, so if you have one after each meal, you will get the 1,500 mg of calcium required by postmenopausal women not taking estrogen.

Viactiv is a new chewable supplement, slightly sweetened like a caramel. Viactiv comes in several flavors, including mocha and chocolate. Each piece contains 500 mg of calcium and 100 units of vitamin D. Many women find these "chews" the most palatable form of calcium supplementation.

▶ Why is cholesterol important?

Cholesterol is a fatty substance manufactured by the body. It is present in foods such as red meat and high-fat dairy products and has been linked to coronary artery disease.

Cholesterol in itself is not harmful. It is used by the body to make certain hormones; it helps in digestion; and it is an important building block of bodily tissues. In the wrong amounts or in the wrong places, however, cholesterol is dangerous. Coronary heart disease, also called coronary artery disease, happens when cholesterol is deposited inside the walls of the arteries that bring the heart its blood supply. These deposits contribute to buildup of fatty blockage called plaque. Deposits of plaque inside the blood vessels are known as arteriosclerosis, or atherosclerosis, or hardening of the arteries.

Until menopause, women are protected by estrogen and do not have to worry as much about cholesterol and the diseases that result from cholesterol deposits. But postmenopausal women, especially those not taking estrogen, should be aware of the importance of controlling blood cholesterol levels.

In recent years, as research has provided new data, beliefs about cholesterol have changed. Fifteen years ago it was considered all right to have a serum cholesterol of 240 (that is, 240 milligrams of cholesterol per deciliter of blood); ten years ago, 220 mg/dl was acceptable; in recent years, however, physicians and researchers have started looking at a cholesterol level of 200 mg/dl or lower as the desired goal.

▶ What are good and bad cholesterol?

It is not merely your total serum cholesterol, the amount of cholesterol in your blood, that counts. Because cholesterol is a fatty substance, it does not mix easily with blood, and in order to be moved around the body via the bloodstream, cholesterol gets packaged into molecules called lipoproteins. Researchers have identified a number of types of lipoproteins, of which two have received a lot of attention, LDL (low-density lipoprotein, bad cholesterol) and HDL (high-density lipoprotein, good cholesterol).

Bad cholesterol is bad because it seems to play an important role in depositing cholesterol on the inside of the artery walls. Good cholesterol is good because it seems to help clean out the cholesterol deposits that have already begun to line the artery walls.

Therefore it is the relative quantities of HDL and LDL that are important to the health of your arteries and your heart. These days an LDL level of up to 130 mg/dl is considered fine, 130 to 160 mg/dl is in a gray zone, and anything over 160 mg/dl is anxiety provoking. So if your total cholesterol is 220 but your HDL is 100, then you are in good shape because your LDL is very low.

People who are at high risk for heart disease—people with diabetes, metabolic syndrome, or those who have had previous heart attacks—should keep their LDL under 100. For many, the only way to do this is with medication, particularly statin drugs.

To complicate this subject still further, levels of HDL and LDL must be taken as relative quantities. It is their ratio that is important. Suppose your HDL is 100 and your LDL is 160, which puts your total cholesterol at something larger than 260 and your LDL at the outer edge of the gray zone. But compare that risk to the risk of someone whose total cholesterol is 190 mg/dl but with an HDL of 20 and an LDL of 170. These people are few and far between, but they are at significant risk for cholesterol problems.

▶ What can you do if your cholesterol levels are high?

Suppose you go to a fair or some public place where cholesterol levels are checked as a public service, and you find that your total serum cholesterol is high. If it is over 300, you should talk soon to your doctor—probably to your internist, since most gynecologists in the country don't feel comfortable prescribing drugs to lower blood cholesterol. Various medicines on the market will lower blood cholesterol levels, but all have side effects and all have some toxicity. If your cholesterol is borderline, the two most important things you can do are start exercising and adjust your diet.

▶ How effective is diet in reducing cholesterol?

Fortunately, you can have a significant impact on your cholesterol levels by controlling your diet. If you are overweight, the main factor seems to be not what you eat but the weight loss that follows a well-designed, controlled diet. The body is able to manufacture cholesterol even though there is no cholesterol at all in your diet. If you live on a diet of all lettuce (which of course you should not) and have an intake of zero cholesterol, your body will still manufacture it for you.

Nevertheless, a diet low in total fat, saturated fat, and cholesterol kills two birds with one stone: it contributes to weight loss (if you need it) and it restricts intake of highly saturated fats, which worsen your blood lipid profile (that is, they increase the relative amounts of bad cholesterol).

Saturated fats, the kind that are solid at room temperature, come chiefly from animal sources. They include the fat in milk, cheese, meat, butter, and lard, as well as a few vegetable products, notably cocoa butter and coconut oil. Researchers now believe that saturated fat in your diet is worse for your blood lipid levels than dietary cholesterol. That is why foods such as shrimp (fairly high in cholesterol but lower in saturated fat) have less fearsome reputations than they formerly did.

A sensible low-cholesterol, low-fat diet includes less than 30 percent of total calories from fat and less than 10 percent from saturated fat, which is the kind found in animal products (meat, poultry, fish) and a few vegetable oils (notably palm oil and coconut oil). Adopting this kind of diet will, on the average, reduce total cholesterol 5 to 10 percent.

One important feature of this kind of dietary restriction is that it reduces total calories. Proteins and carbohydrates have 4 calories per gram, whereas fats have 9 calories per gram, more than twice as much. By concentrating on carbohydrates—for example, fruits, vegetables, and grains—you can eat more food while ingesting fewer calories.

▶ Can you control cholesterol by exercising?

The second important factor both in cholesterol control and in weight reduction is exercise. An appropriate aerobic exercise regimen can increase your HDL as much as 20 percent. If a woman comes into the office with a cholesterol level of 260, I don't automatically ship her off to her internist for cholesterol-lowering drugs. Particularly if she is overweight, I try to get her on a suitable diet. I strongly encourage her to get involved in an exercise program. If she chooses to try hormone therapy, she may notice that her HDL rises as much as 20 percent.

EXERCISE AS A LIFESTYLE CHOICE

The benefits of physical activity are many and well known both to those who exercise and to those who do not. Exercise improves muscle strength, muscle tone, and flexibility. It promotes a sense of well-being and enhances self-esteem. Weight-bearing exercise helps develop and preserve bone. Aerobic exercise helps stave off cardiovascular disease.

If you are trying to lose weight, exercise depresses appetite, which makes it easier to keep your caloric intake low. Exercise together with calorie restriction encourages the loss of fat rather than muscle, so that you look trimmer, fitter, and healthier as you slim down. Exercise boosts metabolism, enabling you to burn calories faster.

So why don't people exercise? Most women say that the problem is time, but you can make time to exercise if you really are determined.

Basically there are three kinds of exercise, which are important all through life and especially as we get older. The first is aerobic exercise, in which the muscles burn oxygen as fuel. Aerobic exercise, which includes fast walking, jogging, running, aerobic dance, and other forms of rhythmic exertion over fairly long periods of time, is important to cardiovascular health and weight control.

The second type, anaerobic or isometric exercise, involves using particular muscle groups in strenuous bursts for fairly short periods of time. As we age, our muscle mass turns to fat and we get weaker. Very elderly people, both men and women, often have difficulty getting up from chairs or lifting bags of groceries. Anaerobic exercise will help maintain muscular strength so that these activities become easier. Calisthenics, tai chi chuan, yoga, weight lifting, and working out on Nautilus machines are examples of this kind of exercise. The benefits of anaerobic exercise include strength, muscle tone, and stamina. If you play golf or tennis, or if you heft grandchildren, improved muscle strength will transfer to these activities. Like aerobic exercise, strength training boosts your metabolic rate, which helps you lose weight, since a trained, muscular body uses more calories than a flabby one, even when sitting still. Furthermore, muscle takes up less space than fat, pound for pound, so if you are more muscular, you will be trimmer.

The third type is exercise for flexibility, which as the years go by becomes increasingly critical to maintaining balance and agility. Muscle stretching before aerobic or anaerobic exercise is important in preventing injury; yoga and Pilates, both of which have a mind-body component, also include stretching.

Although the ideal exercise program includes all three types, for women in the menopausal age bracket, two points are crucial: getting enough exercise to maintain ideal body weight and keep up cardiovascular fitness, and doing the kind of exercise that promotes healthy bone. One commonly used guideline for cardiovascular fitness suggests raising your heart rate into a target zone, which is somewhere between 60 and 75 percent of its maximum, and keeping it there for thirty minutes at least three times a week. To dis-

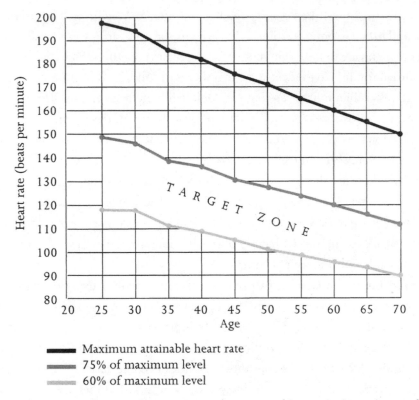

FIGURE 26. Target zone diagram. One way to get adequate aerobic exercise is to raise your heart rate into your target zone and keep it there for thirty minutes at least three times weekly.

cover your target zone, subtract your age from 220, then take 60 and 75 percent of that number.

With exercise, more is better, but less is far better than none at all. Even walking one or two hours a week will help your fitness, but the more briskly you exercise and the longer you keep at it, the more benefit you will receive. The American Heart Association suggests that you expend at least 2,000 calories weekly in exercise.

The American College of Sports Medicine offers exercise guidelines, which suggest that you alternate aerobic and anaerobic types of exercise, doing strength training (anaerobic exercise) for two or three thirty-minute sessions each week, and on alternate days doing aerobic exercise such as walking, jogging, aerobic dancing, or swimming.

HARD-TO-BREAK HABITS

One of the hard lessons in life is that to form a good habit, you seem to have to indulge in hundreds and hundreds of correct repetitions. But do something that is bad for you once or twice, and it seems instantly to become a habit of ferocious tenacity.

Smoking

In terms of aging, smoking is a hugely negative factor. It increases the risk of osteoporosis; it increases the risk of cardiovascular disease by causing injury to blood-vessel walls and apparently also by lowering your good cholesterol; it increases the risk of lung cancer and other pulmonary diseases. And, of course, it contributes to early menopause. In short, smoking is bad for everyone and especially poisonous to a menopausal woman.

Do not despair if you are a smoker; there is evidence that if you stop smoking you will regain the advantage that you have lost—almost immediately in terms of your heart, and somewhat more gradually in terms of your lungs.

Alcohol and Middle Age

A second major risk for women is alcohol. Unfortunately, many middle-aged women turn to drinking, possibly because of the stresses associated with this time of life. Women are at double risk, first because pound for pound of body weight they metabolize alcohol less well than men. Blood alcohol concentration after a given number of drinks is related to the body's ratio of muscle to fat; since men in general are leaner, they have relatively more water into which the alcohol can be distributed. Second, both men and women tolerate alcohol less well as they age than they did as younger people.

Although alleviating stress with prescription medications has a poor reputation, alcohol is much worse for you. Nutritionally, alcohol is worthless; it is full of those fabled "empty calories" that don't bring the benefits of nutrients along with them. When people drink, they feel full and so they don't eat properly; they have ingested plenty of calories but they have not taken in any vitamins, minerals, or protein.

In addition, alcohol puts you at increased risk for all kinds of diseases. It destroys the liver, so that people who are alcoholic have several kinds of liver disease, beginning with fatty liver and continuing on to cirrhosis and carcinoma of the liver.

Heavy alcohol consumption boosts your risk for osteoporosis. Whether this additional risk is nutritional because alcoholic women don't eat properly or attributable to

TABLE 9. Time Needed to Burn Calories from Various Foods

				TYPE OF ACTIVITY (CALORIES BURNED)[a]				
FOOD	CALORIES	SLEEPING (60/HR)	SEDENTARY (80/HR)	LIGHT (110/HR)	MODERATE (170/HR)	VIGOROUS (250/HR)	STRENUOUS (350+/HR)
2 8-inch celery stalks	15	15 min	11 min	8 min	5 min	4 min	3 min
2 medium graham crackers	55	55 min	41 min	30 min	19 min	13 min	9 min
2 tbsp fruit-nut snack	70	1 hr 10 min	53 min	38 min	25 min	17 min	12 min
2 tbsp peanuts	105	1 hr 45 min	1 hr 19 min	57 min	37 min	25 min	18 min
1 cup plain low-fat yogurt	145	2 hr 25 min	1 hr 49 min	1 hr 19 min	51 min	35 min	25 min
1 cup split-pea soup	195	3 hr 15 min	2 hr 26 min	1 hr 46 min	1 hr 8 min	47 min	33 min

Food	Calories						
1 cup fruit-flavored yogurt	225	3 hr 45 min	2 hr 49 min	2 hr 3 min	1 hr 19 min	54 min	39 min
1/3 cup granola with coconut	280	4 hr 40 min	3 hr 30 min	2 hr 33 min	1 hr 39 min	1 hr 7 min	48 min
3-oz hamburger on bun	365	6 hr 5 min	4 hr 34 min	3 hr 19 min	2 hr 9 min	1 hr 28 min	1 hr 3 min
12-oz chocolate milkshake	430	7 hr 10 min	5 hr 23 min	3 hr 55 min	2 hr 32 min	1 hr 43 min	1 hr 13 min

a. All figures are approximate, as energy expenditure varies from individual to individual. The data are calculated on rates for a 123-lb woman; larger, more muscular women will burn calories faster.
Sedentary activity: reading, watching TV, other activities while seated.
Light activity: dusting, ironing, shopping, walking slowly (2½–3 mph).
Moderate activity: housework, walking more rapidly (3½–4 mph).
Vigorous activity: gardening, scrubbing floors, golf.
Strenuous activity: bicycling, running, swimming, chopping wood.
Source: Based on data from USDA Home and Garden Bulletin No. 228, *Food,* pp. 14–15.

some other factor, alcoholic women develop osteoporosis at a faster rate than nonalcoholics.

Some studies in recent years have suggested that very moderate drinking, which for women can be defined as one drink a day, may decrease risk for cardiovascular disease, although the reason is unclear. This research, which has focused only on cardiovascular risk and examined the risks of French wine drinkers and American liquor drinkers, remains controversial. Furthermore, nothing in the scientific literature says that if one or two drinks a day can help you, then three or four can help you more. For many people, particularly those who come from alcoholic backgrounds, drinking one or two often leads to drinking three or four or more. Studies have also suggested that alcohol increases the risk of breast cancer, but this possibility remains ambiguous.

With alcohol, with diet, for that matter with any aspect of your life that you would like to alter, change is certainly possible though usually difficult; replacing destructive habits with healthful ones takes time, discipline, and patience—but it can be done.

THE CHALLENGES AND THE SATISFACTIONS

Biologically, menopause does mark an ending: it signals the close of your reproductive years. Yet it can also be seen as a beginning, a gateway to the second half of your life. Like many women, you may find yourself happier and more content in these middle years than you were as a young woman in your twenties and thirties.

Chances are that you entered adulthood buoyed with energy and youthful optimism. But, lacking in experience, you were probably dependent on parents and mentors, unsure of who you were, of what you wanted to do, of where you belonged in the world around you. By the time you reach the years surrounding menopause, you are a more experienced woman, independent, fortified with knowledge and possibly even wisdom, capable of making the decisions and choices that will shape your future. If you have been a wife and mother, these relationships and the adjustments they require surely have taught you skills of coping and flexibility and have equipped you to distinguish the essential from the peripheral. If you have never married or if you have divorced, you have learned to respect and live by your own values. If you have followed a career, you know how to juggle the demands of other people with your own needs and how to channel your energy where it is most required; you undoubtedly have picked up abilities that serve you beyond the boundaries of your job. Often patients in the menopausal years tell me that while they need reading glasses to check the small print, the big issues in their lives are clear. In their forties and fifties they feel liberated from biological constraints and social expectations. They see this period as a time when they can shape their lives as they want, developing talents and capabilities that were pushed aside earlier in the interest of family or other responsibilities. Other women say that the strands of knowledge they have acquired over the years are suddenly coming together to form a pattern, or that relationships they have cultivated are bearing totally unexpected fruits. No one denies the difficulties of midlife, but for many women the rewards of this stage are extraordinary.

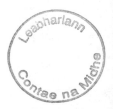

▶ GLOSSARY

ablation (endometrial) Destruction of the lining of the uterus, by different techniques.

acute Sudden, current, not longstanding.

adenomatous hyperplasia Excessive growth of the lining of the uterus; potential precursor to cancer of the endometrium.

adenomyosis A condition in which the glands that line the uterus penetrate its internal muscle walls. Sometimes called internal endometriosis. Often associated with painful and heavy periods.

adhesion Scar tissue that "sticks" one structure or organ to another to which it should not be attached.

agonist A chemical that acts in similar fashion to another chemical.

Alzheimer's disease A kind of dementia, in which destruction of brain cells leads to severe loss of memory and of the ability to think or reason. Alzheimer's is associated with two abnormal brain structures: amyloid plaques (clumps of proteins that accumulate outside brain cells) and neurofibrillary tangles (altered proteins inside brain cells).

amphetamines A class of drugs that make people "speed"; often called uppers. Have been used as diet pills; can be addictive and, with overdose, fatal.

anabolic steroids Drugs of the cortisone family that "build up" tissue. Often used (illegally) by athletes to enhance their performance.

anemia Low red-blood-cell count. In women, can be caused by heavy periods.

angina Chest pain associated with lack of oxygen to the heart, usually caused by narrowed coronary arteries.

anovulatory Associated with lack of ripening and release of an egg from the ovary. Anovulatory menstrual periods are often irregular and heavy.

anterior Referring to the front or top of the body or an organ.

antifungal Referring to substances that act against yeast and other fungi; often used to fight yeast infections.

anti-inflammatory Referring to substances that act against inflammation. Frequently applied to drugs used to treat arthritis (for example, Motrin or Anaprox). Anti-inflammatories are sometimes used to combat menstrual cramps.

antioxidants Chemicals that "eat up" or antagonize free radicals, which are toxic products of cell metabolism. Believed to slow down aging and other toxic cell events.

arrhythmia Fluctuation of the regular, smooth heartbeat. May originate in the atria (upper chambers) or ventricles (lower chambers) of the heart.

ascites Fluid in the abdominal cavity. Often seen in people with liver failure or cancer.

atherosclerosis Thickening of the walls of arteries, primarily composed of fat.

atrophic Aged, inactive. Relative to tissue of the female genital tract, it means thinned out.

atypia Condition of having odd-looking cells; sometimes associated with inflammation, sometimes with precancerous changes.

basal metabolic rate Speed at which the body burns its food. People with a high basal metabolic rate tend to be thin.

basement membrane A thin layer that divides the superficial cells of an organ from its deeper cells, the "skin" of an organ.

benign Not malignant. A tumor that is benign does not metastasize (spread to distant organs), but grows only in place.

beta-blockers A family of drugs that blocks the activity of adrenaline. Used primarily to slow the heart rate and lower the blood pressure.

biopsy A sample; or (as a verb) to take a sample of tissue. Often used to determine whether a tissue is cancerous.

birth control pills Oral contraceptives, also called BCPs. Contain estrogen and progesterone that suppress the release of an egg by the ovary, thus preventing pregnancy.

blood lipids Fats in the bloodstream; usually refers to cholesterol and triglycerides.

board certified Most medical specialties require examinations called board exams that test specific bodies of knowledge. Those who pass are board certified or "boarded." Not every physician who hangs a shingle is board certified.

breakthrough bleeding Bleeding between periods. Usually associated with low-dose usage of birth control pills. Rarely harmful; often a nuisance.

CAD (coronary artery disease) Thickening of the walls of blood vessels to the heart, with obstruction to blood flow. Also known as atherosclerosis. Often leads to angina.

carcinoma in situ A very localized cancer that has not yet penetrated the basement membrane.

cardiac disease Heart problems. Usually either CAD or disease of the valves that control the blood in the chambers of the heart.

CBC Complete blood count, including white and red blood cells.

cerebral cortex The outer part of the brain. Thinking occurs here, as does the processing of complex neurological signals such as vision.

cervix The neck of or entrance to the uterus. Opens, in labor, to let the fetus out.

chronic Long-lasting, not sudden.

climacteric The time frame during which a woman passes from her reproductive to her postmenopausal years; marked by the gradual waning of reproductive function. A more inclusive term than either perimenopause or menopause.

clinical trials Experiments in which some people are given a drug and some people are given a placebo to check the effectiveness of a new medication.

clotting factors Proteins in the blood that bring about clotting.

collagen The substance, which acts like glue, that holds many cells together. Softer than bone, it supports the skin and other structures.

colonoscopy The examination of the entire bowel, using a flexible tube inserted into the rectum.

colposcope A giant microscope used to examine and magnify the cervix and vulva. Used to aid in the diagnosis of precancerous and cancerous conditions of the cervix, vagina, and vulva. Can also be used to examine the penis.

cone biopsy A surgical procedure in which a cone-shaped wedge of tissue is removed from the cervix. Used to diagnose and treat precancerous and cancerous conditions of the cervix.

contraindicated Term for something that is not a good idea, say a medication or treatment that is absolutely wrong for a certain condition and will make it get worse.

corpus luteum Literally, yellow body. The cyst that forms after an egg is released by the ovary. Secretes progesterone and readies the lining of the uterus to receive a fertilized egg.

cryosurgery Freezing. "Cryo" means cold. Usually used in gynecology to treat genital warts and precancerous conditions of the cervix or in endometrial ablation. Also known as cryotherapy.

CT scan Also called CAT scan (computerized axial tomography). An X-ray technique that focuses in at different levels of an organ or body cavity. Allows a three-dimensional visualization of the organ or cavity. Usually fairly expensive.

curettage Scraping. Usually applied to scraping the uterine cavity.

cystic teratoma Medical name for a dermoid cyst; a cyst arising from egg cells in the ovary. Can contain hair, teeth, and other formed body parts. Almost always benign.

cystitis Inflammation of the bladder. Usually causes frequency of and burning with urination.

cystocele Bulging of the bladder into the vagina.

cystoscope A narrow metal tube inserted into the bladder through the urethra to look inside the bladder.

cysts Fluid-filled growths anywhere in the body. Most often benign.

D&C Dilatation and curettage. Stretching of the cervix to permit scraping out the inside of the uterus.

dementia Brain dysfunction, resulting in changes in behavior, personality, and memory. Two important causes are Alzheimer's disease and vascular dementia, in which blood clots in the blood vessels in the brain cause the death of brain tissue.

dermoid cyst See cystic teratoma.

detrusor dyssynergia Irritable or unstable bladder. A condition in which a small amount of urine in the bladder makes the bladder irritable and stimulates the urge to urinate.

diuretic A medication that pushes the kidney to excrete water; increases urine output.

drug trials Comparable to clinical trials, in which patients are randomly given either a new drug or a placebo to assess the the drug's clinical effectiveness.

dysfunction Abnormal working, as of an organ.

dysmenorrhea Painful menstrual cramps.

dyspareunia Painful sexual intercourse.

dysplasia Abnormal cell growth. Not yet cancer, but different from the usual growth of cells.

electrolyte testing Usually refers to three elements present in the bloodstream: sodium (Na), potassium (K), and chlorine (Cl). In good health these elements are found at proper levels. Their presence at abnormal levels generally is an effect of medication or disease.

endogenously Internally; coming from the inside.

endometrial stripe Usually assessed by ultrasound, the thickness of the lining of the uterus.

endometriosis Condition in which endometrial-type tissue is found in locations outside the uterus: anywhere in the pelvis, possibly near the bladder or bowel or, rarely, as far away as in the lungs.

endometrium The lining of the uterus, composed of glandular tissue.

endorphins Chemicals released in the brain that look like opioids (morphine, for example). Give a sense of well-being and are commonly released with exercise.

epidemiological Usually referring to data collected from studies of large populations.

epidural Having to do with the space around the spinal cord. A technique of anesthesia, sometimes used in labor, introducing chemicals into that space.

ERT Also called ET. Estrogen replacement therapy (or estrogen therapy). Given to women in menopause to replace the estrogen they are no longer making. Also called HRT (hormone replacement therapy) when progesterone is also given.

estradiol A steroid hormone and the major estrogen (female hormone) made by women.

estrogen receptors Structures on the surface of tissues to which the hormone estrogen can attach.

euthyroid Pertaining to normal thyroid function and levels.

exogenously Coming from outside the body.

exuberant Very heavy in growth.

fallopian tubes Narrow tubular structures, attached to the uterus, in which fertilization occurs; conduits for eggs to go from the ovaries into the uterus.

false negative A lab test result that indicates there is no problem, when one actually exists.

false positive A lab test result that indicates some problem is present when it is not.

fascia Sturdy connective tissue that covers muscle.

fibroid Benign extra growth of the smooth muscle wall of the uterus.

fibroadenoma Usually refers to a solid but benign breast growth, often seen in women with fibrocystic breast changes.

fistula A hole, an opening between two structures that are not normally connected.

follicle The portion of the ovary that surrounds an egg and helps it mature.

follicular Referring to follicles; also to the first half of the menstrual cycle before the egg is released from the follicle.

formication A creeping sensation of the skin, as if it is crawling with ants; sometimes occurs in menopausal women.

free radicals Toxic chemicals produced during cell metabolism; thought to be associated with aging.

FSH Follicle-stimulating hormone. A peptide chemical made by the pituitary gland; stimulates egg development and estrogen production.

gammalinolenic acid An essential fatty acid.

GnRH Gonadotropin-releasing hormone. A chemical produced by the hypothalamus that makes the pituitary gland secrete FSH and LH.

GnRH agonists Chemicals that act like GnRH, but actually cause the pituitary to make less FSH and eventually decrease estrogen production.

gonad The ovary or testis.

gonadotropins Chemicals made by the pituitary gland that stimulate egg or sperm production by the ovary or testis.

granulosa cells Cells that surround the maturing egg in the ovarian follicles.

hematocrit The percentage of blood volume that is composed of red blood cells. In women a normal hematocrit is in the range 38–42.

hemoglobin A measure of the number of red blood cells in the bloodstream. Normal for women is in the range 12–14.

histones Chemicals found in the seminal fluid with sperm.

HIV Human immunodeficiency virus; causes AIDS (acquired immunodeficiency syndrome).

HMO Health maintenance organization.

hot flash (or flush) A sensation of warmth, commonly noted in the upper part of the body, usually associated with dilation of blood capillaries and the rushing of blood through them.

HPV Human papilloma virus; causes genital warts.

HRT Also called HT. Hormone replacement therapy; sometimes used synonymously with ERT (estrogen replacement therapy). Women who have not had a hysterectomy are almost always given HRT, both estrogen and progesterone, to protect them from endometrial hyperplasia.

hyperplasia Benign but excessive growth of tissue, which if left unchecked can occasionally turn malignant.

hypertension High blood pressure.

hyperthyroidism Overactivity of the thyroid gland.

hypotensive Having blood pressure lower than 90/60.

hypothalamus A portion of the brain that sits on top of the pituitary gland and governs much of the hormonal activity of the body.

hypothyroidism Condition marked by an underactive thyroid.

hysteroscope A narrow tube containing a light, which is passed through the cervix and used to look inside the uterus.

incompetent cervix A weakened neck of the uterus (cervix), which during pregnancy allows the cervix to dilate long before it is supposed to. Often associated with loss of pregnancy in the second trimester.

incontinence Involuntary loss of urine (or stool).

ischemic Referring to lack of oxygen. Ischemia (lack of oxygen to tissue) usually gives pain; for example, angina is ischemia of the heart muscles.

IV Intravenous. A small plastic tube inserted into a vein for administering fluids, medications, or anesthetics.

laparoscope A narrow metal tube, inserted into the abdominal cavity, that allows a look around the inside of the abdomen and pelvis. Can be used to operate without making a large incision.

laser A highly focused light that delivers so much energy that it can actually cut tissue.

LAVH Laparoscopically assisted vaginal hysterectomy.

LH Luteinizing hormone. Chemical produced by the pituitary gland that leads to egg maturation and release by the ovary.

lichen sclerosus et atrophicus (LS&A) An inflammation of the vulvar tissue; causes itching.

luteal Referring to the second half of the menstrual cycle, after ovulation has occurred.

malignant Cancerous. The character of tumors that can both grow locally and spread widely (metastasize).

marker Also called surrogate marker. An indirect indicator, something you can measure that tends to correlate with something you can't measure. Bone density, for example, is a marker for fracture risk.

mastitis Inflammation of the breast. Most often seen in women who are breast-feeding, but occasionally in others.

melatonin A hormone manufactured by the pineal gland in the brain. Only some of its functions are known. Levels tend to decrease with age in both men and women.

menarche The onset of menstrual periods at puberty.

menopause The cessation of menstrual periods.

menorrhagia Heavy loss of blood with periods.

metabolic Referring to the fueling of bodily functions.

metastasis The spreading of cancerous tissue.

micronizing process Breaking down a chemical into tiny pieces, usually to enhance absorption of drugs by the body.

MRI Magnetic resonance imaging. Similar to an X-ray study that allows a detailed look at an organ. Usually expensive.

multifocality The condition of existing in several places. Dysplasia or cancer can be multifocal.

myoma Fibroid.

myomectomy Surgical removal of a fibroid from the uterus.

myometrium The muscular wall of the uterus.

neoplasia Literally, new growth. Usually refers to a precancerous or cancerous condition.

neurotoxicity Harm associated with either pain or loss of function of nerve cells.

neurotransmitter A chemical messenger released by nerve cells in the brain or in the peripheral nerves, which communicates with other nerve cells or the cells that respond to them.

obesity Fatness; technically, body weight more than 20 percent above ideal.

omentum Fatty tissue surrounding the intestines.

oophorectomy Sometimes called ovariectomy; removal of the ovaries.

opiates Chemicals such as morphine or heroin, naturally or synthetically produced, that alter mood.

organic depression Sadness, negative outlook, or melancholy caused not by external events but by chemical imbalances in the brain.

osteoporosis Loss of bone or softening of bone, associated with increased risk of bone breakage; weakening of bone through loss of its hard inner structure.

ovaries The female sex organs where eggs are stored and matured until they are released; the primary source of estrogen in the body.

ovulation The ripening, maturation, and release of an egg by the ovary.

Pap smear Often used as a test for cervical cancer; involves scraping superficial cells of the cervix. Named for Dr. George Papanicolaou.

pathological Abnormal, associated with disease.

pathologist A physician who looks at tissue, either through a microscope or with the naked eye, to assess it for health or disease.

PCA Patient-controlled analgesia. A system, usually with a pump, whereby patients can regulate the frequency with which they receive painkillers.

pedicle The supporting tissue for an organ or, in surgery, the tissue from which a structure is released. (The stem of a mushroom could be considered its pedicle.)

perimenopausal Referring to the time "around the menopause." Describes the period when ovarian function and hormone production are declining but have not yet stopped.

perineum One's "bottom." The structure containing the outlets of the urethra, the vagina, and the rectum.

peritonitis Inflammation of the abdominal cavity; occurs with severe appendicitis or pelvic inflammatory disease.

pessary A device, usually made of rubber, placed in the vagina and used to support sagging structures (vagina, uterus, or bladder).

phlebitis Inflammation of the vein wall.

phytoestrogens Plant estrogens.

pineal gland A brain structure whose function is still not completely known. Secretes melatonin and is sensitive to changes in light and dark.

pituitary gland A part of the brain, right behind the bridge of the nose. Secretes hormones that regulate the activity of most of the glands in the body.

placebo A sugar pill. Often used in drug trials to see whether a patient is just thinking herself better or is actually receiving benefits from the specific drug being tested. (Obviously, the patient doesn't know whether she is getting the sugar pill or the real thing.)

placebo effect See above. In drug trials about 30 percent of those taking placebos feel that they are getting help from them.

PMS Premenstrual syndrome.

PMZ Postmenopausal zest. A feeling of liberation and renewed energy experienced by many menopausal women.

polyps Usually benign outgrowths of normal tissue, they stretch out on a stalk. Polyps in the lining of the uterus may be associated with bleeding.

posterior Underneath or behind; the back part of the vagina.

posterior repair The fixing of a rectocele.

potassium An element in the blood necessary for normal cell functioning. Levels may be depleted by diuretic use.

PPD Purified protein derivative. A skin test for tuberculosis.

primary care physician A doctor who takes basic, overall care of a patient, referring the patient to a specialist if necessary. Women's primary care physicians are usually family practitioners, internists, or gynecologists.

progesterone A steroid hormone made by the ovary in the second half of the menstrual cycle; stabilizes the lining of the uterus and prepares it for implantation of a fertilized egg.

progestin One of several synthetic forms of progesterone, made in the laboratory.

prolactin A hormone made by the pituitary gland, which stimulates secretion of breast milk. When elevated in nonpregnant women, may be associated with infertility.

prostaglandins A family of hormones, made by the uterus and many other bodily organs, that stimulate the activity of smooth muscle, including the uterine wall. In women their principal role is in labor; also produce menstrual cramps.

proteomics Also called proteinomics; the science of looking at protein patterns in the blood as a marker of a disease.

pruritus Itching.

psychotropic Having an effect on moods and feelings.

receptors Structures on the surface of cells that bind hormones circulating in the bloodstream.

rectocele A bulging of rectal tissue into the vagina.

reliability In lab tests, the capability to find (that is, not to miss) some disease or abnormality. See *specificity*.

serosa The tissue on the surface of an organ.

serotonin A chemical produced in the brain whose levels may influence moods.

sigmoidoscopy Examination of the lower bowel through a flexible tube inserted into the rectum.

specificity In lab tests, the capability to pick up only true abnormalities or diseases. See *reliability*.

spina bifida A congenital separation of the spinal cord, which can be associated with neurological dysfunction of the lower part of the body.

squamous Referring to superficial cells that line some part of the body. These cells tend to be flat and form the top layer of the skin, vagina, and cervix.

steroids A family of chemicals whose structure and formation come from cholesterol.

supracervical Above the cervix. Refers to a hysterectomy where the body of the uterus (fundus) is removed but the cervix is left in place.

surgicenter An outpatient surgical facility.

systemic Throughout the body.

TAH and BSO Total abdominal hysterectomy and bilateral salpingo-oophorectomy.

testosterone The "male" steroid hormone. Also made by women, but in much smaller amounts than by men.

thrombosis The presence of a clot in a blood vessel.

thyrotoxicosis A very high level of circulating thyroid hormone.

topical Applied to the surface of the body, as opposed to being taken systemically.

transdermal Through the skin. Medications may be absorbed transdermally.

transvaginal Through the vagina. Ultrasound testing may be done with transvaginal probes; cysts may be drained transvaginally.

tricyclics A family of antidepressant drugs that raise neurotransmitter levels in the central nervous system.

ultrasound A diagnostic tool that uses sound waves, not X-rays, to examine the inside of the body. Often used to determine if a mass is solid or fluid filled (cystic). Ultrasound procedures are basically risk free, as they do not involve exposure to radiation.

ureters The tubes that connect kidneys to bladder.

uterine prolapse A condition in which the uterus slips downward into the vagina or, in severe conditions, actually protrudes outside the body.

urethra The opening of the bladder to the outside of the body.

vaginal atrophy The drying and thinning of the vaginal walls because of loss of estrogen.

vaginitis Inflammation of the vagina.

vasodilation An opening up or expanding of the blood vessels. Caused by certain drugs, and also associated with the mechanism of the hot flash.

vestibular vulvitis A painful but benign condition of the outlet of the vagina; associated with nonyeast and nonbacterial inflammation.

vitamin B6 Pyridoxine, a chemical essential for cell metabolism. Has a number of therapeutic uses including diuretic action, decreasing breast discomfort, and treating the nausea of pregnancy and PMS.

vulva The tissue surrounding the opening of the vagina.

vulvitis Inflammation of the vulva.

well differentiated Used to describe a cancer in which the cells look very much like the original tissue. Usually associated with a better outlook than cancers that are poorly differentiated, that is, do not resemble the normal tissue.

▶ RESOURCES

THE INTERNET

The rise of the Internet has altered the way people search for information about health, and although it allows easy access, it also allows widespread dissemination of false or misleading information. The Cancer Information Service of the National Cancer Institute suggests that you consider several key points as you evaluate medical advice or news on the Web.

- The Web site should make it easy for you to learn who is responsible for the site and its information.
- If the organization in charge of the site did not write the material, its source should be identified.
- The site should give information about the medical credentials of the people who prepared or reviewed the material on the site.

• Any Web site that asks for personal information should explain clearly what the site will or will not do with that information.

GENERAL MEDICAL INFORMATION

American College of Obstetricians and Gynecologists
409 12th St., SW
PO Box 96920
Washington, DC 20090-6920
www.acog.org
Professional organization for physicians in these specialties. The Web site has links to scientific articles and press releases on medical issues pertaining to women and a geographical list of obstetricians and gynecologists who belong to the society.

Healthfinder
www.healthfinder.gov
Developed by the U.S. Department of Health and Human Services and other federal agencies, this site is an important resource for finding government and nonprofit health and human services information on the Internet; there are links to Web sites from more than 1,700 health-related organizations.

The National Women's Health Information Center (NWHIC)
www.4women.gov
Maintained by the Office on Women's Health (U.S. Department of Health and Human Services), this site offers information on topics of special interest to women, from menopause and hormone therapy to body image, heart disease, and violence against women. It serves as a gateway to the government's resources for women and has links to organizations outside the government. The NWHIC site includes "What about men's health," to help women learn about health issues that affect the men in their lives.

MedlinePlus
www.medlineplus.gov
This site, a service of the U.S. National Library of Medicine (part of the National Institutes of Health), offers discussions of some 600 health and wellness topics, health news, dictionaries of medical terms, information on prescription and over-the-counter med-

ications, an illustrated medical encyclopedia, and links to other resources, both inside and outside the government.

NOAH (New York Online Access to Health)

www.noah-health.org

This site is a collaboration among New York City organizations that have banded together to create a Web site with reliable health information. Among the organizations are the City University of New York, New York Academy of Medicine Library (NYAM), and New York Public Library (NYPL). Health information is organized by topic, with links to appropriate institutions. For example, a question on weight loss and the supplement chitosan takes you to the Mayo Clinic Web site.

Yale–New Haven Health Center

www.ynhh.org

Yale–New Haven Hospital online health information. Includes a magazine on women's health with all topics of interest to women, everything from the dangers of high heels (they increase your risk of osteoarthritis in your knees) to the benefits of fish with omega-3 fatty acids (they're great for your heart). Articles written by faculty of Yale University Medical School and staff of Yale–New Haven Hospital. Excellent list of links to other health sites.

FURTHER READING

Komaroff, Anthony L., ed. *The Harvard Medical School Family Health Guide.* New York : Simon and Schuster, 1999.

See also the book's companion Web site, www.health.harvard.edu/fhg, where you can search for a specific diagnostic test or look at tests grouped by category. The Web site also includes updated information.

MENOPAUSE BOOKS FOR THE MEDICAL PROFESSION

Lobo, Rogerio, ed. *Treatment of the Post-Menopausal Woman: Basic and Clinical Aspects.* 2d ed. Philadelphia: Lippincott Williams and Wilkins, 1999.

———. *Perimenopause.* New York: Springer, 1997.

Minkin, Mary Jane, and Karen Giblin. *Manual of Menopause Counseling for the Perimenopausal and Menopausal Patient: A Clinician's Guide.* Boca Raton, Fla.: Parthenon, 2003.

ALCOHOL AND SUBSTANCE ABUSE

Alcoholics Anonymous (AA)
General Service Office of Alcoholics Anonymous
PO Box 459, Grand Central Station
New York, NY 10163
Phone: (212) 870-3400
www.alcoholics-anonymous.org
A very successful self-help group, with branches throughout the country; local branches
are listed in the telephone book.

Al-Anon and Alateen
Al-Anon Family Group Headquarters
PO Box 862, Midtown Station
New York, NY 10018
Phone: (212) 302-7240, (800) 344-2266, or (888) 4AL-ANON
www.al-anon.alateen.org
Support groups for families, teenaged children, and friends of alcoholics.

ALTERNATIVE APPROACHES TO MENOPAUSE AND WELL-BEING

American Botanical Council
6200 Manor Rd.
Austin, TX 78723
Phone: (512) 926-4900
www.herbalgram.org
A nonprofit organization for education and research, offering reliable, science-based information on the safe use of medicinal plants. The Web site has links to recent news articles on herbal medicine.

National Center for Complementary and Alternative Medicine
NCCAM Clearinghouse
PO Box 7923
Gaithersburg, MD 20898
Help line: (888) 644-6226
www.nccam.nih.gov

The National Center for Complementary and Alternative Medicine (NCCAM), established in 1998 as part of the NIH, supports long-needed scientific research on complementary and alternative medicine. The agency also seeks to educate the public and health care professionals on which kinds of alternative medicine work, which do not, and why. The Web site has information about different complementary approaches, organized either by disease or by treatment (vitamin supplements, acupuncture, etc.), as well as a section on possible side effects and drug interactions. The NCCAM Clearinghouse has a hotline for scientifically based information on alternative medicine.

The Alternative Medicine Homepage
Falk Library of the Health Sciences
University of Pittsburgh
Pittsburgh, PA 15261
www.pitt.edu/~cbw/altm.html
An excellent index of Internet resources posted by the University of Pittsburgh. The site has sections on herbal medicine, diet and lifestyle, manual healing, mind-body control, and many other topics.

Memorial Sloan-Kettering Cancer Center
www.mskcc.org/aboutherbs
The Memorial Sloan-Kettering Cancer Center has an excellent Web site with information on some 150 botanicals, vitamins, and minerals. In addition to technical monographs for health care professionals, the site includes material to help nonscientists understand the often confusing claims made for many of these products and regimens.

FURTHER READING

Moyers, Bill. *Healing and the Mind.* New York: Doubleday, 1993.
An intelligent exploration of mind-body interactions, written as a companion to the public television series, more than ten years old, but still relevant.

Seibel, Machelle. *The Soy Solution for Menopause.* New York: Simon and Schuster, 2003. Everything you need to know about soy, including its role in lessening menopausal symptoms and lowering risk for breast cancer and other diseases. Copious scientific references plus recipes for including soy in your diet.

Sifton, David W., ed. *The PDR Family Guide to Natural Medicines and Healing Therapies.* New York: Three Rivers Press, 1999.
A comprehensive book, this guide includes useful information about herbal remedies, alternative approaches, nutritional supplements, warnings about side effects and drug interactions, and other precautions. Describes alternative therapies and their goals and suggests when to consult a conventional physician.

Tyler, Varro E. *The Honest Herbal: A Sensible Guide to the Use of Herbs and Related Remedies.* 3d ed. Binghamton, N.Y.: Haworth Press, 1993.
Varro Tyler, who died in 2001, was an internationally known expert in the field of botanical medicine. Only toward the end of his life did his work begin to be taken seriously by the academic establishment. Nor did the "alternative" herbal community hold him in great esteem. But Tyler noted that if both ends of the spectrum were unhappy with him then he was probably holding a fair position. This book, organized alphabetically by herb, is a very knowledgeable and fair assessment of botanicals.

ARTHRITIS

Arthritis Foundation
1314 Spring St., NW
Atlanta, GA 30309
Phone: (404) 872-7100 or (800) 283-7800
www.arthritis.org
This is a national organization with local chapters; it publishes educational materials, including a newsletter. The Web site has information on research, nutrition and supplements, discussion boards, and an online newsletter, as well as a section on fibromyalgia.

FURTHER READING

Nelson, Miriam E., Kristin R. Baker, and Ronenn Roubenoff, with Lawrence Lindner. *Strong Women and Men Beat Arthritis: The Scientifically Proven Program That Allows People with Arthritis to Take Charge of Their Disease.* New York: Putnam's, 2002.
Sensible diet and exercise tips.

BREAST CANCER

National Alliance of Breast Cancer Organizations
9 E. 37th St., 10th floor
New York, NY 10016
Phone: for information (888) 80-NABCO; for the administrative offices (212) 889-0606
www.nabco.org
This site is a source of timely information for media, medical organizations, profession-als, patients, and their families; also a political organization advocating for regulatory change and legislation that benefits women with breast cancer and women at risk. The Web site has general information about breast cancer, news of clinical trials, and a listing of support groups.

Susan G. Komen Breast Cancer Foundation
5005 LBJ Freeway, Suite 370
Dallas, TX 75244
Phone: (972) 855-1600 or 800-I'M AWARE (462-9273)
www.komen.org
This foundation, started by the sister of Susan G. Komen, who died of breast cancer, offers information and support to women who have the disease and supports medical re-search with the goal of eradicating breast cancer: the Race for the Cure is one of its proj-ects. The Web site has an extensive library of articles on developments in the field includ-ing research updates.

Y-ME National Breast Cancer Organization
212 W. Van Buren St.
Chicago, IL 60607-3908
Phone: (312) 986-8338 or (800) 221-2141
www.y-me.org
The Y-ME National Breast Cancer Organization is committed to providing information and support to anyone who has been touched by breast cancer. The Web site includes in-formation on screening and detection, and a profiler for finding treatment options.

FURTHER READING

Kaye, Ronnie. *Spinning Straw into Gold: Your Emotional Recovery from Breast Cancer.* New York: Fireside, 1991.

This account by a psychotherapist who was diagnosed with breast cancer suggests the possibility of seeing in a devastating personal crisis an opportunity for growth and victory.

Schnipper, Hester Hill, and Joan Feinberg Berns. *Woman to Woman: A Handbook for Women Newly Diagnosed with Breast Cancer.* New York: WholeCare, 1999.

————. *After Breast Cancer : A Common-Sense Guide to Life After Treatment.* New York: Bantam Books, 2003.

The author is an oncology social worker and a breast cancer survivor. Her work provides clear and straightforward information on the issues women face as they face breast cancer, its treatment, and life after treatment.

Wadler, Joyce. *My Breast: One Woman's Cancer Story.* Reading, Mass.: Addison-Wesley, 1992.

A journalist diagnosed with breast cancer tells her own story with wit and energy.

CANCER: GENERAL RESOURCES

American Cancer Society National Office
1599 Clifton Rd., NE
Atlanta, GA 30329
Phone: (404) 320-3333 or (800) ACS-2345
www.cancer.org

This is a national organization for research and education. Its publication *Cancer Facts and Figures,* updated annually, contains statistics on all kinds of cancer, including those related to smoking, and information about risk factors, cancer prevention, and screening. The society also publishes *Kicking Butts,* a guide to quitting smoking.

National Cancer Institute
9000 Rockville Pike
Bethesda, MD 20892
Phone: (800) 4-CANCER (422-6237)
To write for information:

NCI Public Inquiries Office

Building 31, Room 10A31

31 Center Dr., MSC 2580

Bethesda, MD 20892-2580

www.cancer.gov

www.cancer.gov/newscenter

This agency, a branch of the NIH, provides news on cancer research and clinical trials, statistics, and links to related sites. You can call the hotline for understandable written information, which will be mailed to you. The Web site offers information on clinical trials, news on research, statistics, and information on different cancers by type, their causes, and treatment.

Gilda Radner Familial Ovarian Cancer Registry

www.ovariancancer.com

Help line: 800-OVARIAN (682-7426)

Part of the Roswell Park Cancer Institute in Buffalo, New York, the registry enrolls families where two or more members have been diagnosed with ovarian cancer. In its research into the genetic basis of familial ovarian cancer, the registry collects family histories, medical records, and tissue samples of people diagnosed with ovarian cancer. The Web site offers information and links to other cancer resources. The help line offers support and information for high-risk women.

CancerBACUP

3 Bath Place

Rivington St.

London EC2A 3JR

United Kingdom

Help line: 0808-800-1234

www.cancerbacup.org.uk

This British nonprofit organization provides excellent information on many aspects of cancer. The Web site has an excellent discussion of chemotherapy drugs and lists support services in the United Kingdom.

FURTHER READING

Weinberg, Robert A. *One Renegade Cell: The Story of How Cancer Begins.* New York: Basic Books, 1998.

An intelligent and readable account of how cancer develops, as well as the history of research into its causes and possible cures. The author is director of the Oncology Research Laboratory at the Whitehead Institute and professor of biology at the Massachusetts Institute of Technology.

BREAST IMPLANTS AND RECONSTRUCTION

U.S. Food and Drug Administration

www.fda.gov

Information on drugs and medical devices, including breast implants, and news about products receiving FDA approval. The FDA has an Office of Women's Health, with news of special interest to women.

FURTHER READING

Berger, Karen, and John Bostwick III, M.D. *A Woman's Decision: Breast Care, Treatment and Reconstruction.* St. Louis, Mo.: Quality Medical Publishing, 1998.

Information on breast cancer and treatment options, including breast reconstruction, along with personal stories and information about communicating with your doctor and the effect of breast cancer on relationships.

Bruning, Nancy Pauline. *Breast Implants: Everything You Need to Know.* Rev. ed. Alameda, Calif.: Hunter House, 1995.

Written by a breast cancer survivor, this book covers the controversial history of silicone gel implants (up to 1995) and explains how to evaluate the issues and risks of implant surgery and implant removal.

CARDIOVASCULAR DISEASES

American Heart Association

7320 Greenville Ave.

Dallas, TX 75231

Phone: (214) 373-6300 or (800) 242-8721

www.americanheart.org

This is the national organization for education and research on heart disease, stroke, and hypertension; local chapters are listed in every phone book. It provides information on diet, exercise, smoking, and other facets of heart-healthy living. The Web site lists publications and gives links to other sites.

CAREGIVING

Children of Aging Parents (CAPS)
1609 Woodbourne Rd., Suite 302A
Levittown, PA 19057
Phone: (215) 945-6900
www.caps4caregivers
This nonprofit organization offers guidance and referrals to social service agencies and support groups. It publishes a newsletter and other educational materials, including a guide to starting self-help groups for caregivers of the elderly.

DIABETES

American Diabetes Association (ADA)
National Service Center
1701 N. Beauregard St.
Alexandria, VA 22311
Phone: (800) 232-3472
www.diabetes.org
This is a national organization with local chapters; it offers educational materials, including *Diabetes Forecast,* a bimonthly magazine established in 1948 with articles on diet, peer support groups, and research advances, and an e-newsletter. The Web site has basic diabetes information, news about research and clinical trials, and publications of the ADA.

DIET AND NUTRITION

Harvard School of Public Health
www.hsph.harvard.edu/nutritionsource/index.html
This site includes links to important articles in scientific journals as well as information for the general public. It provides breaking news on nutritional topics.

Food and Nutrition Information Center
U.S. Department of Agriculture
www.nal.usda.gov/fnic
This government site has information about dietary guidelines, food labeling, nutrient values of different foods, and FAQs.

FURTHER READING

Critser, Greg. *Fat Land: How Americans Became the Fattest People in the World.* Boston: Houghton Mifflin, 2003.
A readable account by a journalist who specializes in health, this book examines the causes of the obesity epidemic; Critser highlights research that points at cheap fats and sugars as an underlying cause and points a scathing finger at institutions—political and social—that lower nutritional standards.

Nelson, Miriam E., with Judy Knipe. *Strong Women Eat Well: Nutritional Strategies for a Healthy Body and Mind.* New York: G. P. Putnam's Sons, 2001.

Price, Weston A. *Nutrition and Physical Degeneration: A Comparison of Primitive and Modern Diets and Their Effects.* New York: McGraw Hill, 1998.
This idiosyncratic book, far ahead of its time, came out originally in 1939 and is currently available in paperback. Dr. Price hoped to change the nation's eating habits by documenting the health effects of diet, comparing health in cultures that retained their traditional foods with that of cultures where "refined" foods, including white sugar, bleached white flour, polished rice, and synthetic fats, had been introduced. A classic.

Schlosser, Eric. *Fast Food Nation: The Dark Side of the All-American Meal.* New York: Houghton Mifflin, 2001.
A best-seller about the industry that has changed the American diet (and roadside landscape) for the worse.

Shell, Ellen Ruppel. *The Hungry Gene: The Science of Fat and the Future of Thin.* New York: Atlantic Monthly Press, 2002.
The author, a science journalist, explores the reasons for the obesity epidemic from many viewpoints: social class, genetics, the food industry, and the pharmaceutical industry. She presents information about scientific research on obesity and treatments for it (from

stomach stapling to the drug Fen-Phen), explaining the biology of metabolism that makes it so difficult to circumvent the body's appetite.

Willett, Walter C., with P. J. Skerrett; contributions by Edward L. Giovannucci; recipes by Maureen Callahan. *Eat, Drink, and Be Healthy: The Harvard Medical School Guide to Healthy Eating.* New York: Simon and Schuster, 2001.
The USDA food pyramid introduced in 1992 needs revision: clearly some fats are heart healthy and many carbohydrates are not. This book, based in part on information from the Nurses' Study, tells you how the pyramid should be rebuilt and what you can do to optimize your diet.

EXERCISE AND LIFESTYLE

Nelson, Miriam E., with Sarah Wernick. *Strong Women Stay Slim.* New York: Bantam Books, 1998.
———. *Strong Women Stay Young.* Rev. ed. New York: Bantam Books, 2000.
———. *Strong Women, Strong Bones: Everything You Need to Know to Prevent, Treat, and Beat Osteoporosis.* New York: G. P. Putnam's Sons, 2000.
Miriam Nelson is an exercise physiologist and nutritionist at Tufts University. Her first "Strong Women" book, which came out in 1997, focused on the benefits of strength training for older women. It became a best seller, and Nelson has followed it up with other books on the value of healthy lifestyles. The programs are intelligent and easy to follow; many women who never exercised have benefited from Nelson's routines.

Siler, Brooke. *The Pilates Body: The Ultimate At-Home Guide to Strengthening, Lengthening, and Toning Your Body—Without Machines.* New York: Broadway Books, 2000.
There are many books about this popular fitness program, whose emphasis on strengthening the back and abdominal muscles makes it an excellent exercise for people with back problems. A clear, well-organized book; the author studied with a disciple of Joseph Pilates.

EARLY MENOPAUSE

Premature Ovarian Failure Support Group
www.pofsupport.org
The Web site has FAQs, links to scientific articles, a reading list, and newsletters.

FURTHER READING

Petras, Kathryn. *Premature Menopause: When the Change Comes Too Early.* New York: WholeCare, 1999.
One of the few books on this subject, written by a woman who experienced it herself.

HYSTERECTOMY

HERS (Hysterectomy Educational Resources and Services)
422 Bryn Mawr Ave.
Bala Cynwyd, PA 19004
Phone: (610) 667-7757 or (888) 750-HERS
www.hersfoundation.com
Educational organization for women who have had or are contemplating hysterectomy; provides information about adverse effects, alternative treatments. Physician referral, newsletter.

MEMORY AND COGNITIVE ISSUES

Alzheimer's Disease and Related Disorders Associations (ADRDA) National Headquarters
919 N. Michigan Ave., Suite 1000
Chicago, IL 60611
Phone: (800) 272-3900
www.alz.org
This national organization publishes a newsletter, pamphlets, and other educational materials, as well as information about current research. Local chapters, listed on the Web site, sponsor support groups for caregivers of people with Alzheimer's disease.

FURTHER READING

Warga, Claire. *Menopause and the Mind: The Complete Guide to Coping with Memory Loss, Foggy Thinking, Verbal Slips, and Other Cognitive Effects of Perimenopause and Menopause.* New York: Free Press, 1999.
Warga, a neuropsychologist, examines the scientific evidence that the decrease in estrogen production at midlife affects verbal memory and learning. The book explores nutrition, discusses behavioral changes, and supplies tips on coping.

MENOPAUSE INFORMATION AND SUPPORT GROUPS

North American Menopause Society
5900 Landerbrook Dr., Suite 195
Mayfield Heights, OH 44124
Mailing address: PO Box 94527
Cleveland, OH 44101
Phone: (440) 442-7550
www.menopause.org
This is a professional organization of physicians and researchers who work in the field of menopause. NAMS conducts annual meetings for professionals and publishes a bibliography and resource list for nonprofessionals. The Web site has information on perimenopause, early menopause, and therapies to enhance health.

PRIME PLUS/Red Hot Mamas
Menopause Management Education Program
23 N. Valley Rd.
Ridgefield, CT 06877
Phone: (203) 431-3902
www.primeplususa.com and www.redhotmamas.com
This organization works with physicians and health care professionals to organize programs for menopause education and psychosocial support. There are chapters throughout the United States.

OSTEOPOROSIS

National Osteoporosis Foundation
1150 17th St., NW, Suite 500
Washington, DC 20036
Phone: (202) 223-2226
www.nof.org
This is a national organization for osteoporosis research, education, and support. It publishes a quarterly newsletter with information on prevention, exercise, nutrition, and rehabilitation.

WOMEN'S HEALTH INITIATIVE INFORMATION
AND THE NURSES' HEALTH STUDY

Women's Health Initiative

www.whi.nbli.gov

The best place to get information on the results of the WHI is the official Web site, maintained by the National Heart, Blood, and Lung Institute, which undertook the study. The site posts updated press releases, which summarize results, as well as links to the articles in scientific journals where the detailed results are published.

Nurses' Health Study

www.channing.harvard.edu/nhs/hist.html

This Web site summarizes the history of the Nurses' Health Study and provides links to the newsletters that are sent each year to the participants.

FURTHER READING

The results of the WHI were published in scientific journals when the information was released to the public. The most important articles are cited here.

Anderson, G., H. L. Judd, A. M. Kaunitz, et al., for the Women's Health Initiative Investigators. "Effects of Estrogen Plus Progestin on Gynecologic Cancers and Associated Diagnostic Procedures: The Women's Health Initiative Randomized Trial." *Journal of the American Medical Association* 290 (2003): 1739–1748.

Cauley, J. A., J. Robbins, C. Zhao, et al., for the Women's Health Initiative Investigators. "Effects of Estrogen Plus Progestin on Risk of Fracture and Bone Mineral Density: The Women's Health Initiative Randomized Trial." *Journal of the American Medical Association* 290 (2003): 1729–1738.

Chlebowski, R. T., S. L. Hendrix, R. D. Langer, et al., for the Women's Health Initiative Investigators. "Influence of Estrogen plus Progestin on Breast Cancer and Mammography in Healthy Postmenopausal Women: The Women's Health Initiative Randomized Trial." *Journal of the American Medical Association* 289 (2003): 3243–3253.

Hays, J., J. K. Ockene, R. L. Brunner, et al., for the Women's Health Initiative Investigators. "Effects of Estrogen plus Progestin on Health-Related Quality of Life." *New England Journal of Medicine* 349 (2003): 1839–1854.

Herrington, D. M., and T. D. Howard. "From Presumed Benefit to Potential Harm— Hormone Therapy and Heart Disease." *New England Journal of Medicine* 349 (2003): 519– 521.

Li, C. I., K. E. Malone, P. L. Porter, et al. "Relationship Between Long Durations and Different Regimens of Hormone Therapy and Risk of Breast Cancer." *Journal of the American Medical Association* 289 (2003):3254–3263.

Manson, J. E., J. Hsia, K. C. Johnson, et al., for the Women's Health Initiative Investigators. "Estrogen plus Progestin and the Risk of Coronary Heart Disease." *New England Journal of Medicine* 349 (2003):523–534.

Shumaker, S. A., C. Legault, S. R. Rapp, et al., for the Women's Health Initiative Memory Study Investigators. "Estrogen plus Progestin and the Incidence of Dementia and Mild Cognitive Impairment in Postmenopausal Women: The Women's Health Initiative Memory Study: A Randomized Controlled Trial." *Journal of the American Medical Association* 289 (2003): 2651–2662.

Wassertheil-Smoller, S., S. Hendrix, M. Limacher, et al., for the Women's Health Initiative Investigators. "Effect of Estrogen plus Progestin on Stroke in Postmenopausal Women: The Women's Health Initiative: A Randomized Trial." *Journal of the American Medical Association* 289 (2003): 2673–2684.

SEXUALITY AFTER MENOPAUSE

Sexuality Information and Education Council of the United States
130 W. 42d St., Suite 350
New York, NY 10036
Phone: (212) 819-9770
www.siecus.org
This nonprofit foundation provides information about sexuality as a positive part of a healthy life and advocates the right of individuals to make responsible sexual choices. The site has a bibliography covering such topics as sexuality in later life and gender identity.

FURTHER READING

Barbach, Lonnie Garfield. *For Yourself: The Fulfillment of Female Sexuality.* Rev. ed. New York: Signet, 2000.
First published in 1975, this book provides support and reassurance, as well as a practical course in freeing up sexuality.

Berman, Jennifer, and Laura Berman, with Elisabeth Bumiller. *For Women Only: A Revolutionary Guide to Overcoming Sexual Dysfunction and Reclaiming Your Sex Life.* New York: Henry Holt, 2001.
This book explores the psychological and physiological aspects of female sexuality throughout life and offers advice on how to achieve a fuller and more satisfying sex life. It includes detailed information about the female sexual response and describes many options for treatment.

▶ INDEX